Risk versus Risk

Risk versus Risk

Tradeoffs in Protecting Health and the Environment

Edited by
JOHN D. GRAHAM
and
JONATHAN BAERT WIENER

HARVARD UNIVERSITY PRESS

Cambridge, Massachusetts
London, England

First Harvard University Press paperback edition, 1997

Library of Congress Cataloging-in-Publication Data

Risk versus risk : tradeoffs in protecting health and the environment
  / edited John D. Graham and Jonathan Baert Wiener.
       p.   cm.
    Includes bibliographical references and index.
    ISBN 0-674-77304-7 (cloth)
    ISBN 0-674-77307-1 (pbk.)
    1. Health risk assessment.   2. Health behavior—Decision-making.
  3. Environmental health—Decision-making.   I. Graham, John D. (John
  David), 1956–   .   II. Wiener, Jonathan Baert, 1962–   .
  RA427.3.R58   1995
  362.1′042—dc20   95-10457

Contents

Foreword

Cass R. Sunstein

Whatever we do, we are likely to encounter risks. A short drive to the grocery store brings dangers, however small. So too with a decision to ride a bicycle or to walk instead. So too with a decision to stay at home. If you play tennis to improve your health, you may endanger your health instead. Whenever you reduce or eliminate one risk, you may simultaneously increase or create another. If this is not so troubling, it is because most of the time the risks we face are, or seem, blessedly low. But sometimes each of us must make judgments about how to avoid significant risks, or how to minimize overall risk, when a genuine danger is unavoidable.

If this can be an issue for each of us, it is an even more serious issue for governments—especially, perhaps, for the national government. In the twentieth century, the reduction of risks to life and health has become one of government's most important tasks. Despite widespread questions about governmental effectiveness, the United States has already accomplished a great deal in lowering risk, especially in the area of environmental quality, and in the process it has saved many lives. But by now we know that when government tries to make things better, it may make things much worse instead. If, for example, government tries to protect human health by imposing fuel economy requirements on cars, it may lead companies to produce smaller and less safe cars, and thus endanger human health. If government imposes environmental regulations on companies, it may decrease some environmental risks. But these very regulations may increase other environmental risks or shift risks to other areas. Reductions in air pollution may cause greater production of solid wastes; protection of consumers may shift risks to workers; banning one substance may invite the use of more dangerous substances. Some cures are worse than the disease.

This pathbreaking book is the first sustained and systematic effort to explore this problem of "risk-risk tradeoffs." To say the very least, the book comes at the right time. At the national and international levels, it is widely understood that risks to life and health—from pollution, from unsafe consumer products, from dangerous workplaces—can exact a high toll on individual and social well-being. At the same time, there is enormous concern that government regulation may be costly, futile, or counterproductive. If nations are to provide good lives for their citizens, they need to know how to come up with regulations that will be effective in achieving their own goals.

Too frequently, risk regulation has been adversely affected by interest-group pressures, sensationalistic anecdotes, political opportunism, and sheer ignorance. Too often, important voices are left out of the regulatory process, and it is the people who are not heard who suffer the consequences of bad risk regulation. The contributors to this book show that risk-risk tradeoffs are an unavoidable aspect of life and an omnipresent issue for government. Consider the fact that when women reach menopause, they face increased risks of hip fractures and chronic discomforts in old age; hormonal replacement therapies can reduce these problems, but they can create cancer risks as well. Consider also the fact that efforts to reduce the risks associated with ozone depletion and global warming may result in other risks, some of them endangering the environment itself.

But the authors are not content just to demonstrate the pervasiveness of the problem. They also offer a diagnosis and a range of constructive suggestions for the future. They explore the phenomenon of "omitted voices"—the fact that some affected people do not play a role in the process of deciding about risk. They show that ordinary people tend to rely on heuristic devices—simplified cognitive strategies for evaluating evidence—that lead to large private and public mistakes in risk assessment. The authors show too that risk-related decision-making is extremely fragmented in government, leading to a failure to treat risk in a coordinated way. They demonstrate that people's behavioral responses to regulation are often unanticipated by government, and that people sometimes react in a way that defeats inadequately considered regulation.

This book offers a number of promising remedies for the existing situation. The authors urge that the risk problem be treated holistically, with efforts to contain risks made not in isolation but in the context of the entire picture. To this end they emphasize the need to compile much more information about risk levels and to act on the basis of that information—rather than relying on guesswork, sensationalism, or interest-group pressures. As they note, the American government provides a great deal of information about social trends, but it does not monitor and measure levels and trends of risks to health, safety, and the environment; it offers no system for assessing "environmental indicators." This is a critical and easily remedied gap in modern policy.

The authors suggest too that Congress should avoid the "risk of the month" syndrome by adopting a more coordinated approach to regulation. They urge the courts to play a constructive role by striking down regulations that create risks larger than those that they control. They suggest that the executive branch should be more attentive to the danger that regulation of one risk will increase another.

The authors are aware that it is important to come to terms with two large questions with continuing significance for government: Why does the public view some risks as serious and others as trivial? Why do public assessments of risk differ so sharply from experts' assessments? It seems clear that people often misunderstand the sheer facts about risks, thinking, for example, that because a recent incident has occurred—involving a contaminated bottle or an airplane crash—the risk is much higher than it is in fact. As the authors show, people rely on heuristic devices that can lead to systematic errors, in the form of both overvaluation and undervaluation of risks. It is important for people in the private and public sectors to try to counteract these errors, mostly through providing better information, but sometimes through regulation.

On the other hand, people's judgments about different risks are sometimes based not on factual errors, but on deep beliefs about fairness and equity. These beliefs deserve respect. Unlike many experts and economists, ordinary citizens do not seek simply to "decrease overall risk." They make qualitative as well as quantitative judgments. They care about a range of contextual factors—whether the risk is voluntarily or involuntarily incurred; whether it is catastrophic; whether it is equitably distributed or whether it is instead faced by discrete, vulnerable groups; whether the risk is faced by future generations. When dealing with risk, we ought to be especially concerned to ensure, to the extent possible, that ordinary citizens have a sense of control over their own environment and a sense of participation in determining risk levels. Thus the authors' valuable discussion of "risk tradeoff analysis" is designed to consider not merely the statistical magnitude of risk, but also a range of qualitative and contextual issues that the public deems important. Hence the important idea of "risk-superior moves" is an effort to ensure regulation that can make things better from all conceivable standpoints.

Much of the importance of this book lies in its exceptionally illuminating discussions of particular problems and in its wide range of provocative and constructive proposals. In my view, however, the book's importance lies above all in the fact that it promises to help stimulate a national and even international discussion that—astonishingly—has yet to occur. Of course that discussion should involve academics and other experts in the area of risk regulation, embodying the kinds of interdisciplinary work (including law, economics, science, public health, and psychology) so well exemplified by this book. But more than that, the discussion should occur among the officials who are entrusted with making and implementing regulatory policy, especially members of Congress and the executive branch. And most important of all, the discussion should involve citizens generally, who make countless decisions about risk both in their daily activities and in their democratic judgments. In our private capacities, and in our role as citizens in a democracy, we could do much better; this book helps to point the way.

Preface

The idea for a systematic study of risk tradeoffs came from discussions at the 1990 annual meeting of the Advisory Committee of the Harvard Center for Risk Analysis. This group of thirty "risk professionals" from academia, government, nonprofit organizations, and business is asked each year to suggest directions for the research efforts of the Center. The Advisory Committee identified risk tradeoffs as a priority topic for Center inquiry, envisioning it as a modest exercise to bring scholarship to bear on some of the fundamental problems in modern risk management, including the "risk of the month" syndrome and the penchant for simple solutions to complex phenomena.

The research staff of the Center, its Director (Graham), and a member of the Advisory Committee (Wiener) then set out to document and analyze risk tradeoffs in diverse decision-making contexts. During the course of the project, the Advisory Committee periodically received briefings on its progress and provided constructive criticisms. Soon the project grew into a full book-length set of case studies, and we developed the first and last chapters to synthesize our findings and provide a unifying analytic approach to the problem. Extremely helpful comments on the manuscript were provided by Carol Barash, Elizabeth Drye, James Hammitt, David Hemenway, Lester Lave, Tim Profeta, Gerhard Raabe, Joanna Siegel, and Cass Sunstein. Our editors at Harvard University Press, Michael Fisher and Mary Ellen Geer, were extraordinarily challenging, constructive, and dedicated; we owe them thanks for many substantive and technical improvements to the text.

Funding for the project came in the form of unrestricted gifts to the Harvard Center for Risk Analysis. Special thanks are due to Patricia Worden (Harvard) and Judy Williamson, Joan Ashley, and Tim Profeta (Duke) for their work in preparing the manuscript for publication.

In addition, our families were inordinately understanding of our immersion in this project. Sue Graham and Ginger Young (and above all Jonathan and Ginger's first baby, Alex, who arrived a week before the due date for the manuscript) were endlessly cheerful and supportive as we struggled to complete the text.

Since this project began in 1990, there has been an explosion of interest in risk analysis. We hope this volume will contribute to the thorough reexamination now under way of how this country's decisions can reduce risk more intelligently and effectively.

J.D.G., Cambridge, Mass.
J.B.W., Durham, N.C.

1

Confronting Risk Tradeoffs

JOHN D. GRAHAM
JONATHAN BAERT WIENER

Good health and a clean environment are among the goals people seek most earnestly. Every day individuals, families, businesses, and governments are faced with important decisions on how best to achieve these goals. Consumers have increasingly sought "lite" and "organic" foods lacking ingredients they find worrisome, cars with airbags and other advanced safety measures, and "green" products that pollute less and can be recycled. Through politics these pro-safety preferences have been expressed in a growing body of laws to combat such hazards as cancer-causing chemicals, traffic accidents, and ecological degradation. In short, Americans are engaged in a national campaign to reduce risk.

Yet confounding this national campaign to reduce risk is the phenomenon of "risk tradeoffs." Paradoxically, some of the most well-intentioned efforts to reduce identified risks can turn out to increase other risks. Though the term "risk tradeoff" may not be familiar to many people, the phenomenon is commonplace in human decisionmaking, reflected in such familiar adages as "out of the frying pan and into the fire" and "the cure is worse than the disease." The general problem is that efforts to combat a "target risk" can unintentionally foster

1

increases in "countervailing risks." Many kinds of counter-vailing risks are commonly known by the terms "side effects" (medicine), "collateral damage" (military tactics), or "unin-tended consequences" (public policy). Other countervailing risks are less obvious, lurking in dynamic feedbacks and be-havioral responses. Unless decisionmakers consider the full set of outcomes associated with each effort to reduce risk, they will systematically invite such risk tradeoffs. It is also conceiv-able that in addition to countervailing risks there are "coinci-dent risks"—dangers which turn out to diminish in tandem with target risks even though that was not intended by the decisionmaker—and though such happy coincidences should also be considered in decisionmaking, they are not likely to be as plentiful as are countervailing risks. The net effect of ac-tions taken to reduce risk is complex; the phenomenon of risk tradeoffs suggests that in the national campaign to reduce risk, not as much health, safety, and environmental protection is being achieved as was intended and expected.

We believe that risk tradeoffs are a pervasive feature of de-cisions people make to protect human health and the environ-ment. As an example of an ordinary risk tradeoff in action, consider a routine decision we all face: what to do for a head-ache. Taking two aspirin will probably make your head feel better, because aspirin is acetylsalicylic acid, which blocks prostaglandins that would otherwise transmit pain signals to the brain. The analgesic properties of salicylic acid in willow leaves were noticed thousands of years ago, and aspirin was first synthesized in the 1800s; now it is the most widely used drug in the world (Wolfson 1985). But at the same time that the two aspirin make your headache feel better, they may well make your stomach feel worse, because a common side effect of acetylsalicylic acid is irritation of the lining of the gastro-intestinal tract. Prolonged use of aspirin may lead to stomach ulcers, and in children with the flu it may even cause the po-tentially fatal Reye's syndrome (Edelson 1991).

This familiar example illustrates several of the key concepts in risk tradeoff analysis. In order to reduce a target risk (the headache), you decide on an intervention (aspirin), but thereby induce a set of potential countervailing risks (stomach pain, ulcers, Reye's syndrome). The fact that Reye's syndrome and certain other countervailing risks are listed on the aspirin bottle emphasizes the importance to sound decisions of being informed in advance about risk tradeoffs. And the aspirin example suggests how a decisionmaker might resolve the risk tradeoff: in the short term, in which the only two options are to do nothing (endure the headache) and to take aspirin, the decisionmaker will need to weigh "risk versus risk": evaluate in light of his or her individual circumstances (and depending on how much aspirin is taken) the likelihood and severity of the countervailing risks as compared to the target risk and make a decision as to the preferred course. In the longer term, the decisionmaker can seek out additional options that both reduce the target risk and avoid countervailing risks. These options would be "risk-superior," reducing overall risk rather than trading one kind of risk for another.

A "risk-superior" alternative to taking aspirin might be to take acetaminophen, a non-aspirin pain reliever which treats the headache with little or no risk of stomach irritation or Reye's syndrome (Wolfson 1985). But acetaminophen does not match aspirin's ability to reduce inflammation, a target risk of concern to those suffering from injuries, arthritis, or premenstrual swelling. Or one might take ibuprofen, another non-aspirin analgesic, which relieves headache and inflammation with modest risk of stomach irritation (Edelson 1991). Indeed, acetaminophen (for example, Tylenol) and ibuprofen (for example, Nuprin) have been advertised as headache- and swelling-relieving treatments that avoid the countervailing risks posed by aspirin (Edelson 1991). And there may be non-drug alternatives, such as massage, to treat headaches. Ultimately, the choice of different headache remedies will depend on the individual's particular health circumstances and preferences—and on information about the target and countervailing risks of each option.

Our aim in this book is to explore risk tradeoffs faced by decisionmakers in all areas of life, from personal medical decisions to global environmental decisions. Our concern is that risk tradeoffs have received scant analytic attention (Keeney and von Winterfeldt 1986). We trust that development of a more rigorous framework for analyzing risk tradeoffs will be valuable in recognizing, understanding, and resolving them. By suggesting such a framework, we seek to ensure that efforts to reduce health, safety, and environmental dangers are more fully thought through and more fully effective—not just well-intentioned, but pragmatically successful in terms of actual outcomes. Recognizing the prevalence of risk tradeoffs is thus an act not of reactionary intransigence but of constructive candor, since we will endeavor to show that much can be done to minimize countervailing risks once they are discerned. Our research indicates that risk tradeoffs are not an imagined inevitable perversity of life (Hirschman 1991) but rather a real consequence of incomplete decisionmaking, and that with attention and effort, individuals and society can wage the campaign to reduce risk with better tools that help to recognize and progressively reduce overall risk.

In this first chapter we propose a framework for "risk tradeoff analysis" (RTA) that decisionmakers at any level can apply to risk problems. RTA can help to illuminate the full range of risks involved in a decision, including potential countervailing risks that might arise through efforts to reduce the target risk of initial concern. RTA suggests ways to resolve risk tradeoffs when resources and technology are limited, through careful weighing of risk versus risk. This process of weighing risks requires ethical as well as scientific contributions. And RTA highlights the opportunities to resolve tradeoffs between target and countervailing risks by reducing overall risk through the development of risk-superior materials, technologies, and ways of organizing activities.

The heart of this book is a set of case studies drawn from the diverse fields of medicine, food, transportation, energy, and environmental protection. Although these case studies are not a random sample of all risk-reduction activity, we believe they are sufficiently rich and diverse to offer insights into the phenomenon of risk tradeoffs and promising directions for reform of decisionmaking. Each case study in the book treats a significant personal, social, or governmental problem from the perspective of an analyst employing RTA. The case studies are intended to be of current interest, but their main purpose is to describe the tradeoffs that have confronted real-world decisionmakers. Thus new scientific discoveries that may have occurred since this volume was completed should not impair the durability of the case studies as insights into the challenge of decisionmaking.

The case studies begin with individual choices about personal health. Chapter 2 examines the choices a woman faces in dealing with menopause, when her changing hormonal balance can lead to osteoporosis and an increased risk of hip fractures and chronic discomforts in older age, but hormonal replacement therapies to ward off these ills can increase the risk of uterine (endometrial) and breast cancers. The case study in Chapter 3 illustrates a different medical tradeoff: the use of clozapine therapy to treat schizophrenia, which involves patients whose ability to decide for themselves is impaired.

Chapters 4 and 5 investigate tradeoffs in the effort to ensure highway safety. First we study the risks of highway fatalities associated with aging, and the tradeoffs that would be occasioned by rules proposed to restrict driving by senior citizens. Then we examine the tradeoff that has occurred as the government's automobile fuel economy (CAFE) rules have increased mileage per gallon but have also encouraged design changes such as downsizing that reduce the crashworthiness of cars.

The next five case studies involve the social regulation of widespread dietary and environmental risks. Chapter 6 examines the issues of whether to eat fish and whether to warn consumers about doing so, given that fish consumption reduces the risk of heart disease compared to other protein sources but that fish in some waterways may also carry carcinogenic contaminants. In Chapter 7 the question is whether to chlorinate drinking water, which helps suppress microbes that transmit acute infectious diseases, but which may add a cancer risk. Chapter 8 traces the risks posed by extracting more lead to make batteries and other products, versus the risks of recycling existing lead in secondary smelters. The system for registering pesticides is investigated in Chapter 9, with a focus on the extent to which regulatory authorities compare the risks of old pesticides with those of proposed newer substitutes when making registration determinations. And Chapter 10 examines several tradeoffs that confront international authorities seeking to protect the global environment against stratospheric ozone depletion and global warming.

In the concluding chapter we explore why risk tradeoffs seem to occur, and we urge a shift in the prevailing decision paradigm from one that concentrates on "target risks" to a paradigm that respects the importance of the entire portfolio of risks. We propose specific changes in risk management institutions to foster this more comprehensive approach.

The National Campaign to Reduce Risk

For at least the last thirty years, Americans have been seeking substantially higher levels of protection against threats to their health, to their safety, and to the environment—a movement that has enormous social breadth and importance. Some analysts attribute this rising concern about risks to America's economic progress, which motivates and enables people to care more about threats to their health status and to environmental quality (NAS 1981). Others point to rising levels of education, public awareness, and scientific ability to detect minute risks, which together stimulate concerns about risks that were previously unrecognized. Citizens may also have become more skeptical about claims made on behalf of new technologies, especially when innovations are perceived as posing new and perhaps mysterious dangers to human health and the environment (Krimsky and Golding 1992). Or media attention to violence and health risks may have spurred public concern.

Whatever its causes may be, a concerted national campaign to reduce risk is apparent both in our nation's allocation of resources and in our changing lifestyles. The fraction of national income devoted to health care and environmental protection has doubled in the past two decades, from about 8 percent in 1970 to about 16 percent today, and is projected to exceed 20 percent by the year 2000 (U.S. HHS 1992; U.S. EPA 1990). In 1990 over $115 billion was expended in the United States on various pollution control programs, and these expenditures are increasing each year at a rate twice the rate of economic growth (U.S. EPA 1990). In the same year the United States spent $600 billion on the delivery of health care services; these expenditures are also increasing much faster than the growth of the economy. Additional expenditures (and further fractions of national income) go to combat violence and other public health risks.

People are also changing their lifestyles to reduce risk. Rates of safety belt use among adults have increased from 10 percent in 1980 to 50 percent in 1990, and among small children from 20 percent in 1980 to 80 percent in 1990 (Graham 1990). Rates of smoking are declining in virtually all age and demographic groups (Bowman and Ladd 1993), although the rates of decline are larger among men than among women. Alcohol consumption per adult, particularly intake of distilled spirits, declined throughout the 1980s. The percentage of teenagers reporting alcohol use declined from 34 percent in 1974 to 25 percent in 1989. Diets are also changing to pursue risk reduction (Taylor 1992). Both meat and egg consumption are declining, and people are eating more fruits, vegetables, and foods with high-fiber content (USDA 1992). As people have begun to eat differently, they have also begun to exercise more regularly to burn calories and fat. Since World War II Americans have increasingly taken up swimming, walking, jogging, hiking, and playing Frisbee, handball, and racquet sports.

Meanwhile, efforts to combat environmental pollution are proliferating. At least since the first Earth Day in 1970, Americans have become increasingly convinced that protection of the environment is not only an aesthetic good but will also curtail human illness and disease (Dunlap 1990). While the first wave of environmental protection legislation in this country (the parks and land conservation systems created in the early 1900s) reflected concern for ecosystems and recreation, it is largely the public health rationale that has galvanized popular support for the goals of the environmental movement in the second wave of environmental legislation (1970 to 1990; see Burger 1990). New laws adopted in this campaign to reduce environmental risk include the major overhauls of the Clean Air Act, the Clean Water Act, the Safe Drinking

Water Act, and the federal pesticide control law (FIFRA); new federal laws on toxic substances and on hazardous waste sites (TSCA, RCRA, and CERCLA/Superfund); and the federal law giving communities the right to know about toxic chemicals emitted by local industries (EPCRA). Indoor air pollution, acid rain, radon, lead paint, asbestos, hazardous wastes in groundwater, ozone-depleting chemicals, and greenhouse gases are recent targets of environmental policies. The Clean Air Act Amendments of 1990, which were advocated primarily on public health grounds, will add another $25 billion per year to the nation's growing investment in environmental protection (Rice 1992), and cleanup of waste sites may add another $30 billion per year (Russell et al. 1991). Federal and state laws are increasingly giving workers and communities a "right to know" about toxic materials in their vicinity (Roe 1988; Viscusi 1993). Some environmental advocates are urging "pollution prevention" and "toxics use reduction" (Geiser 1991), and even a goal of "zero-discharge" of wastes (potentially quite a challenging objective—imagine if it were applied to human beings!).

How Successful Is This Campaign?

By many accounts, the campaign to reduce risk has shown impressive results. Americans today face lower overall risks of early mortality, illness, and injury than at any time in the country's history (U.S. HHS 1992). The average American's life expectancy at birth has increased from 47 years in 1900 to 78 years in 1990. Deaths as a result of infectious diseases have dropped precipitously, from about 20 percent of annual deaths in 1900 to under 5 percent today (CDC 1991). And the risk of a fatal or disabling accident in the workplace fell by 50 percent between 1970 and 1990 (Bureau of the Census 1992, table 665, p. 419).

The most likely causes of these long-term health improvements are not medical care services (Fuchs 1986) but public water and sanitation systems, immunizations, and improved nutrition. Nevertheless, risk factors treated by medical care have improved as well. For example, while progress against infant mortality accounts for much of the gain in life expectancy over this century, the risks faced by senior citizens have also declined. Average life expectancy at age 65 has increased from 12 years in 1900 to 18 years in 1990. Not only are Americans living longer, but they are facing declining risks of various forms of nonfatal illness. The incidence of nonfatal heart attacks, strokes, and trauma has declined steadily since the 1960s. In the last decade alone, senior citizens have experienced a 25 percent decline in the number of days of restricted activity due to illness.

Many forms of pollution have also dropped markedly over the last three decades, even while total U.S. economic output grew by 70 percent (CEA 1994, table B-2, p. 270). Between 1970 and 1989, many air pollutant emissions were significantly reduced: total suspended particulates were cut over 60 percent, sulfur oxides fell almost 30 percent, volatile organics dropped 25 percent, and carbon monoxide fell nearly 40 percent (though nitrogen oxide emissions rose 7 percent over the period) (U.S. EPA 1990). Management of airborne lead has been a major success: the phaseout of lead in gasoline reduced lead emissions into the air by 96 percent between 1970 and 1989 (U.S. EPA 1990), and, most likely as a direct result of that phaseout, the level of lead detected in children's blood fell by 77 percent over that period (Pirkle et al. 1994). On the other hand, management of airborne ozone has been troublesome on two fronts: ozone at the ground level (the major component of urban smog, posing risks of injury to human lungs and vegetation) continues to exceed national standards in many cities, while the ozone layer high in the upper atmosphere (the earth's shield against harmful ultraviolet radiation) has been thinning. As for water pollution, industrial point-source discharges of suspended solids and of materials creating biological oxygen demand fell by over 90 percent between the mid-1970s and mid-1980s, but discharges of those pollutants from non-point sources—such as farms and parking lots, which are largely outside the scope of clean water laws—increased over the period, contributing to a net increase in overall water discharges (U.S. EPA 1990). Meanwhile, even though more species are alive today than probably ever before, the rate of species extinctions appears to have increased significantly in this century (Wilson 1992).

Measuring the overall success of the nation's efforts to reduce risk is hampered by two key factors. First, the United States has no coherent system for monitoring and measuring levels and trends of risks to health, safety, and the environment. Although we do collect statistics on human mortality and morbidity, there is no comparable system of data on environmental indicators (Portney 1988). Second, our measurements of success do not tell us how well we could or should be doing in light of our efforts; they do not show the effectiveness or ineffectiveness of our interventions to reduce risks. Could life expectancies be even longer? Should people be even healthier? Could pollution be even lower? Consideration of risk tradeoffs suggests that we could be doing better than we are.

The Phenomenon of Risk Tradeoffs

Despite the record of successes (and some failures) in reducing risks, we suspect that risk tradeoffs are quietly hindering the effectiveness of the national campaign to reduce risk. The campaign to reduce target risks may in effect be at war with itself: it may be clearing away target risks but cultivating a new crop of countervailing risks. The gains in life expectancy and freedom from illness and injury, while encouraging, may be smaller than those we should have experienced if countervailing risks were not eroding the gains of policies against target risks. Or the increased life expectancy might be accompanied by increases in other types of countervailing risks, such as psychological stress (Taylor 1992). Or, as some environmentalists argue, increases in human activity might be coming at the expense of the survival of other species (Wilson 1992), or of long-term ecological viability in general, perhaps foreshadowed by the mysterious recent worldwide disappearance of frog and other amphibian populations (Yoon 1994). Or the overt improvement in our longevity might mask subtle increases in latent countervailing risks, as hinted perhaps by the recently reported long-term decline in male sperm counts and increase in breast cancer rates (Hileman 1994), or the alarming decreasing effectiveness of antibiotics against infectious microorganisms (Fisher 1994).

Writ large, the implications of risk tradeoffs are potentially quite grave. First, we may be getting much less protection from risk than we expect. Medical treatments, products, and government regulations may be protecting people and the environment less than advertised and less than needed—and might even, in some cases, be doing more harm than good.

Second, the credibility of the entire social movement for protection against risk could be at stake. Unless risk tradeoffs are acknowledged and addressed forthrightly, the national campaign to reduce risk may ultimately come to be viewed as oversold, or even viewed with a cynicism that forfeits its legitimacy and public support.

Because there are no coherent data on overall trends in risks to environmental quality and human health, it cannot (yet) be proven that risk tradeoffs have offset some quantified percentage of the success of the national campaign to reduce target risks. Our effort in this book is therefore based on case studies rather than broad statistics of risk levels. Unlike the economic indicators reported every night on the national news (such as the gross national product and the Dow Jones Industrial index), we do not have many broad indicators of overall risk levels in society. Life expectancy is a useful measure, but an incomplete and imperfect one: it abstracts from the types of risks being faced; it ignores nonfatal illness and distress; and it omits risks to other forms of life besides humans. Most important, it is retrospective—it cannot forecast the effect on future well-being of risks being sown today. Improved measures of social risk levels should be high on the national research agenda, for use in concert with financial economic indicators as a gauge of society's standard of living (Portney 1988; Sen 1993). Meanwhile, case studies such as those in this book can help illuminate the subtle details of risks reduced and risks increased.

Unfortunately, there are reasons to believe that the prospect of risk tradeoffs is growing. First, our progress in reducing target risks in the past suggests that America has already conquered many of the most obvious and easily preventable risks. Future efforts to reduce overall risk may encounter diminishing returns, comprised in part of increasing tendencies toward countervailing risks. To put it another way, as we try to squeeze out more and more risk, the pressure leading to side effects may grow. Second, as we address ever smaller target risks, the importance of countervailing risks *relative* to the target risks is likely to increase (Whipple 1985). Third, as a society grows steadily more well-off, it may place more value on countervailing risks which would be of less immediate concern to destitute societies plagued by basic problems. Finally, as we tackle problems rooted in more complex systems and technologies, such as the global atmosphere, the pathways for feedbacks and tradeoffs to occur may multiply.

Experience with Risk Tradeoffs

Historical experience offers ample reason to suspect that risk tradeoffs are ubiquitous. The following examples provide some evidence of the diversity of risk tradeoffs in the national campaign to reduce risk. In each case, it is important to keep in mind that recognizing that a risk tradeoff is occurring simply shows the existence of the phenomenon; without further analysis one cannot say that the countervailing risks necessarily outweigh the reduction in the target risk.

- Hospital care can reduce risks from trauma and illnesses, but can also lead to other illnesses. This is the general problem of iatrogenesis (injury due to therapy). For example, before the advent of antiseptics and antibiotics, surgery to repair acute traumas lost many lives to infections of the incision wound. Today hospital admission and surgery still carry with them a general risk of nosocomial (hospital-acquired) infection that, though much reduced, is still often higher than the risk in the general population (Bunker et al. 1977)—and may rise again as microbes gain resistance to antibiotic drugs (Fisher 1994). Specific therapies such as radiation treatment for cancer and anesthesia for surgery (Brown

1992; Bunker et al. 1977; Keeney 1994) continue to pose significant countervailing risks of morbidity and mortality. Iatrogenesis remains a key problem in the effort to improve medical care (Brennan et al. 1991; Leape et al. 1991).

- The major policies adopted to control pollution in the United States have been aimed at one target environmental medium (air, water, or land) at a time, with the result that pollution has too often been merely shifted from one medium to another instead of reduced overall (Hahn and Males 1990; Hornstein 1992). For example, the 1977 Clean Air Act requirement that all coal-burning power plants install scrubbers to remove sulfur dioxide from their smokestacks has generated tons of sulfur sludge that must be disposed of elsewhere (Harrington 1991), and has ironically also increased emissions of other pollutants such as the greenhouse gas carbon dioxide because scrubbers reduce energy efficiency, thus requiring extra fuel to be consumed to produce the same amount of electricity (Dudek, LeBlanc, and Miller 1991).

- Prohibiting drug use can reduce the number of people suffering addiction and its concomitant social ills, but may increase violent crime as competition for underground drug markets is waged among illegal gangs. This was the experience with the prohibition of alcohol in the 1920s, and with the effort to restrict illegal drugs such as cocaine and heroin in the 1980s and 1990s (Duke 1993; Moynihan 1993; Kleiman 1992), and it is one of the concerns surrounding proposals to ban or restrict cigarettes. In contrast, legalizing such drugs may reduce crime but concede increasing addiction rates.

- Disposable diapers create solid waste at the landfill, but cloth diapers create air pollution because they require energy-intensive washing and often household visits by the washing service in an energy-consuming truck (Poore 1992).

- The ban on the fungicide EDB removed its cancer risk, but in turn may have left on grains and nuts a fungus that promotes aflatoxins more carcinogenic than the fungicide (OMB 1990–1991; Ames et al. 1987).

- Child safety caps on certain medicine bottles were required beginning in 1970. Yet this requirement was associated with no observable reduction in poisoning rates from the regulated bottles (for example, aspirin), and with a significant increase in poisonings from related but unregulated bottles (such as antibiotics and unregulated cleaning and polishing agents), yielding a net increase in poisonings. Evidently the supposedly "childproof" safety caps had the effect of lulling parents into leaving the bottles within children's reach or even uncapped (for the parents' own convenience), and into leaving other bottles more accessible as well (say, by leaving the entire medicine closet unlocked) (Viscusi 1992, ch. 13).

- Mandatory minimum or life sentences for criminals (such as "three strikes you're out") may or may not keep those likely to be violent off the street (Neff 1994; Kaminer 1994b). Meanwhile, such lifetime sentencing rules may end up keeping geriatric inmates occupying prison cells that could be used to incapacitate younger and more violent felons (Kaminer 1994b).

- Cyclamates, used as artificial sweeteners, were banned on the ground that they were carcinogenic. This invited consumers to turn to the artificial sweetener saccharin, which was itself later banned for the same reason (but Congress suspended the ban). Meanwhile, prohibiting artificial sweeteners to reduce cancer risk may increase consumption of sugar, with attendant risks of weight gain in some consumers and particular risks for diabetics (Lave 1981; Keeney 1994).

- The anti-depression drugs Prozac and Elavil, widely used to treat depression among cancer patients, ironically may increase the incidence of cancer tumors (Nemecek 1994).

- The ban on ocean dumping of industrial wastes may have encouraged disposal or incineration of such wastes on land, closer to human populations and fragile freshwater ecosystems (Schneider 1993).

- Policies to stop chlorination of drinking water, in order to reduce the risk of cancer associated with chlorine, may increase more immediate risks from water-borne microbial diseases that the chlorine was meant to kill. For example, the largest outbreak of cholera in recent history, which killed nearly 7,000 people and afflicted over 800,000, was apparently unleashed in 1991 in part as a result of Peru's decision to cease chlorinating its drinking water, spurred by U.S. risk assessments classifying chlorination as carcinogenic (Anderson 1991).
- Tamoxifen, a medication that helps prevent recurrence of breast cancer and is taken by over half of women who have surgery for breast cancer each year, may meanwhile increase the risk of uterine cancer, according to the U.S. Food and Drug Administration (FDA). In 1994 the FDA, weighing the risks in this tradeoff, concluded that because breast cancer is more prevalent and more often fatal than uterine cancer, the warning on tamoxifen should be upgraded but it should still be prescribed for breast cancer patients (AP 1994).
- "Toxics Use Reduction" policies, which mandate restrictions or bans on the use of certain substances on a list, may encourage shifts to off-list substitutes that pose other (possibly greater) risks (Graham and Gray 1993).
- Reducing logging in American forests, in order to safeguard wildlife in old-growth areas, may raise world timber prices and thus encourage increased logging of sensitive forests overseas (Sedjo 1993).
- In 1989 the EPA banned asbestos in many uses in order to reduce the risk of cancer from its inhalation. Partly in light of evidence that substitute substances might also be carcinogenic, and that the use of asbestos in brake linings helped prevent accidents by reducing the stopping distance of automobiles, a federal court instructed the EPA to reconsider its proposed ban (*Corrosion Proof Fittings v. U.S. EPA* 1991).
- Spraying hot water to clean oil off the beaches of Prince William Sound, Alaska, after the Exxon Valdez oil spill in 1989, removed the oil from the beach surface and

thus reduced the risk to nearby otters and migratory birds which might land on the beach, but also killed the marine organisms that live on and under the beach, thereby harming the ecosystem's longer-term ability to support life of all kinds and even wiping out particular microbes that would in time have digested the oil residue themselves. Scientists supervising the Prince William Sound cleanup later reflected that by "sterilizing" the beaches, the hot water spraying may actually have done more harm than good (Schneider 1991; Lancaster 1991; Loy 1993).

- Repeated scrubbing of the Lincoln and Jefferson Memorials has turned out to cause the monuments to crumble more seriously than did the dirt and graffiti that were the target of the scouring process (Angier 1992).

- Restricting the use of potentially toxic synthetic chemical pesticides may induce farmers to use plants bred to harbor pest-resistant properties; the plants' pesticides may be more toxic than the regulated synthetic pesticides. Recent examples include pest-resistant strains of celery (containing 6,200 parts per billion carcinogenic psoralens, compared with 800 ppb in normal celery), potatoes (containing 75,000 ppb toxins such as solanine and chaconine), and cassava root (a major food crop in Africa and South America, containing cyanide) (Ames and Gold 1993).

- Removing asbestos from buildings to protect residents may increase the risk of asbestos exposure to removal workers (HEI 1991).

- Cleanup of hazardous waste sites can reduce risks of chemical contamination of soil and groundwater, but the cleanup activity also creates increased risks of accidental fatalities, especially in construction and transportation jobs. For a hypothetical typical site, the accident fatality risk from cleanup appears to be several times larger than the health risk from not cleaning up (Hoskin, Leigh, and Planek 1994). Still, the accident risk may be viewed as voluntarily undertaken (and may be compensated by market wage premiums) while the chemical risk may be viewed as more involuntarily incurred; relative risks may vary by site and by type of cleanup; and the cleanup may also provide ecological benefits.

- Keeping a gun at home to defend against the risk of criminal intruders turns out to increase the risk of being killed by gunshot nearly threefold, largely because the gun is more likely to be used in a family dispute (Kellerman and Reay 1986; Kellerman et al. 1993).
- The body's own defense mechanisms may generate countervailing risks. "Those white [blood] cells that guard against our demise from infection use nasty mutagens to incinerate their targets," protecting us from disease in the short term but increasing our long-term risk of cancer (Brody 1994, quoting Dr. Bruce Ames).

In researching this book, we found these examples of risk tradeoffs scattered throughout both the scholarly literature and print media sources. Readers may be aware of other examples, or of reasons why the examples cited above are less (or more) worrisome than they appear; our point is simply that the phenomenon is widely observable. Indeed, various analysts over the last few centuries have decried the problem of well-intentioned programs causing perverse outcomes, though many of these critics have exaggerated the inevitability and inescapability of risk tradeoffs (Hirschman 1991). In any event, these examples provide only anecdotal evidence. Far less evident are systematic efforts to understand risk tradeoffs as a general property of behavioral and technological choices. However, there do exist some pioneers in the emerging field of risk tradeoff analysis—a small but potent array of scholars who have helped to shape our thinking on the role of decision-making frameworks in fostering risk tradeoffs. Table 1.1 describes these thinkers, whose technical contributions have been made in disciplines ranging from biochemistry, physics, and engineering to economics, political science, and law. The theme that ties their writings together is a broad view of the phenomenon of risk tradeoffs.

Table 1.1 Pioneers of risk tradeoff analysis

Scholar	Area of study	Key insight
Lester Lave	Regulation	Risk-risk decision framework can be used to compare policies
Stephen Breyer	Regulation	"Mismatch" between social goals and regulatory strategy can be counterproductive
Allen Kneese	Environmental protection	Narrow pollution control measures may simply shift pollution from one medium to another
Sam Peltzman Kip Viscusi	Auto safety, consumer products	Requiring installation of mechanical safety devices may induce drivers/consumers to be less cautious
Aaron Wildavsky	Societal risks	Additional social resources enable greater overall risk reduction
Chauncy Starr Chris Whipple John Holdren Herbert Inhaber Richard Wilson	Energy technology	Risk comparisons of energy system fuel cycles
Robert Crandall Peter Huber Howard Gruenspecht	Technological innovation and regulation	Regulating risks of new technologies and practices may keep older, riskier technologies and practices in use longer
Barbara Tuchman	National defense	Strategies to expand a government's power can lead to its own defeat
Bruce Ames Renae Magaw Lois Swirsky Gold	Food safety	Carcinogens occur in both synthetic and natural foods
Terry Davies	Environmental protection	Effort to draft a single unified, integrated environmental law

Our aim in this book is to build on these insights and offer a conceptual framework to systematize the identification, evaluation, explanation, and resolution of risk tradeoffs. Because no such systematic framework is currently in use, decisionmakers may approach problems of countervailing risks in an ad hoc, often casual manner, or sometimes not at all.

A Framework for Risk Tradeoff Analysis

The development of a more systematic, rigorous method for recognizing and resolving risk tradeoffs begins with the realization that there is no magic recipe. Weighing risk versus risk will often require both objective information and personal judgment, both expert analysis and ethical values. Some countervailing risks may be deemed sufficiently unimportant that it is worth tolerating them; at other times the countervailing risks may rival, or even outweigh, the net benefits from the reduction in the target risk. In many cases the countervailing risks will be important enough to affect the decision—warranting a modification of the intervention so that it addresses the countervailing risks as well as the target risk—but not so grave that addressing the target risk is wholly undesirable.

The method of risk tradeoff analysis (RTA) that we have developed attempts to illuminate and characterize risk tradeoffs and to aid in their resolution. In part we seek to build on the concept of "risk-risk analysis" described by Lave (1981). Our development of RTA begins with a typology of risk tradeoffs (described in the following section) that defines terms and helps decisionmakers *recognize* the tradeoffs that might result from an intervention. Second, RTA posits a set of factors for decisionmakers to evaluate in *weighing* the comparative importance of target risks and countervailing risks when hard choices must be made. Third, RTA analyzes the possibility of *overall risk reduction* through "risk-superior" moves.

In RTA, the challenge is to consider and assess explicitly the impacts of interventions on important countervailing risks as well as on the target risk. For doctors and patients, for example, this means balanced consideration of a drug's efficacy and side effects, and those of alternative therapies. For energy and environmental policy, RTA calls for a modest form of "general equilibrium" analysis of target and countervailing risks rather than exclusive focus on the target risk. In the evaluation of the economic impacts of a policy, general equilibrium analysis refers in essence to the assessment not only of the costs within the regulated sector, but of the ripple effects on other sectors of the economy as well. RTA extends that approach to the evaluation of the benefits of policy, examining the ripples made by the intervention not just in the target area but in the broader range of consequences it may affect. These ripples may extend into non-environmental domains (for example, highway safety) and to international effects, given the increasingly integrated nature of world economic markets and the recognition that risks do not stop at borders; the point is to discard the categorical boundaries that constrain current thinking and encompass more of the comprehensive whole. RTA can thus be one tool in the shift toward a more integrated, comprehensive approach to environmental risk-reduction policies (Haigh and Irwin 1990; Guruswamy 1991; Stewart and Wiener 1992).

In this book we are analyzing the effectiveness of decisions designed to secure risk reduction, not the financial costs imposed on taxpayers, regulated industries, and consumers by efforts to reduce risk. Thus we do not address the economic losses imposed by risk management, or the risks to human health that such economic hardship may entail (Viscusi et al. 1994; Keeney 1990; Wildavsky 1980). Those health risks may be significant, but they relate to economic losses resulting from *all* government policy (or from other more general causes) and are not uniquely related to policies aimed at risk reduction. In contrast to the literature analyzing the *costs* of regulation and how to design regulatory tools so as to minimize those costs, we want to explore the comparatively unexamined issue of the *effectiveness* of risk reduction policies. We want to ask the question whether, at given cost, risk reduction policies are being designed so as to minimize overall risk.

Urging that decisionmakers employ RTA nonetheless obliges us to articulate some way to judge which countervailing risks are worthy of concern: how many ripples in the pool should analysts investigate? This question asks about the value of more information (to better decisions) and the cost (including delay of decisions) of obtaining that information (Finkel and Evans 1987; Hammitt and Cave 1991). The answer, unsurprisingly, is that it depends—on the importance of the countervailing risk and hence the value of amassing information about it, compared to the cost of gathering that information (Morgan and Henrion 1990). As we hope the case studies demonstrate, not all countervailing risks are of equal seriousness, and efforts to remedy target risks should not always be held up while countervailing risks are being addressed. There will be situations in which the costs of learning more about countervailing risks do not justify the resulting gains in overall risk reduction. But there will also be cases where the costs of obtaining additional information are well worth it, rewarded by the reduction in countervailing risks. And the use of RTA may help identify opportunities to reduce both target and countervailing risks—a net gain for society.

Moreover, there may well be attractive efficiencies in the use of RTA. RTA may not be increasing the total informational and analytic resources required so much as front-loading those resources in analysis accompanying the decision. The more holistic approach taken in RTA may thus help avoid the subsequent conflicts, delays, and course reversals that would occur if countervailing risks were excluded from the initial decision and the victims of those countervailing risks later returned to the table to demand changes in settled policies.

The decisionmaker being urged to think about a larger portfolio of risk consequences is not being asked to do the impossible, to know what cannot be known or to foresee the unforeseeable. There is certainly a difference between unintended consequences and unforeseeable consequences. The former category encompasses many countervailing risks which might have been considered in the effort to reduce the target risk, but which were either ignored or considered and dismissed. And the latter category is not immutable but is itself determined by the investment made in gathering information; the horizon yields as research presses ahead. A guideline that obliged only consideration of foreseeable risks would beg the question; why not encourage decisionmakers to look further? Thus, the challenge remains one of weighing not only risk versus risk, but also the value versus the costs of learning. In the present situation, where countervailing risks are plentiful but appear to be so often ignored, rejecting RTA on this ground would be like worrying about whether to slide at home plate while still standing on first base. We are starting with the first, nearest and biggest ripples.

Recognizing Risk Tradeoffs

Like all complex phenomena, risk tradeoffs are difficult to describe coherently and comprehensively. In order to articulate more systematically the kinds of tradeoffs that may occur in response to an intervention, we present in Table 1.2 a conceptual matrix that has been helpful to us in describing the phenomenon.

This typology defines risk tradeoffs along two dimensions. One dimension considers whether the adverse outcome resulting from the countervailing risk is the same as or different from the adverse outcome resulting from the target risk. The other dimension considers whether the population bearing the countervailing risk is the same as or different from the population bearing the target risk. The magnitudes of the risks are not addressed by this typological matrix, but are addressed below in terms of the factors to be weighed in RTA.

Table 1.2 Typology of Risk Tradeoffs

		Compared to the Target Risk, the Countervailing Risk is:	
		SAME TYPE	DIFFERENT TYPE
Compared to the Target Risk, the Countervailing Risk affects:	SAME POPULATION	Risk Offset	Risk Substitution
	DIFFERENT POPULATION	Risk Transfer	Risk Transformation

The terms used in our discussion of RTA require some definition. While the term "risk" is used differently in various disciplines, we define risk as the chance of an adverse outcome to human health, the quality of life, or the quality of the environment. This definition is intentionally quite broad, encompassing the full range of injuries to humans—accidents, illnesses, loss of mobility or enjoyment of personal freedoms—and injuries to other life forms, such as ecological disruptions. "Chance" of an outcome implies some degree of uncertainty about the outcome, which may be due to variability in responses among the affected population (for example, some people are more susceptible to disease than others) or due to incomplete information about how many individuals will incur the adverse outcomes under consideration. By "quality of life" we mean not only material well-being but also more intangible facets of life such as happiness, privacy, and mobility.

We define a "target risk" as the risk that is the primary focus of risk-reduction efforts. For example, the "target risk" in hypertension control is usually the chance of a heart attack or stroke due to elevated blood pressure. The "target population" is the group of individuals who are intended to benefit from reduction in the target risk. In contrast to the target risk, we define a "countervailing risk" as the chance of an adverse outcome that results from an activity whose ostensible purpose is to reduce the target risk. Perhaps the classic illustrations of countervailing risks are the side effects of a medication, or the risk of death from anesthesia during surgery. Note that the target risk in one context could be a countervailing risk in another context; for example, elevated cancer incidence is a target risk of policy to control toxic chemicals, but a countervailing risk of estrogen treatment to reduce osteoporosis after menopause.

A "risk tradeoff" is the change in the portfolio of risks that occurs when a countervailing risk is generated (knowingly or inadvertently) by an intervention to reduce the target risk.

The cells of the matrix in Table 1.2 define four qualitatively different types of risk tradeoffs. When the same risky outcome is shifted from one group to another, we say that a *risk transfer* has occurred (Whipple 1985). For example, toxic air emissions from an industrial facility can be reduced by accumulating hazardous wastes that are disposed in landfills, but the risk of adverse health outcomes from chemical exposure may simply be shifted from people who breathe air near the facility to people who ingest drinking water from wells contaminated

Table 1.3 Synopsis of case studies

Decision context	Decisionmakers	Target risks	Countervailing risks	Risk tradeoff
Estrogen therapy	Patients Physicians	Osteoporosis fractures Heart disease	Uterine cancer Breast cancer	Substitution
Clozapine therapy	Patients Physicians Families Insurers	Schizophrenia Suicide	Agranulocytosis Seizure Infection	Substitution
Elderly drivers	Government Physicians Elderly Families	Crash injuries	Depression Falls Crime Nutrition	Substitution Transfer Transformation
Auto fuel efficiency	Government Manufacturers Consumers Insurers	National security Economics Pollution	Crash injuries	Transformation
Eating fish	Consumers Government	Heart disease	Cancer	Substitution
Chlorine in drinking water	Government	Cancer	Infection	Substitution
Recycling lead	Government	Lead poisoning	Lead poisoning	Transfer
Registering pesticides	Government	Cancer	Cancer Reproductive problems Nutrition	Offset Substitution Transfer Transformation
Global environmental protection	Governments International agencies	Ozone depletion Global warming	Global warming Food Illness Biodiversity	Substitution Offset Transfer Transformation

by the groundwater. Or emissions to the air could be reduced by sealing the facility more tightly, with a potential increase in exposure to workers inside.

When the same adverse outcome is created in the target population, we label the result a *risk offset*. For example, banning the use of a fungicide on foods because it increases the risk of cancer when consumed (the target risk) may free a fungus which promotes other carcinogenic compounds (such as aflatoxins) in the food. Restricting one type of emissions that may cause global warming, only to induce increased emissions of another greenhouse gas, likewise poses a risk offset.

When one type of adverse outcome is replaced by another adverse outcome in the same target population, we observe a *risk substitution*. In the effort to treat hypertension, for example, medication for adults with elevated blood pressure may reduce the target risk of heart attacks and strokes but increase the countervailing risk of nausea for the same people. Banning cancer-causing chemicals may encourage use of chemicals which are less carcinogenic but which pose greater neurotoxic and reproductive effects.

Finally, when the countervailing risk is different in both outcome and affected population, we describe the situation as a *risk transformation*. For example, banning DDT, a persistent yet mildly toxic pesticide, may indeed have protected wildlife but at the expense of the health of farmers, who must now handle the less persistent yet more toxic organophosphate products (Ottoboni 1991).

This typology of risks can be particularly useful in recognizing risk tradeoffs and identifying countervailing risks, and in illustrating the difficult choices and ethical issues that can arise when considering risk tradeoffs. The case studies in this book illustrate each of these four types of tradeoffs; in some situations, more than one type of tradeoff is evident in a single case study (see Table 1.3).

Modeling Risk Tradeoffs

A risk tradeoff can be modeled, albeit simplistically, as a move from one set of risks to another. In Figure 1.1 we present a

simple model of two risks, the Target Risk and a Countervailing Risk. Moving outward on each axis increases the level
of protection against that risk. For example, moving upward
on the vertical axis would decrease the probability of adverse
consequence from the Target Risk. In our simplified illustration, the probability of the Target Risk occurring is one (1) at
the origin (point O) and declines toward zero as one moves
upward along the vertical axis. Similarly, the probability of the
Countervailing Risk occurring is one (1) at the origin (point O)
and declines toward zero as one moves outward to the right
along the horizontal axis. Thus at the origin (point O), it is
certain that both the Target Risk and the Countervailing Risk
will occur.

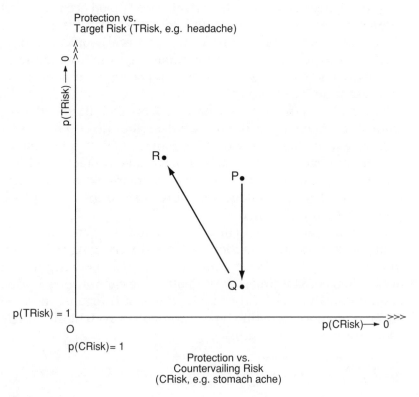

Figure 1.1 Risk tradeoff.

To model the aspirin example with which we began this chapter, we define the Target Risk as a headache and the Countervailing Risk as a stomach ache. Before the headache, the person is at a point like P, with low but non-zero likelihood of both risks. The onset of a jackhammer outside one's window moves the person to point Q, with high probability of headache but still low probability of stomach ache. A decisionmaker who considers only the change in the Target Risk will look only at the vertical dimension of Figure 1.1: whether protection against the Target Risk is going up or down. Taking aspirin moves the person from point Q to point R—vertically increasing the protection the person receives against the Target Risk (that is, reducing the headache). But while the move to point R reduces the Target Risk (headache), it also increases the probability of the Countervailing Risk (stomach ache), by moving leftward on the horizontal axis relative to points P and Q. Note that the move from Q to R depicts a "risk substitution" in the terminology of the matrix in Table 1.2. Obtaining more and more protection against the Target (headache) Risk by taking additional aspirin would move the person farther up the vertical axis, but farther left on the horizontal axis, increasing the Countervailing (stomach ache) Risk.

The set of situations in which any increase in protection against one risk means a decrease in protection against the other risk, using the maximally effective available interventions, traces out a "Risk Protection Frontier" (Figure 1.2). Along the Risk Protection Frontier the risk tradeoff occurs, in a general sense, because the intervention available to the decisionmaker to reduce risk is limited (here, we have defined the available intervention as taking aspirin). Subject to that limitation, resources devoted to increasing protection against the Target Risk mean reduced resources to combat (or increased agents causing) the Countervailing Risk (and vice versa). As we will discuss below, improved interventions which could reduce both risks can ease the tradeoff. All along the Risk Protection Frontier, the decisionmaker is achieving maximum risk protection with available resources and technologies. Each point represents the maximum protection against one risk for any given level of protection against the other risk. Choices to increase protection against one risk mean reductions in protection against another risk.

The shape of the Risk Protection Frontier will depend on the relationship between protecting against one risk and reducing protection against the other. We have drawn the Frontier as concave to the origin to suggest that as more and more protection against the Target Risk is obtained (that is, moving toward the vertical axis, say from point P toward point R and beyond), relatively larger and larger increases in Countervailing Risks must be tolerated. To put it another way, we depict diminishing marginal returns to protection against each risk. The Frontier could be shaped in other ways, including a linear (straight line) relationship, curved, or even discontinuous. The shape will depend on the real-world relationship

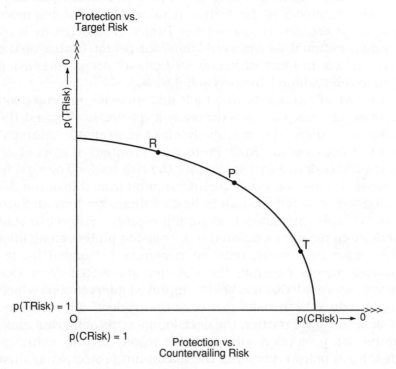

Figure 1.2 The Risk Protection Frontier.

between the particular risks posed and the particular intervention used to address them.

Moreover, in the real world there may be numerous countervailing risks (Risks C_1, C_2, C_3, and so on), each on its own axis orthogonal to the axis of a Target Risk. Thus the Risk Protection Frontier is a multidimensional surface. A decisionmaker faced with choosing the ideal point in n-dimensional risk space may find his or her information-crunching capabilities well tested. Suffice it to say that someone looking at a problem in only one dimension—the Target Risk axis alone—is likely to miss a great deal.

Weighing Risk versus Risk

The Risk Protection Frontier depicts the decisionmaker's ability to produce protection against different risks. Given the limits of this capability, the decisionmaker must weigh risk versus risk—compare the severity, likelihood, and other factors characterizing each risk—in order to choose a best outcome. For example, how should the decisionmaker choose among points on the Risk Protection Frontier, such as points P, R, and T in Figure 1.2? The choice will depend on the decisionmaker's preferences for (avoiding) different risks, and thus will require both valid assessments of the quantitative parameters of each risk (probability, magnitude, and so forth) calculated by expert scientists, and conscious and explicit value judgments. (These preferences for risk avoidance could be depicted as "risk indifference curves," convex to the origin; see Viscusi, Magat, and Huber 1991.)

Using the typology described in Table 1.2 helps illuminate the kinds of risk tradeoffs that may occur, but does not determine how risk tradeoffs in any particular case should be resolved. Faced with a choice of moving along the Risk Protection Frontier (Figure 1.2)—a choice among different options with different risk portfolios—the decisionmaker must exercise judgment to determine the best course of action. In essence, the decisionmaker must make the hard choice of selecting among risks. These are difficult decisions that people make all the time, such as the choice in the headache example, the choice of whether or not to undergo intrusive surgery for a life-threatening disease, the decision of where to live, whether to drive on the highways or fly in an airplane, and many others described earlier in this chapter. There is evidence that people are quite capable of expressing consistent preferences for (avoiding) different health risks across a range of tradeoffs (Viscusi, Magat, and Huber 1991). And to handle extremely complex comparisons of multidimensional risk portfolios, computer-graphics tools just short of virtual reality are now being developed for use by financial brokers (*Economist* 1994) and could be adapted for use by risk managers as well. But today people seldom make these hard choices with a systematic analytic approach; hence we seek to develop a set of factors that decisionmakers can use to guide their comparisons of different risks.

Decisionmakers faced with risk tradeoffs must have some basis on which to weigh risk versus risk and come to a decision about the best course of action. In the case studies, we found that several key factors were relevant in weighing risk versus risk: chief among them are magnitude, degree of population exposure, certainty, type of adverse outcome, distribution, and timing. Note that the decisionmaker must consider not just the characteristics of the target risk, but these characteristics *relative* to those of the countervailing risk(s).

Magnitude (Probability) of Risk. Recall that risk is defined as the probability of an adverse outcome. When target and countervailing risks are compared, the magnitudes of probabilities often differ. If the adverse outcomes are similar or identical (for example, fatal cancer vs. fatal cancer), as in a risk offset or risk transfer (see Table 1.2), the relative probabilities of the adverse outcomes become critical.

Although people appear to have difficulty comprehending small probabilities (Fisher, McClelland, and Schulze 1989), it is important for decisionmakers to recognize the difference between a lifetime probability of, say, 1 in 100 and a lifetime probability of 1 in 100,000. For example, the elevation in the probability of death from contaminants in fish appears to be far smaller than the estimated reduction in the probability of death associated with eating fish instead of meat.

One of the virtues of RTA is that it exposes the logical fallacy of using any uniform probability (for example, 1 in 1,000,000) as a threshold for action or inaction. There is no magic threshold that can tell us what risks are worth reducing through interventions—the answer depends, in part, on what countervailing risks, if any, would be incurred to reduce the target risk (Graham 1991).

Size of Population. If we hold constant the probability of adverse outcome to a specified individual for the target and countervailing risks, the relative size of the exposed populations is an important consideration. Statistics such as aggregate cancer incidence (sometimes called "population risk" in contrast to "individual risk") are useful in capturing the importance of the size of an exposed population. If 1,000 citizens each face an incremental lifetime cancer risk of 1 in 1,000,000, the population risk (0.001 cases of cancer) seems negligible. If 200,000,000 citizens are exposed to the same individual risk, the resulting population risk (200 cancers) may not be so negligible. By recognizing the size of exposed populations, RTA can help decisionmakers avoid perverse "risk transfers" where a small individual cancer risk is shifted from a small population to a large population (Goldstein 1989).

Certainty in Risk Estimates. Estimates of risk are often uncertain because of gaps in scientific knowledge. Hence, consideration needs to be given to the scientific basis or credibility of the target and countervailing risks. Some risk estimates are amply supported by science, while others are supported only by speculation.

When the degree of scientific uncertainty about the target and countervailing risks differs, RTA calls for the analyst to characterize the uncertainty for risk managers. Where relative certainty can be quantified objectively, the risk estimates can be adjusted with classical statistical methods to reflect this knowledge (Finkel 1990; Bogen 1990). But the extent of scientific uncertainty is sometimes not objectively quantifiable, in which case it will be necessary to obtain subjective yet quantitative technical judgments from experts. Using Bayesian methods, these subjective probabilities can be combined with objective probabilities in reporting estimates of individual and population risk (Morgan and Henrion 1990).

In making such comparisons, RTA calls for symmetrical reporting of the degree of scientific uncertainty about target and countervailing risks. If worst-case estimates are reported for target risks, worst-case estimates should likewise be reported for countervailing risks. When expected-value estimates are reported for target risks, countervailing risks should by analyzed similarly. Ideally, RTA calls for both target and countervailing risks to be analyzed in distributional form (Frey 1992), where risk distributions reflect both variability (that is, differences in susceptibility and exposure among people or generations) and uncertainty (that is, extent of knowledge). Ultimately, the risk manager must decide whether to favor the mitigation of well-proven risks or of more speculative risks.

Type of Adverse Outcome. Because risks do not come in a single flavor, countervailing risks are often of a different character from target risks. "Risk substitutions" and "transformations" (see Table 1.2) both exhibit changing kinds of risk. For example, estrogen therapy may prevent hip fractures but induce cancer; eating fish may prevent heart disease but induce cancer; replacing CFCs may prevent stratospheric ozone depletion but accelerate global warming. Similarly, reducing the risk of cancer by smoking less may (for some people) increase the risk of obesity from overeating; "clean" fuels that eliminate the carcinogenic air pollution associated with burning gasoline may introduce a new spectrum of chemical emissions and adverse health effects (Adler 1992); reducing the risk of terrorist attacks may require increased restrictions on personal liberty.

Can these risks be usefully compared? For some types of risks, endpoints are similar enough that an aggregate calculation of the "net risk" posed by an intervention is currently possible. For example, in the case study on estrogen replacement therapy in Chapter 2, the patient and her physician may be able to compare and calculate the net change in life expectancy resulting from reducing the target risk of osteoporosis-induced hip fracture and the countervailing increased risk of uterine cancer. Or the mortality risk of eating fish (Chapter 6) might be calculated as the net risk due to carcinogens delivered in the fish, minus the risk of heart disease avoided.

But are equal probabilities of death by cancer and death by

accident, or by heart disease, really equivalent? For some kinds of risks, such net-risk calculations will be incomplete or impossible with current methods of evaluation. For example, patients may have different subjective attitudes toward the risk of uterine cancer versus the risk of hip fracture, or versus the risk of breast cancer. This factor will be important to their decision even at equal calculated expected mortality rates from the accident and the two cancers. For risks that seem very "dissimilar," risk cannot (yet) be measured on a unidimensional scale, and the exercise of informed value judgments becomes all the more central. For example, it is currently rather difficult to quantify on the same scale the risk of highway fatality and the risk of international entanglement resulting from dependence on foreign supplies of oil (Chapter 5), or the risk of harm to humans versus the risk of harm to non-human species (Chapter 10). But it is chiefly our lack of methods of comparison—of ways of seeing commonality among these risks—that makes these risks seem "dissimilar" or noncomparable, not an inherent incommensurability. As we improve methods of risk analysis, the idea of calculating the "net risk" of a risk portfolio, or the change in net risk due to a risk tradeoff, may become more meaningful. The theory of multiobjective decisionmaking has been explored (Keeney and Raiffa 1976), and research has demonstrated the ability of questionnaire respondents to weigh and trade off risks of two quite different health effects (chronic bronchitis versus sudden death in an automobile accident) (Viscusi, Magat, and Huber 1991). Indeed, people appear able to quantify their relative dislike of equally probable but dissimilar causes of mortality: Tolley, Kenkel, and Fabian (1994, pp. 339–344) find that avoiding death by cancer is generally viewed as about twice as desirable as avoiding sudden accidental death.

The case studies in this volume cover a diverse range of adverse outcomes including cancer, heart disease, hip fracture, head injury, personal immobility, depression, war, famine, and ecological dysfunction. One qualitative difference among risks commonly noted in psychological research is that some risks are felt to be controllable and voluntarily assumed, while others seem uncontrollable by the individual and involuntarily imposed (Slovic et al. 1985). Other qualitative differences include the degree of dread the risk inspires, and the extent to which it afflicts special members of society such as children.

To say that people do place different weights on different ways of incurring risk is not to say that they should, or that public policy should necessarily validate these subjective attitudes. Dread of the unfamiliar may reflect an irrational fear of the new or the foreign, a fear we discount in other areas of social policy (for example, immigration). But because reasonable people can disagree about how onerous these outcomes are (relative to one another), the case studies in this book describe the various outcomes without drawing hard conclusions about their relative importance. The case studies do provide several illustrations of risk substitution and risk transformation, situations where the adverse outcome from the target risk is qualitatively different (at least with current comparison methods) from the adverse outcome from the countervailing risk. Chapter 2 compares cancer risks to fracture risks; Chapter 6 quantifies the relative mortality risk from cancer and heart disease; Chapter 7 highlights the difference between microbial disease and cancer; Chapter 10 examines the risks of cancer, famine, and ecological disruption. These problems provide a vivid account of the need to weigh different types of adverse outcomes.

Distributional Considerations. Even when the risk tradeoff involves equal probabilities of two similar outcomes that are equally uncertain, risk managers may also be interested in distributional issues: who incurs the risks. When risks are unequally distributed among the population, they may be perceived as more onerous than when risks are distributed equally. Moreover, risks that are incurred disproportionately by disadvantaged groups in society may be perceived as less fair than risks that are incurred by all groups in society. Just as the distributions of wealth and income in society are ethically significant, so can the distribution of risks be a matter of ethical concern. RTA would provide such distributional information to risk managers.

Ethical issues are often raised by "risk transfers" or "risk transformations," situations where risks are shifted from one population to another. Indeed, some environmental policies appear to be designed not so much to reduce pollution as to shift the burden from one population group or region to another. The 1977 Clean Air Act, for example, shifted sulfur pollution from local areas to long-range downwind deposition, and protected high-sulfur Eastern coal mines at the expense of low-sulfur Western mines (Ackerman and Hassler 1981). The ban on disposal and incineration of wastes at sea may protect ocean biota, but may shift risk to land-based human and freshwater communities.

Ethical questions may be particularly sensitive when the populations to whom risks are shifted have not been represented in the deliberations that led to the policy to address the target risk. The affected population may lack a voice because it consists of groups with disproportionately less power, wealth, or social standing. The phenomenon of countervailing risks thus provides some insight into contemporary concern about the siting in disadvantaged neighborhoods of potentially risky facilities such as waste disposal sites and incinerators (Hamilton 1993), and the call for "environmental justice" on behalf of disadvantaged (often minority) population subgroups (Bullard 1990; Anderton et al. 1994; Zimmerman 1993). These questions need to be analyzed carefully, however, since discrimination may turn out to be in education, employment, housing, and other arenas rather than in the siting decision itself (Been 1993), since choices of definition and measurement can exaggerate or conceal inequity (Zimmerman 1994), and since what appears to be an inequitable distribution of risk may prove to be otherwise when the full range of target and countervailing risks is analyzed (Hird 1993).

Similarly, political incentives may systematically encourage governments to try to shift risks away from citizens or the environment within a political jurisdiction at the expense of citizens or the environment of other, unrepresented jurisdictions. The current debate over whether U.S. environmental laws apply extraterritorially can thus be seen in terms of risk tradeoffs. In other situations, the victimized population may lack a voice in the debate because it does not yet exist: concern about imposing risks on future generations—such as by causing latent illnesses manifested in offspring, or changing the earth's climate over the next century—partly reflects this problem. Or the population at risk may lack a voice in the policy dialogue because it is not human, but consists of non-voting forms of life sharing the global ecosystem. RTA cannot easily resolve these sensitive issues, but application of RTA can highlight such distributional shifts for resolution by accountable risk managers.

The Timing of Risks. The timing of target and countervailing risks may differ. The risks of trauma are often more imminent than the risks of cancer; the latter may occur only after a long latency period. Analysts are making progress in estimating the implicit discount rates that citizens assign to future as opposed to present health effects (Cropper and Portney 1990; Cropper et al. 1991; Viscusi 1992). In RTA, risks to future generations are distinguished from risks to the current generation. Once again, our case studies document temporal differences in risks and ask readers to struggle with the tradeoff between reducing risks now versus reducing future risks. In this area RTA is just beginning to illuminate choices, and will benefit from more social science research on citizens' preferences about the timing of risky outcomes.

Thus, through the process of RTA, risk managers and the public will begin thinking not just about an ideal risk-free existence, but about what types of risks should be accepted and what types avoided, who should incur which risks when, and who should have the power to decide these matters. Though these questions may be uncomfortable to discuss and difficult to resolve, we believe that America's campaign against risk will be improved in the long run by a scientific and ethical dialogue that confronts the phenomenon of risk tradeoffs.

Reducing Overall Risk

Beyond choosing among points along the Risk Protection Frontier, can we do better and reduce overall risk? We believe the answer is yes. The prevalence of countervailing risks does not imply their inevitability or invincibility. We do not posit some kind of thermodynamic law of conservation of risk, nor an inescapable "perversity thesis" (Hirschman 1991) in which one risk-reducing action is always matched by an equal and offsetting increase in other risks. The feasibility of overall reductions in risk is partly illustrated by the indicators of decreasing risks to life and health documented in the first section of this chapter. Contrary to theories of "risk homeostasis" (Wilde 1985), we believe that contemporary social systems leave room for improvement and that, with intelligent efforts, superior choices can be found through which overall risk can decline. "Risk reduction" is thus a meaningful goal: choices can be made that, on balance, make the world safer for humans and for other life forms.

The possibility of overall risk reduction is illustrated in our simple model by a "risk-superior" move to a point on a *higher* Risk Protection Frontier. As shown in Figure 1.3, moving from point P to point S enables greater protection against both risks than points along the original RPF. Since moves along a given RPF were constrained by limited resources and technology, such "risk-superior" moves are made possible by increases in the total supply of resources devoted to risk reduction, or by innovations in technologies, practices, and scientific understanding. There can also be "coincident risk reductions"—unintended bonuses of efforts to reduce a target risk (see, for example, Shelef 1994)—but for reasons we explore in Chapter 11, these are likely to be rare.

The first implication of this simple model is that there is an important symbiotic relationship between economic growth (in its true sense of increasing social well-being, not increasing industrialization or physical consumption levels) and risk reduction. Empirical evidence indicates that a growing resource base can and often does contribute to decreasing manifestations of at least some risks, such as human mortality (Graham, Chang, and Evans 1992; Wildavsky 1980) and air pollution (Grossman and Krueger 1991).

The flip side of this implication is that moving to risk-superior frontiers may entail opportunity costs. If newer technologies are safer in terms of overall risk, but more costly, society will need to devote more resources to this purpose or

choose to forgo those risk-superior moves whose costs exceed
their benefits. The incremental social cost of shifting the Risk
Protection Frontier further and further out from the origin,
closer and closer to zero risk on all axes, may rise (that is,
there may be increasing marginal costs of protection).

Furthermore, if government policy requires new equipment
to incorporate costly risk-control technologies, consumers
may be encouraged to keep their older equipment in use longer
(that is, remain on a lower Risk Protection Frontier), thus in-
hibiting (and in some cases even reversing) the aggregate net
reduction in risk that would have been obtained had consumers more readily retired old equipment and adopted new
equipment (moved to a higher frontier) (Huber 1983; Gruenspecht 1992). For example, differential standards for new
versus old equipment have been imposed by the government
on automobile mileage (CAFE), pesticides (FIFRA), and certain
emissions from electric power generating stations (CAA § 111),

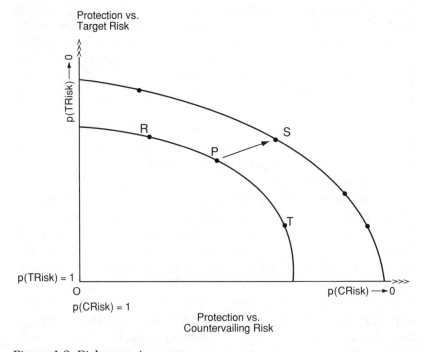

Figure 1.3 Risk-superior moves.

thus encouraging owners to keep older cars, pesticides, and utility boilers in use longer even though faster turnover toward newer models would have contributed a larger reduction in overall risk (considering both the regulated endpoint and other endpoints such as auto crashworthiness, worker exposure, and electric utility emissions of other pollutants). One solution to this new-old dilemma is to tax or limit risk-producing activities regardless of the vintage of the equipment—for example, to tax air pollutant emissions from sources of all ages rather than requiring only new facilities to incorporate tighter controls.

The second major implication of this simple model is that scientific research and technological change (in its broad sense, encompassing not only new hardware but also new ways of organizing work and lifestyles, and the diffusion of those ideas into practice) play an extremely important role in risk reduction, perhaps the fundamental role. Progress in knowledge and technical abilities can elucidate or devise better ways to reduce target risks and countervailing risks in concert (Huber 1983). Because of the cost of shifting to risk-superior frontiers, society will put great value on devising risk-superior technologies and practices that are low-cost, or more precisely, highly cost-effective (offering a greater degree of risk-improvement per unit of opportunity cost).

With effort and ingenuity, risk-superior moves are achievable. For example, in the headache problem, we noted that analgesics that reduce headaches without causing stomach distress (such as acetaminophen) have been developed as alternatives to aspirin. New vaccines are being developed which immunize children without causing harmful side effects (New York Times 1994). In the oil spill example noted earlier in this chapter, potential alternatives that both clean the beaches of oil (the target risk) and reduce the collateral damage to beach bacteria (the countervailing risk) include fertilizing the existing bacteria to accelerate their own digestion of the spilled oil—an idea that was tested in Prince William Sound—and the use of genetic engineering to develop new bacteria that will digest oil-spill residues on beaches. In the problem presented in Chapter 5, newer automobile engine systems and

lighter but stronger construction materials might make possible more fuel-efficient vehicles that do not increase risks to
motorists in highway crashes. Still, such moves typically
come at some cost—for example, acetaminophen and ibuprofen typically cost more per dose than aspirin—and it must
be asked whether the added risk-reduction benefits justify
that use of resources.

The development of new science and technologies often allows risk-superior moves, but that result is not preordained.
Much innovation is the product of brilliant scientists, given
support for basic research, who serendipitously invent a new
way of doing things or devise a new paradigm for looking at
and solving current problems (Wiener 1993; Kuhn 1970).
Other innovations are introduced by energetic entrepreneurs
who see an opportunity to reinvent an industry or a technology
(Schumpeter 1942). Whether a particular innovation will be
risk-reducing, however, is not certain. Without needing to
imagine mad scientists bent on wreaking havoc, it is plain that
even well-intentioned innovations can pose countervailing
risks. For example, chlorofluorocarbons (CFCs), touted as the
wonder chemical of the 1930s, did provide refrigeration (to
limit the risk of food-borne infectious disease) in a way that
eliminated the risk of toxicity posed by ammonia-based cool-
ants, but ultimately the CFCs proved to increase the risk of
ultraviolet radiation by thinning the stratospheric ozone layer
(see Chapter 10).

The path of science and technology is determined by human
choices, at the individual (inventor/entrepreneurial) level and
at the societal level. Its direction depends on several factors,
including the professional culture and personal commitment
of researchers and their institutions, the freedom provided to
scientists to research fundamental problems, and the incentives provided to entrepreneurs to make risk-reducing technologies and ideas more widely available. These incentives derive chiefly from the market demand for risk reduction and
from risk-reducing laws and regulations. If risks are not priced
in markets—whether by informed consumer choice or by government interventions to internalize risks in market decisions—then the entrepreneur will earn no reward for her in-

vestment, and newer, better methods of reducing risk will be either left undeveloped or developed but left unused.

Applying RTA

We attempt in this book to document the significance and complexity of risk tradeoffs through in-depth case studies of a variety of real-world choices. Our framework and case studies are designed to help decisionmakers identify risk tradeoffs, and to structure their decisionmaking so that these tradeoffs are intelligently resolved and overall risk reduction is better achieved. Thus, these case studies (summarized in Table 1.3) illustrate both successful and unsuccessful efforts to recognize and respond to countervailing risks.

In the concluding chapter of this book we explore the vexing question of why risk tradeoffs occur. On the basis of insights from our case studies as well as current examples of creative risk management, we suggest institutional reforms to improve the handling of risk tradeoffs. Our hope is that through the systematic application of risk tradeoff analysis, society can escape the cycle of target and countervailing risks that now plagues the national quest for health, safety, and a clean environment, and can begin to move to a risk-superior future.

2

Estrogen Therapy for Menopause

EVRIDIKI HATZIANDREU
CONSTANCE WILLIAMS
JOHN D. GRAHAM

There are few if any medical therapies that cure the target malady without producing unwanted side effects. Drugs administered to kill an infection may also traumatize related tissues; remedies for problems in one organ or body system may affect the functioning of other organs or body systems; any surgical procedure involving anesthesia presents patients with a non-zero probability of dying on the operating table. In medicine, analyzing risk tradeoffs is simply essential to making sound therapeutic decisions.

If the physician-patient relationship is functioning well, the physician gives the patient an objective assessment of the risks of going without treatment and the risks that may be induced by each potential therapy. The final decision about therapy is a balancing of risks made by the patient in consultation with her physician.

Although the necessity of making risk tradeoffs is commonly recognized in medicine, that does not make the process easy, even when physicians are well informed about the latest biomedical science and patients are well equipped to comprehend such complex information. As an illustration of this phenomenon, we consider the dilemma faced by a woman at the onset of menopause: Should she take hormone replacement therapy as a preventive therapy for conditions such as heart disease and osteoporosis? If so, for how long and with what frequency, doses, and mixes of hormones? This is a highly salient question now faced by more than 40 million women in the United States and many others throughout the world (Ubell 1993; Brody 1992).

The Health Risks of Menopause

A woman's production of estrogens begins to decline at about age 35. Menopause refers to the complete cessation of ovarian function, the termination of a woman's menstrual cycles, and a resulting condition of chronic estrogen deficiency. For most women, menopause occurs between the ages of 45 and 55. Since the average American woman's life expectancy at age 50 is about 40 years and is increasing, the post-menopausal phase is approaching one-half of a grown woman's expected lifetime.

As they pass through menopause, women experience temporary discomforts. Almost 90 percent of menopausal women experience hormonal effects in the form of "hot flashes," which vary in duration (30 seconds to 5 minutes) and frequency (once a week to three times daily). The discomforts of hot flashes may persist from one to five years and frequently result in interrupted sleep, leaving some women less productive and more depressed than normal. Hot flashes are disruptive enough to cause 10 to 20 percent of menopausal women to seek medical attention.

The genito-urinary effects of menopause are also significant. Without stimulation by estrogen, the vagina and vulva shrink and the vaginal walls become thinner, drier, and more sensitive, which can result in itching, inflammation, infection, and pain during intercourse. The bladder and urethra also become prone to infections and may weaken to the point that urination becomes more frequent and less controllable.

In the longer run, estrogen deficiency has serious adverse effects on the skeletal system. When the amount of estrogens circulating in the body declines, the bones begin to lose calcium faster than they incorporate it. The ultimate result may be osteoporosis, a common metabolic disorder in the elderly that is caused by accelerated breakdown in bone mass and a resulting drop in bone density (Hillner 1992). Osteoporosis is believed to be the cause of 50 to 60 percent of the 300,000 hip fractures that occur each year in the United States. Hip fractures are very expensive to treat, often render victims permanently disabled, and lead to premature death in 10 to 15 percent of cases.

Perhaps the most devastating long-term effects of estrogen loss are experienced by the woman's heart and blood vessels. Prior to menopause, rates of coronary heart disease in men are much higher than in women of the same age. During and after menopause, however, the risk of coronary heart disease among women approaches the elevated rates of men. Although the biological mechanisms of this effect are not fully understood, estrogen deficiency causes blood cholesterol problems in many women as well as a variety of cardiovascular disorders. The result is a sharp increase in the rate of heart attacks among postmenopausal women.

Estrogen Replacement Therapy

By prescribing estrogens to supplement the body's natural rate of production, physicians can prevent, mitigate, or delay the adverse sequelae of menopause and estrogen deficiency. For many women, estrogen therapy has led to marked improvements in quality of life. As a cure for hot flashes, estrogens are virtually 100 percent effective. Moreover, even if a woman has given up intercourse for several years because of pain and bleeding, estrogen therapy can help restore the lining, depth, and secretions of the vagina, which are integral to sexual enjoyment. There is also some evidence (though it is controversial) suggesting that estrogen therapy promotes a woman's psychological well-being by reducing bouts of anxiety and depressed mood (Ditkoff et al. 1991).

The mortality and morbidity prevention effects of estrogen treatment are no less dramatic. Estrogen therapy appears to increase a woman's life expectancy by 20 to 30 percent, primarily by cutting the death rate from osteoporosis and coronary heart disease. The best available estimates are, for the average 50-year-old woman, that estrogen therapy decreases the lifetime probability of coronary heart disease by 25 percent, from 0.461 to 0.342, and the lifetime probability of hip fracture by 17 percent, from 0.153 to 0.127 (Grady et al. 1992).

Therapeutic norms have changed significantly in recent decades in response to greater knowledge of the efficacy of estrogen therapy. Two decades ago, estrogens were prescribed for the sole purpose of relieving the temporary discomforts experienced by women during menopause. The mean duration of estrogen therapy was only two years, and therapy was almost always terminated within five years. In recent years, as physicians have begun to recognize the long-term health benefits of estrogen replacement, it has become more common to prescribe estrogen continuously for up to twenty years.

Countervailing Risks of Estrogen Therapy

Endometrial Cancer. In 1975 women and the medical community were startled by the discovery that estrogen therapy increases a woman's risk of endometrial cancer, which is a slow-growing yet life-threatening cancer of the lining of the uterus. This cancer can arise as estrogens stimulate tumor formation on the endometrium, the lining of the uterus. Effective treatment usually requires hysterectomy.

Each year in the United States, 35,000 cases and 2,900 deaths are reported from endometrial cancer. At age 50, a woman's baseline risk of contracting this form of cancer in the remainder of her lifetime is 1 to 2 chances in 1,000. Chronic use of estrogen therapy (that is, more than five years of continuous use) is estimated to increase the baseline risk seven- to eight-fold, to an elevated level of 7 to 16 chances in 1,000 (Grady et al. 1992).

When this cancer risk was recognized, the doses of estrogen prescribed for postmenopausal women were reduced. From years of experience, physicians have learned that the doses of estrogen necessary to prevent hot flashes and achieve long-term health benefits are smaller than previously thought. A smaller dose may reduce the risk of endometrial cancer. Instead of receiving daily doses of 2.5 milligrams, most women on replacement therapy now take only a fourth as much (0.625 milligrams), which is also believed to be adequate to offer long-term health benefits (American College of Physicians 1992).

Recognition of the countervailing cancer risk also made physicians more cautious about prescribing "unopposed" estrogens for long periods of time. They instead began to prescribe estrogen together with a second hormone, progestin, to protect the lining of the uterus and minimize the risk of endometrial cancer. Although the protective effects of progestin are not firmly established, it appears that it counters the growth-stimulating effects of estrogen on the endometrium.

Unfortunately, taking this second hormone introduces a new spectrum of risks, such as weight gain, swelling of tissues, lower abdomen cramps, and irregular vaginal bleeding. Many women on progestin also experience dose-dependent increases in depression, irritability, loss of energy, loss of libido, and breast pain. These are all symptoms of premenstrual tension which become more severe with an increase in the duration of progestins (Studd 1992).

Physicians often find it necessary to reduce the recommended twelve-day course of progestins down to seven days in order to minimize these side effects. But returning toward "unopposed" estrogen stimulation of the lining of the uterus can induce heavy or irregular bleeding, and this may result in the need for invasive and somewhat painful diagnostic endometrial evaluation. To prevent bleeding and other side effects, some success has been achieved with the use of continuous, combined preparations of estrogen and progestin.

Concern has been expressed that long-term use of progestin may diminish or eliminate the cardiovascular benefits of estrogen therapy. This concern has arisen because progestin tends to aggravate the blood cholesterol problems that estrogen therapy reduces, by reversing the favorable alteration in the lipid (fat) profile induced by estrogen therapy. The most recent indications are that the net effect of both hormones on cardiovascular health is beneficial (Nabulsi et al. 1993), but more long-term study of patients treated with combination therapy is needed.

Breast Cancer. Perhaps the most salient yet controversial side effect of estrogen therapy is breast cancer, the form of cancer that women tend to fear most (Grady and Ernster 1991). The short-term use of estrogen to combat menopausal symptoms (that is, less than five years) is not associated with a detectable increase in the incidence of breast cancer (Hillard et al. 1991). However, several studies of long-term estrogen therapy (that is, ten to twenty or more years of use) have reported increases in the risk of breast cancer. Women with a family history of breast cancer appear to be particularly susceptible to the carcinogenic activity of estrogen. Taken together, the available studies suggest that long-term estrogen therapy is associated with an approximate 25 percent increase in the risk of breast cancer, though some scientists doubt the presumed cause-effect relationship (Gambrell 1992). Controlled animal tests have shown that high doses of estrogen cause mammary tumors and breast cancer, although the relevance of these results to humans is unclear.

Since progestin appears to curb the risk of endometrial cancer, it was hoped that this hormone might also reduce the risk of breast cancer associated with estrogen therapy. Preliminary biological evidence, however, suggests otherwise. Progestins increase mitotic (cell division) activity in breast cells, which suggests that progestin with estrogen may be associated with a larger risk of breast cancer than occurs with estrogen alone. The findings of some (but not all) of the available human studies support this hypothesis (Harlap 1992). Since the human studies on this question are inadequate to draw a firm conclusion, large-scale studies with long-term follow-up of women are urgently needed and have been undertaken recently by the federal government. Some authors urge large-scale human trials even among patients with a history of breast cancer (Wile et al. 1993).

To summarize, an average 50-year-old woman's probability of contracting breast cancer in the remainder of her life is about 10.2 percent. Long-term therapy with estrogens alone is estimated to increase this lifetime probability to about 13.0

percent. The combination of both hormones (estrogen with progestin) is associated with lifetime breast cancer probabilities in the range of 13.0 to 19.7 percent (Grady et al. 1992), a range that reflects the paucity of definitive study.

Weighing Risk versus Risk

Although the American College of Physicians recently developed guidelines regarding estrogen replacement therapy (American College of Physicians 1992), no guidelines in this area are universally accepted. A medical consensus exists that all women at menopause should be considered for therapy, yet clinical practices vary. Gynecologists tend to prescribe estrogen more often than do internists, but mainly for relief of the acute menopausal symptoms, while internists are more inclined to prescribe estrogen for long-term protection against osteoporosis and coronary heart disease. Despite therapeutic advances, it is estimated that only 15 to 20 percent of the 40 million women eligible for estrogen treatment are currently undergoing therapy (Baber and Studd 1989).

Uniform treatment recommendations are of questionable value because what is appropriate for some women may be inappropriate for others. It is important to emphasize the individualized nature of the risk tradeoffs. For example, women who have already had a hysterectomy (and are thus not susceptible to endometrial cancer or bleeding) may be inclined to take long-term "unopposed" estrogen therapy rather than combination therapy or no therapy. Women with a family history of breast cancer may be more reluctant to undergo long-term estrogen therapy than women without such a history. The adverse side effects of progestin therapy, holding constant dose and regimen, appear to be more severe in some women than in others.

Women faced with the same objective probabilities of the target mortality risks (osteoporosis and heart disease) and the countervailing mortality risks (endometrial cancer and breast cancer) may make different choices, reflecting their value judgments about how risks should be weighed. Some women may have a greater subjective aversion to a given risk of a particular ailment than do others. Thus they may, for example, choose to tolerate an increase in total mortality risk if the risk of a particularly dread disease, such as breast cancer, is reduced. Some women feel that estrogen therapy is "unnatural" or "unnecessary" in the absence of discomforting symptoms (Studd 1992). And since the decision about menopause and its treatments can significantly involve non-mortality risks to the quality of life—such problems as hot flashes, itching, bleeding, swelling, cramps, sexual dysfunction, and emotional depression—the patient's participation in clinical decisionmaking is crucial.

The decisionmaking process for women and their physicians is further complicated by the uncertainty surrounding each of the risk estimates, as a result of the absence of definitive data. Until large epidemiological studies (some of which are now under way) are complete, women must decide (and physicians must recommend) therapies without knowing for certain whether or to what degree the chances of contracting cancer or cardiovascular disease will be influenced by these choices. Since the currently advancing generation of women have already witnessed other unexpected calamities in the medical treatment of reproductive systems (for example, the unexpected risks of DES and the Dalkon Shield), they may be more cautious and have a heightened demand for information about the risks of alternative therapies.

All of these factors underscore the importance of individualized treatment plans that take into account a woman's profile of risk factors and her personal preferences regarding types of risks and health states (Birkenfeld and Kase 1991). Even if the biomedical science were crystal-clear to all women and physicians, the decisions to be made would not be easy. Patients and physicians need to approach these medical choices in an open-minded and thoughtful manner. Unless patients grapple with the probabilities of both short- and long-term consequences, both positive and negative, they will not really face the dilemmas. Meanwhile, physicians need not only to understand the latest biomedical science and provide patients with accurate probabilistic statements about the risks of taking and not taking different therapies, but equally to acknowledge and respect the subjective aspects of the patient's decision problem, including quality-of-life issues and strong fears of particular maladies.

Conclusion

The increasing use of estrogen therapy among postmeno-pausal women has proved to be a large-scale exercise in re-solving a "risk substitution" (see Table 1.2), in which reducing the target risk creates new risks for the same population. Women in their early fifties appear to be choosing to incur modest elevations in the risks of cancers in exchange for di-minished risk of heart disease and osteoporosis and enhanced quality of life. On the basis of this case study, we raise here some broader themes for sound management of risk tradeoffs, themes which are elaborated further in the first and last chapters of this book.

Ethics. The ethics of coping with risk substitution, as con-trasted with risk transfers and transformations, are simplified here because the same individuals incur both the target risks and the countervailing risks. In this case, the target popula-tion is postmenopausal women who are eligible for estrogen therapy. It is certainly true that the lives of a woman's spouse, family, and friends may be affected by her choice to undergo or forgo therapy, but the great majority of the risks faced are personal and ultimately it is the woman's choice to make (in collaboration with others she chooses to consult). Thus, the key to making ethically sound decisions about risk substitu-tion is informed choice by members of the target population after careful consideration of (1) the objective probabilities of experiencing various health states with and without interven-tion, and (2) the subjective aspects of how these different health states affect the quality of life.

Comparing Risks. Given the subjective complexities, anal-ysis of risk substitutions needs to go beyond quantitative com-parisons of the length of life and embrace quality-of-life con-siderations. The adverse health effects of menopause are numerous and are qualitatively different from the carcinogenic risks and other side effects of estrogen and progestin therapies. The numerical comparison of life expectancy with and without estrogen therapy—which for the average woman favors long-term therapy by a considerable margin, because the mortality risks of heart disease and osteoporosis-induced fracture reduced by estrogen therapy are of greater magnitude than the mortality risks of endometrial and breast cancer it creates—is a useful statistic but should not necessarily override the less quantitative yet real concerns about quality of life and living with elevated fears of breast cancer. In order to combine subjective concerns and unquantified quality issues with objective data on life expectancy, risk analysts are making greater use of measures such as "quality-adjusted life-years" that have been devised by the decision science community (Torrance 1986).

Evaluation Studies. Well-intended measures taken to reduce target risks need to be accompanied by evaluation research programs that search systematically for countervailing risks. In the case of estrogen therapy, a good argument can be made that women have been subjected to a large-scale therapeutic experiment without adequate monitoring of potential side effects. When treatment was begun, thorough studies were not initiated. The discovery of the link to endometrial cancer was somewhat fortuitous, while the facts about breast cancer are still not fully understood. Since countervailing risks (like target risks) may be low-incidence (yet serious) outcomes, they may escape detection in the absence of carefully designed and implemented studies.

Scientific Progress. If scientific expertise is mobilized to identify risk tradeoffs, new strategies may be devised that can minimize or eliminate countervailing risks without lessening progress against the target risk. Once the dangers of endometrial cancer were recognized by physicians, they were soon reduced by more precise doses of estrogen and by a decline in the practice of prescribing estrogen unopposed by progestin. Of course, scientific advances are not risk-free, as women are now faced with the challenge of determining the long-term risks of combining estrogen and progestin treatments.

Treat the Whole Patient. Critical to sound decisions about therapy for menopause has been an understanding of the risks to the whole patient, not just to the woman's reproductive organs as though they were a separate system. The target risks of menopause include uterine and vaginal dysfunctions, but also heart disease and calcium deficiency in bones throughout the body. Similarly, the countervailing risks of estrogen therapy include cancer of the endometrial lining of the uterus, but also cancer in the breast. Decisions by patients and physicians, and the research conducted and advice given by the medical community, need to encompass the whole patient if they are to recognize and fully resolve the risk tradeoffs presented.

3

Clozapine Therapy for Schizophrenia

MIRIAM E. ADAMS
HOWARD CHANG
HOWARD S. FRAZIER

When deciding whether to undergo a promising new drug therapy with known risks of side effects, a patient normally makes a decision in consultation with his or her physician. What happens, however, if the patient is incapable of making such a decision? In this chapter we explore the complex issues surrounding the prescription of a new drug, clozapine, for treatment of the symptoms of severe schizophrenia. This case study is encouraging because it demonstrates how, even under constrained patient choice, biomedical progress and medical monitoring have reduced a serious target risk while identifying and minimizing the chance of risk substitution.

To illustrate the course of chronic severe schizophrenia, we begin with a case vignette about "Margaret Thompson," a composite of the lives of several real people who suffer with this disease. This vignette describes schizophrenia's effects on many aspects of life, and some of the benefits and risks of available treatments. We then provide a brief description of schizophrenia followed by a discussion of the risks of the disease and of its treatment alternatives—primarily the traditional antipsychotic drugs and the atypical drug clozapine. We discuss the various decisionmakers who must consider the risk tradeoffs: the Food and Drug Administration (FDA), drug companies, physicians, families, and patients. We conclude with the results of interviews of patients who have been treated with clozapine, to provide some insight into their knowledge and concerns about being treated with this drug.

Case Vignette: Severe Chronic Schizophrenia

Margaret Thompson was first diagnosed with schizophrenia when she was 16 years old and a sophomore in high school. Until that year she had been a superior student who was quiet, withdrawn, and had few friends. Her academic performance declined markedly during that year, as her behavior became increasingly unusual. She heard voices that discussed her every action, and she believed that the teachers at school were writing articles about her that were published in the local newspaper. She stopped bathing, and her appearance became disheveled. She stopped socializing at school and spent her time outside of school sitting alone in her bedroom. Her papers and exams became disorganized and incoherent, and in class her responses to questions from her teachers were rambling; she rarely completed an idea before jumping to something else quite unrelated.

Margaret's first hospitalization lasted for six weeks. She was given the diagnosis of schizophrenia and was started on Haldol, an antipsychotic medication. By the time she returned home, she had begun to improve: the voices no longer bothered her, she spent less time alone, and she took better care of herself. Her thoughts and speech became more organized and coherent. As the symptoms of her illness diminished, the side effects of her medication became most troublesome. Her arms and legs felt stiff, and her hands often trembled involuntarily. Because of muscle rigidity, her movement and posture looked rather awkward. She was given another drug to help counteract these side effects.

Margaret eventually returned to high school and was able to graduate despite a second hospitalization during her senior year. Over the next six years she lived with her parents, completed a bachelor's degree at a local college, and led a very limited social life. She was hospitalized repeatedly during that period, usually after she had stopped taking her medication because the side effects were becoming more troublesome. When started again on medication, Margaret would again improve enough to be discharged from the hospital.

After college, Margaret worked for one year as an assistant librarian at the public library. She moved out of her parents' house and rented a small studio apartment within walking distance of the library. She did well for the first six months of this job, but then started to deteriorate and was hospitalized again with active psychotic symptoms. Her medication was again changed with some success, and she was able to return to work after about eight weeks. She did not return to her own apartment, but moved back in with her parents. Unfortunately, Margaret continued to have trouble with unclear thinking and strange speech, which hampered her ability to do her job. After one year at the public library she was asked to resign. She was unemployed for five months before finding a job reshelving books in the university library. She lost that job after nine months of frequent absences and poor work performance.

After that, Margaret did not find another job. Over the next four years, from age 27 to 30, Margaret's condition continued to deteriorate, and she cycled between the hospital and her parents' home. Although with each hospitalization she improved enough to be discharged, her improvements were not as marked as they once were, and her episodes of illness were more debilitating. Moreover, from her most recent medication, Thorazine, she had developed constant involuntary facial twitching and lip-smacking movements, characteristic of an adverse drug effect called tardive dyskinesia. Thorazine seemed to be more effective at quieting her symptoms of schizophrenia than the several other drugs that she had taken over the years, but because of the bad side effects, Margaret frequently stopped taking the Thorazine. This would be followed by a rapid reappearance of her psychotic symptoms, requiring rehospitalization within a week or two.

In March 1989, at the age of 31, Margaret was hospitalized

for the twenty-third time. The hospital had just started to enroll patients in a clinical trial testing a new drug, clozapine, for treatment of severe schizophrenia. Margaret was included in this clinical trial and started taking clozapine in April of 1989.

By June 1989, Margaret had moved from the inpatient unit to a supervised residence on the hospital grounds. In January 1990, she moved to a halfway house in the community. She volunteered on a part-time basis in an elementary school library. In September 1990, she entered a six-month program in floral design at a local community college. In October 1990, she moved to her own studio apartment near the college. In April 1991, after completing her studies, Margaret was hired by a local florist to work as a floral designer. Though still bothered by some problems with concentration and memory, Margaret had few symptoms of schizophrenia. She no longer heard voices, and her thinking had cleared. The delusions from which she had suffered seemed to have lifted. As her symptoms dissipated, so did the movement disorders that were side effects of her previous antipsychotic medications. She no longer suffered from rigidity in her limbs, from awkward posture and gait, or from involuntary movement of her face and hands. Socially, Margaret's life improved dramatically. She had a small circle of friends from school and began to date a man she met there. As she started to feel better and more confident, her engaging personality began to emerge, along with an excellent sense of humor.

Margaret noticed a few side effects from the clozapine. She felt tired most of the time, needed at least ten hours of sleep each night, and often fell asleep in church, at the movies, or in class. This became quite embarrassing to her because of another side effect, hyper-salivation, which caused her to drool during sleep. The only other aspect of clozapine treatment that bothered her was having her blood drawn every week, but she tolerated it, knowing that it was very important to have her white cell count monitored.

The Risks of Schizophrenia

As Margaret's story illustrates, chronic schizophrenia is a devastating illness that can affect all aspects of a person's life. It produces psychosis with severe disruptions of perception, cognition, emotion, and behavior (Tsuang et al. 1988). The illness generally appears during adolescence or young adulthood, and affects equal numbers of men and women. It is a relatively common affliction, affecting 1 to 2 percent of the U.S. population (Neale et al. 1982, p. 179; Kane et al. 1988; Bromet et al. 1988). The manifestations of schizophrenia are quite diverse; in fact, schizophrenia is often described as a group of disorders.

Schizophrenia has biological roots, probably related to neurotransmitters in the brain. One popular theory is that an excess of dopamine is responsible for the symptoms of schizophrenia; drugs such as Thorazine block the dopamine receptors in the brain. Other biochemical and social factors (as yet poorly understood) may also play a causative role.

The symptoms of schizophrenia include delusions, auditory hallucinations, unclear or markedly illogical thinking, bizarre speech and behavior, inappropriate displays of emotion, blunted emotions, emotional and social withdrawal, a blank and expressionless face, slowed speech and movement, and, at the extreme, catatonic stupor. Studies show tremendous variability in the outcomes for people with schizophrenia, ranging from excellent adjustment to total impairment. Approximately 50 percent of patients experience a very unfavorable outcome or course of illness, while about 25 percent of all patients can be expected to experience complete or total remission (Westermeyer and Harrow 1988). The chronic course tends not to be steady, but rather to go through periods of improvement and relapse.

Approximately 80 percent of all schizophrenics are hospitalized at some time during their lives; 40 to 50 percent are rehospitalized during the first year after initial hospital discharge, and 65 to 85 percent of those discharged will be rehospitalized eventually (Westermeyer and Harrow 1988). In the current health care climate, few schizophrenics are hospitalized continuously. Many patients are rehospitalized at frequent intervals ("revolving door" patients), interspersed with periods of being discharged back into the community.

For people with schizophrenia, the illness poses risks both to the quality and to the continuation of life. Quality-of-life problems encompass such areas as the living situation, family and social relations, leisure activities, work, finances, personal safety, and health (Lehman 1983). Schizophrenia limits the individual's ability to enjoy and to participate in all aspects of life. An important goal of treatment is to improve substantially the quality of life.

In addition to its effects on quality of life, schizophrenia carries an increased risk of mortality. Numerous studies have shown that people with schizophrenia have higher mortality rates than the general population (Alstrom 1942; Niswander et al. 1963; Babigian and Odoroff 1969; Lindelius and Kay 1973; Tsuang and Woolson 1977; Tsuang 1978; Tsuang et al. 1980; Herrman et al. 1983; Martin et al. 1985a, 1985b; Black et al. 1985a, 1985b, 1985c; Allebeck and Wistedt 1986). Premature mortality from all causes in the schizophrenic population is approximately twice that of the general population, and the mortality rate from suicide is about 10 or more times the rate in the general population. The rate of suicide for females with schizophrenia is especially high, at 18 times the rate for females in the general population (Allebeck 1986). Overall, about 10 percent of schizophrenics die by suicide (Drake et al. 1985). Other causes of death, such as cardiovascular, respiratory, and gastrointestinal, show rates approximately twice those of the general population.

The elevated mortality risks due to schizophrenia appear to be clustered in the younger age groups; after 60 years of age, the schizophrenic population shows no greater mortality rate than the general population (Allebeck 1986). Moreover, it is not clear whether successful treatment and control of the symptoms of schizophrenia reduce excess mortality. The patients followed in mortality studies had received treatment for their schizophrenia, consisting at least of hospitalization, often coupled with drug therapy, but when considering the cause of the elevated mortality rates, it was not possible to separate the possible effects of schizophrenia from those of treatment. It seems likely, however, that successful symptomatic treatment will reduce the risk of suicide. Together with improved quality of life, these are important benefits of treatment.

Traditional Therapies for Schizophrenia

There are no known preventive or curative treatments for schizophrenia. The traditional treatments affect only the symptoms of the illness. Antipsychotic drugs provide the main form of symptomatic treatment, often coupled with psychosocial interventions to help the patient live with his or her illness. Electroconvulsive therapy (ECT) has been used in some patients for relief of psychotic symptoms when antipsychotic drugs are ineffective, especially if the patient's behavior is violent or uncontrollable. Hospitalization is often used during severe bouts of illness, and supportive living environments, such as residential care and halfway houses, are frequently the next step for patients trying to make the transition from hospital to independent living.

The traditional drug treatments for schizophrenia include chemicals that, in essence, block the dopamine receptors in the brain, thereby reducing the psychotic symptoms produced by excess dopamine. These antipsychotic drugs, such as chlorpromazine (Thorazine) and haloperidol (Haldol), are effective in reducing psychotic symptoms to some degree in up to 70 percent of treated schizophrenics (Tsuang et al. 1988). Without such drug treatment, 17 to 40 percent of schizophrenics will show spontaneous improvement (Hastings 1958; Beck 1968; Langfeldt 1969; Bleuler 1978; Tsuang et al. 1988). Once patients have shown improvement on an antipsychotic drug, about 19 percent will relapse while still being treated with the drug, as compared to 55 percent of patients who are maintained on a placebo (Davis et al. 1980).

Countervailing Risks of the Traditional Therapies

The dopamine-blocking mechanism of the antipsychotic drugs also produces side effects that range from mildly uncomfortable to life-threatening. Common mild side effects include sedation, weight gain, dry mouth, blurred vision, constipation, low blood pressure, and fast heart rate. More debilitating are the so-called "extrapyramidal" side effects: neurological effects that produce disorders of movement. Such effects include parkinsonism (tremors of the hands, slow movement, an awkward shuffling gait, muscular rigidity, drooling) and restlessness (constant pacing, fidgeting, and movement of the fingers, lips, and legs). More severe and less common extrapyramidal effects include dystonia (sustained muscular contractions that produce abnormal postures and difficulty in swallowing) and tardive dyskinesia (involuntary, repetitive movement of the face and mouth, producing lip-smacking, chin-wagging, and sucking motions). Tardive dyskinesia develops in 10 to 15 percent of patients who take antipsychotic drugs over long periods of time (Davison and Neale 1982, p. 663).

The traditional antipsychotic drugs also carry a small risk of mortality from a rare systemic reaction called neuroleptic malignant syndrome. This syndrome carries a 20 percent risk of mortality when it develops.

The greatest risk from the traditional antipsychotic drugs is one of morbidity rather than mortality. Quality of life may be severely affected by the debilitating side effects of these drugs. As patients show symptomatic improvement of their schizophrenia while taking these drugs, they often must contend with the onset of the extrapyramidal side effects. As a result, patients often stop taking their medication, precipitating the return of the symptoms of schizophrenia.

Clozapine Therapy

The antipsychotic drug clozapine was introduced to the U.S. market in 1990 for the treatment of severe chronic schizophrenia. Clozapine is manufactured by Sandoz Pharmaceutical Corporation, under the trade name Clozaril.

Clozapine works through a somewhat different dopamine-blocking mechanism than the other antipsychotic drugs on the market, and it has antipsychotic efficacy with less risk of the adverse effects that accompany other antipsychotic drugs (U.S. FDA 1990). Its major drawback is a countervailing danger: a bone marrow disorder that leads to a severe lack of white blood cells (agranulocytosis) in 1 to 2 percent of patients. This condition leaves the patient vulnerable to infection and subsequent death. Because of this serious mortality risk, clozapine's use is limited to patients with chronic schizophrenia who have been treated unsuccessfully with other available drugs.

Clozapine is not a new drug; its history spans nearly three decades of testing and clinical experience throughout the world. The story of clozapine in the United States illustrates the weighing of risk tradeoffs by many different players: the pharmaceutical manufacturer, the Food and Drug Administration (FDA), providers of psychiatric care, as well as individual patients and their legal guardians. The initial marketing of clozapine also included a unique approach by the pharmaceutical company and the FDA to minimize the countervailing risk of the drug: a blood monitoring system closely tied with drug dispensing.

Several clinical trials have shown significant improvement in schizophrenic patients treated with clozapine as compared to those treated with traditional antipsychotic drugs, such as chlorpromazine (Thorazine) or haloperidol (Haldol) (Fischer-Cornelssen and Ferner 1976; Honigfeld et al. 1984; Marder and Van Putten 1988; Shopsin et al. 1979; Claghorn et al. 1987). In particular, one key study, a six-week multicenter trial, established that clozapine was more effective than chlorpromazine in a group of 268 severely ill schizophrenic patients (Kane et al. 1988a, 1988b). These patients had previously failed to respond to at least three different antipsychotic drugs, and a six-week trial of haloperidol was also ineffective for them. After six weeks of treatment with either clozapine or chlorpromazine, 30 percent of clozapine recipients but only 4 percent of chlorpromazine recipients were classified as having improved.

In addition to the clinical manifestations of schizophrenia, researchers have used a Quality-of-Life Scale (Heinrichs et al. 1984) to assess the effects of clozapine among hospitalized patients with schizophrenia (Meltzer et al. 1990). The researchers measured several aspects of functioning before and after clozapine treatment, including sense of purpose, motivation, curiosity, lack of enjoyment, aimless activity, empathy, emotional interaction, interpersonal relations, social activity, occupational role, work functioning, and engagement in commonplace activities. Using these measures, they found that as psychopathology decreased after six months of clozapine treatment, quality-of-life measures on all aspects increased significantly, and the rehospitalization rate decreased markedly (82.6 percent decrease in rehospitalization rates after 12 months). Twenty-one of the thirty-eight patients in this study (55.3 percent) took paying or volunteer jobs or returned to school. On the basis of this kind of data, clozapine is considered a very effective drug for some patients.

Overall, the clinical benefits of clozapine include improvement in behavior and in display of emotion. The delusions and fragmented and bizarre thoughts may remain, although patients may be less bothered by them (Green and Salzman 1990).

Countervailing Risks of Clozapine

Clozapine produces minor side effects in up to 40 percent of patients. Sedation and excess salivation are common. Also frequently reported are constipation, fast heart rate, dizziness, low blood pressure, headache, tremor, fainting, nausea, and fever.

A more serious adverse effect of clozapine is seizure. The risk of seizure appears to be dose-dependent, with convulsions occurring in up to 2 percent of patients treated with less than 300 mg per day, and in 5 percent of patients treated with 600 mg or more per day.

The most serious side effect is the mortality risk from agranulocytosis, a lack of white blood cells. As of February 28, 1991, 55 cases of clozapine-related agranulocytosis had been reported in the United States, with 1 resulting death. By March 23, 1992, approximately 20,000 patients had received clozapine since it had been introduced to the U.S. market in February 1990. In all, 110 cases of agranulocytosis had been reported, with a total of 7 clozapine-related fatalities (Sandoz Pharmaceutical Corporation, personal communication). All fatalities are believed to have been related to the concomitant use of other medications also known to suppress bone marrow function. Thus, these fatalities may not be attributable solely to the effects of clozapine.

Death from infection can be averted if agranulocytosis is detected early. The bone marrow recovers and begins producing white blood cells again after clozapine treatment is discontinued. Once an episode of agranulocytosis has occurred, however, the patient cannot be treated again with clozapine, since it is highly likely that the bone marrow disorder will recur.

Evidence about rates of adverse effects from clozapine comes from Sandoz Pharmaceutical's drug development experience in the United States and Europe. Safety data were reported for 1,742 patients treated with clozapine through August 1989 (U.S. FDA 1990, p. 20). These were mostly American patients, with approximately 150 European patients included. This experience yielded 15 reported cases of agranulocytosis, with a cumulative incidence at one year of treatment of 1.3 percent (with a 95 percent confidence interval of 0.6 to 2.1 percent). All of these patients recovered fully once clozapine treatment was withdrawn (U.S. FDA 1990, p. 23). Data on the incidence of seizure in the 1,742 patients showed a cumulative incidence at one year of 5.4 percent, with a 95 percent confidence interval of 3.9 to 6.9 percent (U.S. FDA 1990, p. 24).

Other data on mortality rates from agranulocytosis come from limited use of clozapine in thirty (mostly European) countries. From 1973 through 1987, 182 cases of agranulocytosis were reported, with 43 of those cases resulting in death. Of importance to the future approval of clozapine was the observation that 42 of those 43 deaths occurred in cases where clinical complications of agranulocytosis, primarily infection, had already developed at the time of detection. Only half of those who recovered following withdrawal of clozapine had clinical complications at the time that agranulocytosis was detected. This observation indicated that early detection of agranulocytosis, before infection set in, could reduce the risk of mortality. A second key observation was the sharp decrease in the rate of fatal cases of agranulocytosis since the late 1970s. Of the 43 deaths from agranulocytosis, 32 occurred from 1973 through 1980. From 1981 through 1987, only 11 deaths occurred, while the rate of agranulocytosis remained stable. This reduction in the rate of fatal cases of agranulocytosis seems to be related to increased monitoring of the white blood cell count of all patients treated with clozapine, resulting in earlier detection of agranulocytosis.

The FDA's Approval of Clozapine

Concerns about the risk of death from agranulocytosis slowed clozapine's path through the FDA approval process. Clozapine was introduced in clinical trials during the 1960s but was suspended from further testing in the United States in 1975, after 13 cases of agranulocytosis and 8 fatalities occurred in patients treated with clozapine in Finland. Sandoz Pharmaceutical finally applied for FDA approval of clozapine in 1983. After reviewing the evidence, the FDA asked Sandoz for more data, stating that it would reconsider clozapine if clinical trials demonstrated it to be more effective than the standard antipsychotic drugs for severely psychotic schizophrenic patients who were resistant to or intolerant of the standard drugs (U.S. FDA 1990, p. 15).

Sandoz submitted a new application to the FDA for approval of clozapine in 1987. This application contained evidence from the six-week multicenter randomized trial comparing the use of clozapine with chlorpromazine in severely psychotic treatment-resistant schizophrenics. This study found clozapine to be more effective than chlorpromazine in treating all measured symptoms of psychosis except hallucinations (U.S. FDA 1990, pp. 16–18; Kane et al. 1988a, 1988b).

On the basis of these new data for severely ill treatment-resistant patients, clozapine was approved by the FDA in February 1990 for clinical use for such patients in the United States. This decision to approve clozapine only for those very sick patients who were untreatable with other available drugs indicates that the FDA found the countervailing risks of the drug to outweigh the potential benefits for all other patient groups; in the FDA's view, only for the sickest patients did the potential benefits of clozapine treatment outweigh its risks. An unusual move by Sandoz helped to clinch the FDA's decision:

the pharmaceutical company offered to market clozapine with a mandatory blood monitoring system that might help to minimize the risk of death from agranulocytosis.

Blood Monitoring of Patients

The Clozaril Patient Monitoring System (CPMS) developed by Sandoz required that patients have their blood drawn once a week for a white cell count before receiving their weekly clozapine supply. This would help to ensure that agranulocytosis would be detected early, before complications such as infection set in. The system was designed to prevent patients with unacceptably low white cell counts from receiving more clozapine. In addition, all cases of agranulocytosis would be recorded in a registry, to prevent patients from later receiving clozapine after recovering from a bout of agranulocytosis. Sandoz contracted with Caremark Homecare Inc., a national home health care company, to coordinate all blood testing services, and Roche Biomedical laboratories to do all laboratory work.

The FDA approved clozapine for marketing with the CPMS in place, although the FDA did not require that the blood monitoring be done through the CPMS. It was Sandoz that required providers to use the CPMS in order to dispense clozapine to their patients. Sandoz sold the drug and the blood monitoring service as a package priced at a hefty $8,900 per year for each patient.

Adverse publicity about these high bundled costs, and an antitrust suit filed by 23 states against the firm (Robb 1991), induced Sandoz in early 1991 to change the blood monitoring requirement somewhat, allowing institutions and physicians to use alternative monitoring systems as long as they complied with Sandoz's criteria and registered the systems with the pharmaceutical company. The cost of clozapine, unbundled from the monitoring costs, declined to about $4,000 per patient per year. The cost of blood monitoring varies depending upon the provider, but it is probably substantially lower when testing is done by individual providers rather than through Caremark's services. In May 1991 the federal government mandated that state Medicaid programs pay for clozapine and blood monitoring for eligible patients.

The CPMS appears to have worked effectively to identify most patients at risk of death from agranulocytosis early enough for clozapine treatment to be stopped before complications set in. An important concern of Sandoz and some providers was whether the separate monitoring systems used by individual providers and institutions would be as effective at preventing agranulocytosis-related fatalities as the Sandoz CPMS was. Some providers worried that if the new blood monitoring systems were less effective, the resulting increase in fatalities could cause Sandoz or the FDA to pull clozapine from the market (Safferman 1991).

Providers also worried that deaths might increase when other pharmaceutical companies gained the right to manufacture clozapine in 1994. Until then, Sandoz maintained fairly tight control through its system to track cases of agranulocytosis.

Who Should Be Eligible to Receive Clozapine?

The FDA approved clozapine only for treatment of the severely psychotic patient whose illness does not respond to the traditional antipsychotic drugs, or who suffers from severe adverse reactions to those drugs. About 20 percent of people with schizophrenia fulfill these criteria (see Figure 3.1). Approximately one-third of these patients, or roughly 7 percent of all patients with schizophrenia, will have a meaningful clinical improvement on clozapine (Kane et al. 1988). The National Alliance for the Mentally Ill estimates the potential clozapine market to number 100,000 in the United States (*Medicine & Health* 1991, p. 2). Another estimate ranges from 133,000 to 189,000 eligible individuals, depending on the selection criteria (Terkelson and Grosser 1990).

Some have suggested that a trial of clozapine is appropriate for *inpatients* who have had a suboptimal response to the traditional antipsychotic drugs. This includes a large group of patients who receive only slight benefit from the traditional antipsychotic drugs and who might receive greater benefit from clozapine. Because of the need for careful weekly blood monitoring, more caution in prescribing clozapine for *outpatients* has been urged (Marder and Van Putten 1988).

Rationing clozapine is necessary not only because of clinical factors but also because of the limited funds available to public hospitals for purchasing clozapine (Pelonero and Elliott 1990). Despite their clinical eligibility, many people with severe chronic schizophrenia are not receiving clozapine, apparently because of the high economic cost of the drug. For example, by mid-1992 only 1,300 of 60,000 potentially eligible patients in California had received clozapine, and only 300 of 9,000 eligible patients in U.S. Veterans hospitals had received it (Wallis and Willwerth 1992).

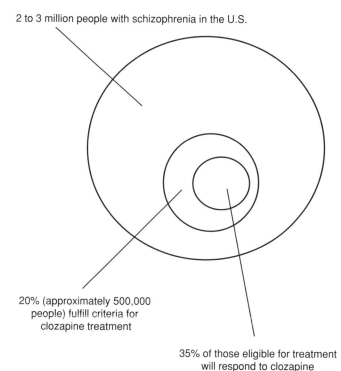

Figure 3.1 Population eligible for clozapine treatment in the United States.

The clinical criteria for allocating clozapine suggested by some physicians emphasize treating patients who fail to respond to traditional antipsychotic drugs or who develop severe side effects on those drugs. Severity of illness is not necessarily a criterion, since patients should have the ability to give informed consent and to comply with the weekly blood monitoring requirement. Some physicians suggest giving priority to patients for whom the fewest treatment alternatives are available. Using a lottery system to select patients is not considered ethically satisfactory, because it would not necessarily maximize benefits to the greatest number of patients. It is also not considered ethical to give priority to those patients whose families most actively request treatment.

Do Patients Understand the Risk Tradeoffs?

When the risks and benefits of clozapine and alternative treatments are being weighed, the patient's views are crucial but problematic. For a devastating chronic illness like schizophrenia, quality-of-life concerns may weigh very heavily in favor of an effective treatment, even in the face of mortality risks. The patient's viewpoint and priorities need to be considered, but schizophrenia hampers cognitive functioning, making it difficult to determine how well a patient has understood and weighed the tradeoffs.

Does this result in the patient not being fully informed about the risks and potential benefits of therapies such as clozapine treatment? How well do patients remember and understand what they are told about the risks and potential benefits of this treatment? Do patients know why they must have their blood tested every week while taking clozapine? Overall, how do patients feel about taking this drug?

We explored these questions by talking with patients who were taking clozapine for severe chronic schizophrenia. Patients were sampled at random from a list of twenty-one patients enrolled in a hospital-based clinical trial of clozapine in Massachusetts. These twenty-one patients had the most severe cases of chronic schizophrenia in the hospital. At the start of the trial, all were unable to function outside of the hospital.

The patients had received clozapine for at least eight months at the time of our interview, and all had tried at least two different traditional antipsychotic drugs without success before being enrolled in the clozapine trial. We interviewed four patients who gave their consent, for about 30 minutes each.

When these patients were asked whether clozapine had helped them, the responses varied but were generally positive. Memories were sketchy about the decision to start on clozapine. All four patients seemed not to worry very much about side effects, and remembered little about being informed of the risks of clozapine treatment. All of these patients were well aware of having their blood drawn, and most seemed to understand what kind of blood test was being done. None mentioned the risk of death from a lack of white blood cells.

Although informed consent is required in such a clinical trial, these patients may have been judged incompetent to provide such consent, with the result that formal consent was provided by a legal guardian. Even so, it is likely that these patients did receive an explanation of the risks at the start of the trial and then subsequently forgot. Recall is a problem in this situation because of the long time frame since the start of clozapine treatment (over two years for some patients), as well as the memory problems related to schizophrenia or to other treatments.

Even when these patients did have some knowledge of the risks posed by clozapine treatment, there were two important gaps in their reported knowledge: none volunteered knowledge about the risk of seizure and none mentioned the mortality risk related to the risk of developing an episode of agranulocytosis. Perhaps these patients had lost their concern about risks because they had been treated successfully (without adverse effects) for many months. It may also be that the patients focused more on the potential benefits of the drug than on the risks, because the illness itself was so devastating. Or it may be that they trusted their physicians or legal guardians to weigh the risks for them. According to their descriptions, these patients were not very involved in weighing the risks for themselves. This pattern may of course hold for all treatments of schizophrenia, including but not limited to clozapine. And, of course, our small sample size of four interviews makes it difficult to generalize.

Conclusion

The clozapine story illustrates how scientific progress, if managed intelligently, can curtail target risks without inducing unacceptable countervailing risks. If the "risk substitution" posed by clozapine therapy—agranulocytosis—had not been managed carefully, the result could have been either excess deaths or premature rejection by the FDA of the therapy, with adverse consequences for schizophrenia patients (and Sandoz) in either case. The weekly blood monitoring program minimized the danger of risk substitution to the point where clozapine's clinical benefits could be safely provided to a sizable number of schizophrenic patients. Now most patients who develop agranulocytosis are quickly diagnosed and recover once clozapine is withdrawn. Agranulocytosis may still develop in patients receiving clozapine at the rate of 1 to 2 percent per year, but perhaps a better metric for risk assessment is the rate of death from agranulocytosis: in the 1970s, several deaths due to agranulocytosis did occur; now, with blood monitoring, deaths due solely to clozapine's effects are rare or nonexistent. By incorporating concern about countervailing risks into the design of clinical policy, Sandoz and the FDA acted as relatively successful practitioners of risk tradeoff analysis.

A case can be made, however, that Sandoz and the FDA became overly concerned about the countervailing risks of clozapine therapy. The mortality risk from agranulocytosis was substantial, but it slowed the FDA's approval of clozapine, caused the FDA to adopt a fairly narrow definition of the eligible patient population, and led to a high-cost product (because of the requirement for weekly blood monitoring of patients). Today it appears that a larger fraction of the schizophrenic population might benefit from clozapine therapy. This drug is so effective that many patients, were they able to choose, might be willing to face a substantial risk of earlier death in exchange for the opportunity to live more independently and with a markedly improved quality of life. But even if clinical eligibility were expanded, the economic cost of moving to a "risk-superior" frontier could continue to keep many eligible patients from receiving the drug.

One of the obstacles to a more generous policy in this case was the FDA's posture toward quality-of-life benefits. In clinical trials of drugs, the traditional measures of effectiveness are mortality and morbidity rates. Quality-of-life measures are not explicitly and formally used in the FDA's drug approval process, although they may be considered to some extent in the definitions of efficiency and safety. For devastating chronic diseases such as schizophrenia, mortality and morbidity appear to be incomplete measures of effectiveness. Objective and subjective measures of emotional, cognitive, social, and occupational functioning need to be weighed along with the risks of mortality and morbidity.

More explicit consideration of quality of life often occurs at the level of physician-patient decisions. This emphasizes the need for the FDA to allow use of therapies with profound quality-of-life benefits, and to enable physicians and patients to conduct their own risk tradeoff analyses. The process of informed consent by patients does not appear to be fully viable among many schizophrenics who might be eligible for clozapine therapy, but legal guardians and physicians may be in a better position than the FDA to evaluate the risks and quality-of-life benefits of clozapine and its alternatives. Their evaluations would in fact be enhanced if FDA procedures made more rigorous information available on quality-of-life issues.

In the years ahead, several new drugs that are effective treatments for schizophrenia and safer than clozapine will probably be brought to the market. This progress to further "risk-superior" frontiers illustrates that risk tradeoff analysis must be a dynamic process that responds to (and stimulates) innovation in technology and practice.

4

Licensing the Elderly Driver

CONSTANCE WILLIAMS
JOHN D. GRAHAM

In medicine, the risks of taking or not taking a prescribed therapy are typically incurred predominantly by the patient. While the process of weighing these risks is often difficult, and there can be impacts on family members or others (for example, in the case of vaccines to prevent epidemics), the legitimacy of final decisions usually derives from the informed consent of the patient or a legal guardian who is supposed to act in the patient's best interests.

In this chapter we introduce a new dimension of complexity: a case in which the countervailing risks of taking protective action are imposed on people different from those who experience the benefits of reducing the target risk. We examine the phenomena of "risk transfer" and "risk transformation" (defined in Chapter 1) and the associated ethical challenges of allocating risks to different populations without express consent.

In particular, this case study considers the relative risks of extending driving privileges to the elderly or withholding them under narrow or broad conditions. The changing demographics of the U.S. population highlight the significance of this question. At the beginning of the 1990s about 16 million

Americans, or 10 percent of all drivers, were over the age of 65. During the next thirty years, as the baby boomers grow older, the number of drivers over age 65 will increase to 50 million. Of these senior citizens, more than half will be over the age of 75 (NRC 1988).

With the rapid growth of the elderly population in recent years, concern has increased about the dangers posed by larger numbers of elderly drivers on the roads. Studies indicate that older drivers are more frequently involved in automobile crashes than the average adult driver. This fact has led some to advocate that the driver's licenses of older Americans be restricted in some way; proposals have ranged from tougher retesting requirements to automatic revocation at a certain age threshold.

Such policies, however, would impose important countervailing risks on the elderly themselves. For many people, acquiring their first driver's license represents their entrance into the adult world. A driver's license enables us to go where we want, when we want, for whatever period of time we choose. With a driver's license, any American can go anywhere across the continental United States without having to show identification or report one's itinerary—a freedom that may not be available on any other continent. Indeed, the mobility conferred by the driving privilege has come to be perceived as a vital ingredient of American personal freedom. Almost every adult American has a driver's license (167 million), and the average American (children included) travels over 8,000 miles per year in a car (NHTSA 1991).

Now imagine that license being taken away, simply because of age, from someone who has had the freedom to drive for decades and who uses it every day to pursue his or her way of life. To go somewhere, to shop, to get medicine, to visit friends would require either walking (if the older person is capable), relying on the vagaries of public transportation (if it is accessible), or relying on the kindness of friends and relatives who still can drive. Without a driver's license, independence and personal freedom would be seriously compromised.

Today many elderly citizens face the potential loss of driving privileges. The families of elderly drivers often exert subtle or overt pressure on them to give up their licenses and their cars. Some physicians regularly recommend that certain older patients curtail or stop driving. Other physicians, after diagnosing specific physical or mental impairments, report impaired drivers to licensing authorities. Such reports are either mandated by law or reflect a physician's professional responsibility to the safety of these patients and the safety of other road users. Some states have become more restrictive in the relicensing of elderly drivers through a variety of techniques ranging from more frequent vision tests to mandatory driving tests. And some states have considered imposing automatic license cancellation at a certain age. Similar challenges are being confronted in Europe (Hakamies-Blomqvist 1993; Schlag 1993).

If the elderly driver were the only person affected by such decisions, then one might be tempted to approach this dilemma using the doctrines of informed consent. But this approach is not viable because older drivers may pose some danger to other road users. Indeed, all drivers, including elderly ones, can represent a hazard not only to themselves but to their passengers and other road users; and driving itself is a means to avoid other risks. Any societal decision that is made concerning licensure will affect risks to some citizens in society without their direct consent. The question becomes how to weigh the risks—to both the elderly and other citizens—of extending versus withholding the privilege to drive.

Unsafe at Any Age?

How large is the target risk of automobile accidents caused by elderly drivers? Traffic crashes are not a major cause of premature death among the elderly. The probability that a premature death will result from a traffic crash decreases markedly from 0.48 at age 20 to 0.01 at age 85 (Evans 1988a). This decline reflects not only changes in driving behaviors but also the growing importance of other causes of death, such as chronic diseases, later in life.

When expressed as the number of deaths per 100,000 population, the traffic death rate is actually higher for those older than age 74 than it is for any age group except for those between the ages of 15 and 24 years (CDC 1991). Although these data are interesting, they do not speak directly to the safety of the elderly as drivers because they include the deaths of elderly passengers and pedestrians as well as of elderly drivers, and because they reflect the pattern of increasing frailty with age—an 80-year-old male is four times as likely to die as a 20-year-old male in a crash of the same severity (Evans 1993, p. 774).

To assess the risks to others posed by elderly drivers, it is instructive to consider crash involvement statistics, which are based on crashes severe enough to cause a report to be filed with the police. When crash involvement rates are computed by age of driver and adjusted for the number of vehicle miles of travel, a general U-shaped pattern emerges, as shown in Figure 4.1. Crash rates are elevated for the young and the old. Of all age groups, drivers over age 85 have the highest rate of crash involvement: 40 crashes per 100 million vehicle miles of travel. Even the notoriously risky-driving youth age group has a lower rate of crash involvement than the oldest Americans.

The mileage fatality rates by age group exhibit a similar pattern. Teenagers have a fatality rate of 5.6 deaths per 100 million vehicle miles of travel, while drivers in their forties have a rate of less than 1.0. As Figure 4.1 illustrates, the rate rises sharply after age 75 and reaches a high of 31 deaths per 100 million vehicle miles of travel for drivers over the age of 85 (NHTSA 1989). Part of this elevated fatality risk reflects the relative frailty of older drivers, as mentioned above; the number of fatalities per crash begins to rise rapidly after age 70 (Evans 1988b).

Similar patterns, though much less pronounced, are revealed in longitudinal studies of cohorts of male drivers: as a group of male drivers born in the same year ages, its fatality rate falls dramatically after age 20 and then begins to rise slowly around age 75 (Evans 1993, figs. 2 and 5). This relationship is forecast for a currently young cohort in Figure 4.2. The lower fatality rate for elderly drivers relative to youth drivers shown in the longitudinal estimate (Figure 4.2), as compared to the cross-sectional snapshot data in Figure 4.1,

most likely reflects in part the different denominators employed (fatalities per mile traveled versus fatalities per population) and in part the fact that each successive cohort of male
drivers in this century has had lower accident rates than the
preceding cohort (Evans 1993, p. 771). This steady trend, with
the fatality rate per mile traveled falling over 90 percent since
the 1920s (while total miles traveled have increased many-
fold), is the result of improvements such as better roads and
better vehicles as well as better driving behavior (Evans 1993,
p. 775).

For female driver cohorts, the fatality rate per million population has historically fallen after age 20 but has not risen
appreciably in older age (Evans 1993, p. 771). But as growing
percentages of women born in more recent years tend to drive,
their predicted age-risk profile may begin to mirror that of men
as shown in Figure 4.2, with increasing fatalities in later years
(Evans 1993, p. 773).

Crashes involving an elderly driver, unlike those involving
young drivers, are not significantly caused by alcohol or high

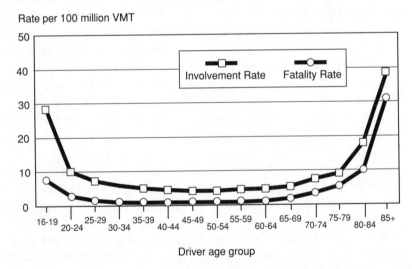

Figure 4.1 Crash involvement and fatality rates per vehicle mile
traveled (VMT), by age group, 1986. *Source:* Adapted from NHTSA
1989.

speed (Stephens and Schoenborn 1988). Compared to young drivers, older drivers are more likely to crash in the daytime and at urban intersections. They are also more likely to be charged with a traffic violation, especially one involving right-of-way and traffic signal violations (NHTSA 1989; Williams 1989). Older drivers are more likely to be involved in multi-vehicle crashes than are younger drivers. But notably, elderly drivers are less likely to kill pedestrians than are younger drivers (Evans 1993, p. 774), which suggests that elderly drivers may be less reckless or careless than younger drivers.

It is important to remember when interpreting these statistics that elderly drivers take steps that reduce their overall exposure to traffic crashes. While younger drivers travel over 10,000 miles per year, the average elderly driver travels an

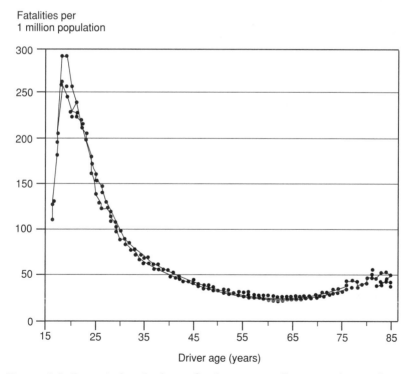

Figure 4.2 Projected male driver fatalities per million population, by age. *Source:* Evans 1993.

average of 7,000 miles per year (Graca 1987). The elderly also tend to drive in less hazardous conditions by avoiding rush hours, heavily congested conditions, poor weather, and night-time conditions (Reuben 1988). Some analysts have suggested that the elevated crash involvement rates of elderly drivers may simply reflect the fact that they tend to travel on city streets with no access restrictions whereas younger drivers accumulate miles on safer divided multi-lane freeways with limited access (Janke 1991). More work is needed to estimate the relative crash probabilities for younger and older drivers in identical driving situations.

Why Older Drivers Might Pose Greater Risks

The most important sensory function in driving is vision. Between the ages of 35 and 45, distance vision, binocular depth perception, and color sensitivity begin to decline. Between the ages of 55 and 65, one's visual field narrows, one's sensitivity to light decreases, and one's sensitivity to glare increases. This does not even begin to take into account such age-related diseases of the eyes as cataracts and glaucoma (Doege 1986).

In addition, aging is associated with cognitive impairment. Dementia and stroke are among the age-related neurological diseases that impair cognitive functioning (Aronson et al. 1991). Among the very old, dementia is a common impairment, with prevalence rates of Alzheimer's disease as high as 47 percent among community-residing elderly persons who are 85 and older (Evans et al. 1989). Dementia is characterized by deficits in memory, visual-spatial functions, language, and orientation. Studies show that elders suffering from dementia often continue to drive (Graca 1987; Gilley et al. 1991; Friedland et al. 1988; Carr et al. 1990). One survey administered to patients referred to a dementia clinic found that 30 percent had had at least one automobile accident since the onset of symptoms, and that 11 percent were reported to have "caused" crashes (Lucas-Blaustein et al. 1988).

Diseases characterized by loss of consciousness result in cognitive, sensory, and motor deficits. It has been estimated that by age 80, 10 percent of the population will have had some type of seizure (Krumholz et al. 1991). Every state in America has regulations pertaining to driving and seizures, although they differ on how long a person must be "seizure-free" before resuming driving. Six states mandate that doctors must report patients with seizures to licensing authorities. Others either encourage doctors to do so, or rely upon drivers to report themselves when they apply for license renewal.

Other conditions associated with lapses or alterations of consciousness include diabetes mellitus, which occurs in about 9 percent of the elderly (Hansotia and Broste 1991), cardiac arrhythmias (Strickberger et al. 1991), sleep apnea (Findley et al. 1991), and the use of prescribed, illicit, or over-the-counter drugs. The elderly clearly have an increased exposure to medications; although they represent only 12 percent of the population, they consume one-third of all prescription medications (Avorn 1988). Unfortunately, definitive studies linking the effects of drugs on crash counts involving the elderly have not yet been performed. It will be important to investigate the extent to which elevated risks can be attributed to subgroups of the elderly (Hakamies-Blomqvist 1993).

Reducing the Risks of the Older Driver

Like most Americans, senior citizens try to avoid driving risks. Along with the adaptive behaviors noted above (decreased mileage and limiting driving to the least hazardous conditions), many older drivers sign up for special senior driver education programs that review the rules of the road and advise older drivers of practices that minimize traffic risks. In some states, lower insurance premiums are offered to graduates as a financial incentive to take these classes. Unfortunately, the efficacy of these courses in reducing crashes has not been established (Waller 1985). Since enrollment is voluntary, they are likely to attract the more risk-averse drivers while failing to recruit those who are potentially more dangerous.

A primary focus of licensing programs has always been to qualify beginning drivers. Only seven states have restrictions specifically pertaining to elderly drivers (Reuben et al. 1988). But today licensing authorities face a dilemma. Despite anecdotal testimony and conventional wisdom, there is no simple and consistent connection between advanced age per se and driving impairment, and no well-accepted protocol for testing and identifying impaired elderly drivers. Advocacy groups for senior citizens have effectively opposed solely age-based restrictions as arbitrary and discriminatory (Meier 1992). Yet states are increasingly concerned that they will be held financially liable for those drivers whom they license and who are later involved in crashes. The question before a court may focus not just on motorists' competence to drive, but also on the competence of the authorities who license them.

In response to this dilemma, the National Highway Traffic Safety Administration and the American Association of Motor Vehicle Administrators have sponsored research and made preliminary recommendations to guide license renewal reform—all of which primarily seek to place limitations on elderly drivers. Some of these proposals include the following:

Counseling and education of older drivers. License renewal offers an ideal point for educational interventions, though the types of training that will benefit older drivers the most are not well established. In an innovative program, Oregon offers driving improvement counseling to drivers who have been reported to have functional limitations. Counselors reassure drivers that their goal is to try to help them keep their driving privileges. These drivers perform simple reaction time tests, review medications and medical history, and perform vision tests. A short oral quiz and a road test prepare the driver for the formal state evaluation (Frisbee 1991). A 1990 survey found that six states had programs to counsel elders about alternative forms of transportation (Popkin and Little 1990).

Expanded use of graded, restricted driver's licenses. Just as teenagers often begin with driving permits that stipulate certain restrictions, support is growing for graduated driving restrictions for older drivers (Waller 1988). Special licenses can restrict driving to certain areas or particular times under conditions thought to be safest without being unduly restrictive.

Developing systems for reporting impaired drivers. In some states, mechanisms exist that allow private citizens, health providers, and police officers to report potentially dangerous drivers to licensing authorities. Family members are often the first to notice a decline in an elder's ability to drive. Many develop ingenious methods to limit their relatives' access to their car. Yet often family members do not want to be responsible for taking away the driving privilege (Gillins 1990). It may be easier to turn to an authority outside the family, who frequently is the physician.

Physicians routinely see patients with medical conditions that may contraindicate driving. The medical literature is evolving to deal with this area of clinical decisionmaking (Reuben et al. 1988; Underwood 1992; Drachman 1988; Holton 1990; Doege and Engelberg 1986). Unfortunately, good clinical research is still quite limited, and there are virtually no controlled studies that can accurately distinguish safe from "accident prone" drivers. Thus, clinicians make these important and essentially social determinations based on "medical judgment."

Legal guidelines that assist physicians in knowing when to report impaired drivers have been developed (Gregory 1982; California DHS 1990), but preliminary research suggests that physicians are generally unaware of reporting opportunities or requirements. For instance, of the drivers referred to Oregon's counseling program, only 2 percent were referred by physicians despite that state's mandatory reporting law (Frisbee 1991). In a survey of cardiologists randomly chosen from each state, 74 percent did not know their state law concerning driving by individuals with cardiac arrhythmias (Strickberger et al. 1991).

Reducing Risks without Using Age as a Criterion

Some experts, and a few states, have begun to experiment with measures to reduce traffic risks that focus on impaired skills rather than on age as a proxy for impairment. These measures include the following:

Routine renewal of licenses with heightened testing based on driving records. Some states allow drivers with clean records to renew by mail, but require drivers with moving violations to take written or road tests. This helps to target testing to those who may be worse drivers and saves the expense of needlessly testing safer drivers, without an adverse effect on traffic safety (Waller 1988). There is evidence that more frequent license renewal requirements significantly reduce accident fatalities (Keeler 1994).

Improved vision screening tests to detect impairments of nighttime and dynamic visual acuity. Although impaired vision is intuitively a likely cause of any increase in accident rates among the elderly, testing for such impairments has not been implemented widely. Research on vision testing is a growing field of endeavor, but results are still too preliminary to warrant implementation.

Improved design of road tests and knowledge tests using validated psychometric principles. The evidence to date indicates that road and knowledge testing "are not effective in meeting the objectives of identifying and licensing drivers who can operate a vehicle safely. Immediate concern should be in developing more valid procedures. Unfortunately, the tests would be longer and more costly" (Popkin and Little 1990).

The Countervailing Risks of Withholding Driving Privileges

Policymakers seeking to enhance the safety of the roads by restricting the driving privileges of senior citizens need to consider the countervailing risks that removing those privileges would entail. Although there are no studies that specifically document the risks of license restriction or revocation for elderly drivers, one can to some extent extrapolate from existing studies on the adverse effects of social isolation on physical and mental health. Drivers are the only elderly group who report satisfaction with their ability to get around, and automobile ownership is a powerful correlate of general life satisfaction (Carp 1988). For example, the inability to drive may reduce one's access to employment opportunities, thus imposing an early and semi-forced retirement with its attendant negative financial and psychological consequences. Taking away a person's driver's license may limit his or her access to formal and informal support systems and recreational opportunities, resulting in social isolation and concomitant depression.

Limiting driving may also impose significant barriers to performing essential tasks such as shopping for medicines, food, and clothing, or obtaining timely medical care. Limiting shopping opportunities to those stores within walking distance may result in an individual being forced to purchase higher-priced, lower-quality goods. And losing the ability to drive can strike at one's self-esteem.

Forcing senior citizens to walk itself invokes a range of risks. Walking, although widely promoted as a healthy, low-impact form of exercise, may actually increase the chances of debilitating falls. Of those elderly persons who do fall, 10 percent experience serious injuries, including fractures. Indeed, roughly 10,000 deaths from falls are reported each year, the vast majority among those 65 and older (National Safety Council 1993). The fear of falling among elderly persons is already so widespread that 12 to 20 percent of older individuals currently say they limit their social activities to avoid the risk of falling (Tinnetti and Speechley 1989). Although most elders' falls currently occur inside the home, that might change if the safer modes of transport currently available to the elderly were restricted.

Senior citizens using public transportation also face an increased risk of falls because of the stairs that often need to be negotiated when getting on or off buses and trains, because of sidewalk hazards such as potholes and ice, and because of the jostling that invariably occurs when traveling by public conveyances. One study found that persons older than 65 using public transportation were five times more likely to be injured than those aged 6–17 years (Hundenski 1992).

In addition to increasing their risk of falling, walking and public transportation increase elders' exposure to crime. An older person carrying a grocery bag in one hand and a cane in the other may be a particularly vulnerable target. For some seniors, the fear of crime—real or not—may induce isolation.

When an older person is forced to rely upon family and friends for transportation, it can feel as though the declaration of independence that came with the driver's license has been revoked. The emotional toll of this event can be significant. Recovering stroke patients who stopped driving, for example, had a higher incidence of depression than those who continued to drive, despite the fact that 80 percent of the ex-driver stroke patients had relatively easy access to alternative means of transportation (Leigh-Smith et al. 1986). Public transportation, friends, and relatives do not easily replace the convenience and feeling of independence conveyed in this country by a driver's license and car ownership (Persson 1993).

Any calculation of the change in traffic safety achieved by restricting the elderly driver needs to take account of the increased miles driven by friends and relatives to chauffeur the elderly passenger. Furthermore, the person or persons upon whom the new non-driver is now forced to rely for transportation may feel burdened by this new responsibility. The degree to which caregivers feel overburdened may be a predictor of their long-term willingness to continue to provide care, and that, in turn, may be a predictor of nursing-home placement. Thus, in determining the countervailing risks to society of restricting elders' driving privilege, the risks and costs of increased long-term institutionalization may be relevant.

Advocacy groups for the elderly are well aware of the risks to elders when their ability to drive is circumscribed or removed entirely. These groups lobby vigorously to prevent the enactment of regulations that discriminate by age. They also work for the passage of laws, such as the Americans with Disabilities Act and the Older Americans Act, supporting alternative forms of transportation. However, with limited public resources, truly accessible and effective alternative transportation expressly designed for the elderly remains scarce. In rural communities and small towns, the automobile often remains the exclusive mode of transport.

Rational Tolerance of Involuntary Risk?

There are not very many examples of involuntary risks that are deemed tolerable by the American public. Despite the involuntary risks to other road users that may be posed by the elderly driver, however, we have been reluctant in this country to curtail the driving privileges of the elderly.

It is certainly difficult to make the case that the elderly will be better off—all things considered—without the privilege to drive. The countervailing risks of immobility, including diminished freedom, independence, self-esteem, and psychological and physical health, are substantial. Given the countervailing risks of falls, crime, depression, and institutionalization, it is not even clear that society's overall age-adjusted mortality rates would be reduced if the elderly were barred from driving. The tradeoff would be especially adverse for elderly women, who pose less increased risk of crash fatalities but who would face the panoply of countervailing risks if their licenses were restricted.

New technology could change the practices of licensing authorities dramatically (Schlag 1993). The elevated accident rates observed among younger and older drivers may result from specific impairments in such factors as vision, reaction time, experience, and intoxication, and licensing authorities could probably be more effective at reducing accident rates if they could somehow target those factors rather than discriminating by age. Although automobile insurance policies do make past accident history a factor in future premium rates and thus do help discourage risky driving, there is currently no validated test that can forecast the riskiness of drivers. Since old age per se is considered a discriminatory basis for license restrictions, policy is unlikely to change until a valid driving test is developed that pinpoints the physical, mental, and behavioral impairments that are associated with substantial elevations of driving risk. Given the burgeoning size of the elderly population and the growing demand for science-based licensing policy, state agencies and the National Highway Traffic Safety Administration can expect increasing pressure to develop such a test (Barr and Eberhard 1994). The prospect that such a test might be developed highlights the need for flexible public policies that reconsider the proper balance between target and countervailing risks.

Conclusion

This case study shows that a target risk, even one that is well-documented and to some extent involuntary in nature, should not necessarily be eliminated without regard to countervailing risks. The potential problems of "risk offset" and "risk substitution" are apparent in this case. Given current technology, any effort to eliminate the risks that elderly drivers pose to themselves and others is likely to entail serious countervailing risks for the elderly. Moreover, blanket restrictions on all elderly drivers could pose a particularly harsh risk tradeoff for safer older drivers, such as (in general) elderly women.

By declining to revoke licenses on the basis of age alone, most states have in effect made the implicit judgment that the involuntary dangers that older drivers impose on other road users are not of sufficient magnitude and severity to justify the risks that immobility would impose on senior citizens.

This judgment may reflect the voice of the victims of countervailing risks being heard by decisionmakers. The objections of politically active, organized senior citizens to the countervailing risks of age-based license restrictions may have been sufficiently influential to block such policies. But if the elderly were not so politically active, would the countervailing risks be taken so seriously? This underscores the importance of conducting risk tradeoff analysis when the population exposed to countervailing risks has less political visibility.

5

Saving Gasoline and Lives

JOHN D. GRAHAM

The countervailing risks of well-intended actions designed to reduce a target risk are not always analyzed or openly discussed in public policy debates. Because advocacy groups, elected officials, and bureaucracies may benefit from an exclusive focus on a target risk, they may choose to ignore—or even suppress discussion of—the countervailing risks of proposed policies. The systematic tendencies of decisionmakers to slight consideration of countervailing risks are explored in more detail in Chapter 11. In this chapter, we consider a case study in energy policy where initial efforts to ignore or downplay a countervailing risk were exposed in public debate by the concerted actions of risk analysts, interest groups, and the federal judiciary. The case study examines the federal government's program to conserve energy by requiring car companies to build more fuel-efficient vehicles.

The Risks of Oil Consumption

Since the world oil crisis of 1973–1974, the U.S. Congress has sought to establish an energy policy that would reduce the nation's dependence on foreign oil while preserving domestic

nonrenewable energy resources such as petroleum. Congress
has maintained this policy out of concern for the country's national security, economic security, and environmental quality.
Automobile fuel-efficiency rules have been a key element of
this national policy. But overly ambitious fuel-efficiency rules
may pose a countervailing risk: compromising the safety of vehicle occupants by inducing manufacturers to build smaller,
lighter new vehicles that are less crashworthy.

The national security risks posed by automobile fuel consumption arise from America's dependence on foreign oil,
which now accounts for 40 to 50 percent of annual petroleum
consumption (OTA 1991). The human and economic losses of
the recent war in the Persian Gulf are seen by some observers
as a cost of America's heavy dependence on Middle East oil.
Dependence on insecure oil supplies may also create opportunities for other nations to blackmail the United States,
thereby threatening our national interests.

Reliance on foreign oil sources also creates dangers to America's economic security. An economy heavily dependent on foreign oil leaves producers and consumers vulnerable to unexpected price increases and supply disruptions. Instabilities in
world oil supplies were significant causes of the two recessions
experienced by the United States in the 1970s. If the American
economy had been less dependent upon oil, critics point out,
these recessions might have been less severe.

Several environmental risks are associated with petroleum
consumption. Automobile emissions are a major contributor
to persistent levels of smog (ground-level ozone) and volatile
aromatics (for example, benzene) in America's cities. And the
prospect of global warming may be aggravated by fossil fuel
combustion processes that release the "greenhouse gas"
carbon dioxide (CO_2) into the atmosphere. In addition, importing oil for automobile fuel may increase the risk of coastal
oil spills.

Congress Regulates Detroit

The transportation sector of the economy accounts for about
25 percent of U.S. energy use and about 63 percent of U.S.

petroleum use (OTA 1991). Policymakers have therefore sought to reduce the consumption of gasoline by the nation's growing fleet of motor vehicles, which nearly doubled (from 111 million vehicles to 193 million) between 1970 and 1990 (NHTSA 1991). Before the Arab oil embargo of 1973–1974, the average fuel economy of new cars sold in the United States was estimated at about 14 miles per gallon (mpg). Today new car fuel economy is about double the 1973 value, or about 28 mpg (NAS 1992). These fuel efficiency improvements reflect a combination of regulatory and marketplace forces.

One of the more popular energy policies in Congress is the national program to reduce oil consumption by compelling automobile manufacturers to produce more fuel-efficient vehicles. In 1975 Congress responded to the tripling of world oil prices by passing the Energy Policy and Conservation Act, which established "Corporate Average Fuel Economy" (CAFE) standards for each vehicle manufacturer, starting at 18 mpg in 1978 and increasing to 27.5 mpg for the 1985 model year. Since 1985 the CAFE standard has remained at about 27.5 mpg.

While some analysts attribute the doubling of new car fuel economy to CAFE standards, consumer fears of rising gasoline prices, particularly from 1974 to 1983, also contributed to the pressure on manufacturers to improve fuel efficiency (Greene 1990). Most of the improvements in new car fuel economy were achieved before 1985, and progress has since slowed as the real price of gasoline has declined and interest in energy conservation has waned (NAS 1992).

Recently, Congress has responded to energy conservation advocates by considering new legislation designed to compel further boosts in the fuel economy of new motor vehicles. The most prominent bill, introduced by Senator Richard Bryan (D–Nevada) calls for a 40 percent improvement in new car fuel economy (to about 40 mpg) by the year 2000. Despite opposition by the Bush administration and automakers, the Bryan bill came close to passing the Congress in both 1990 and 1992 (Graham 1992). The same question was hotly contested in the 1992 presidential election campaign, but the Clinton administration has backed away from stricter CAFE standards—re-sisting calls to raise CAFE as part of its 1993 "action plan" to reduce greenhouse gas emissions—in favor of a large-scale R&D program aimed at producing a "clean car."

The Impact of CAFE on the Target Risks

Does CAFE Really Save Oil? CAFE regulation is designed to save oil by inducing manufacturers to sell fuel-efficient vehicles. More fuel-efficient new vehicles can be expected to reduce petroleum consumption per mile traveled. For example, increasing average new-car miles per gallon from 27.5 to 40 would cut fuel use by about 45 percent, per mile traveled, in those cars. But the impact of CAFE on national fuel consumption is very gradual: because the nation's vehicle fleet turns over at a rate of only about 7 percent per year, it would take about fifteen years for the nation's automobile fuel use, all other things equal, to decline by the same 45 percent per mile traveled.

In practice, the energy savings from raising CAFE may be even further diminished. First, by reducing the amount of fuel needed to drive a vehicle each mile, improved fuel efficiency lowers the driver's cost of operating a vehicle per mile of travel, and thereby encourages drivers to travel more miles. More total miles of driving thus offsets some of the energy conservation gains achieved by the lower fuel use per mile of more fuel-efficient vehicles. The magnitude of this offsetting effect is uncertain, but it is estimated that somewhere between 10 and 30 percent of the potential fuel savings from increased CAFE standards will be lost to increased driving during the lifetime of vehicles (OTA 1991; NAS 1992).

Second, CAFE standards may discourage new vehicle sales and encourage vehicle owners to hold onto their existing vehicles longer. CAFE rules have this effect if they compel manufacturers to offer vehicles whose price-quality combination is less attractive to consumers than the offerings that would occur without tighter fuel economy standards (Crandall et al. 1986)—that is, if the rules push the market to produce and buy more fuel-efficient cars than the market would otherwise have chosen to buy. (If not, CAFE is having no effect at all.)

Measures taken to improve fuel efficiency, such as use of new technology, provision of less engine horsepower, and downsizing of vehicles, can make the new vehicles less attractive (or more expensive) to some consumers than they would otherwise be. Since new vehicles are more fuel-efficient than old ones, this perverse effect on the turnover rate of the vehicle fleet can be expected to dampen the energy savings expected from CAFE policy (Crandall et al. 1986; Gruenspecht 1992).

Thus, the net effect on national fuel consumption of raising CAFE is likely to be significantly smaller than even the small gradually increasing effect estimated from the increase in fuel efficiency per mile.

National Security Risks. In the area of national security, the primary concern is America's heavy dependence on *imported* oil, particularly from oil reserves in the Middle East/Persian Gulf area. This region has been plagued by political instability and hostility to American interests. Unlike other sectors of the U.S. economy, the transportation sector is almost 100 percent dependent on petroleum, about half from foreign sources, with little ability to engage in immediate fuel switching in the event of a crisis.

World oil production has diversified since the 1970s, leading to relatively less reliance on Middle Eastern sources for America's import needs. Some short-term protection from foreign supply shortfalls may also be offered by the U.S. Strategic Petroleum Reserve and the increased levels of strategic storage in Europe and Japan, though this approach is more controversial. Despite these encouraging developments, the national security of the United States and numerous allies continues to hinge significantly on access to low-priced oil from the Middle East (OTA 1991).

But CAFE policy may not directly aid America's security interests. First, CAFE's impact on overall fuel consumption, as just discussed, is small and incremental. Second, CAFE reduces demand for all oil, not just for imported oil. Insofar as lower demand for oil leads to less production of oil in the United States (rather than less importation of oil), the national security benefits of CAFE policy may be less than expected. Third, even if oil imports are reduced, it matters which countries reduce their exports to the United States. Unless reliance on suppliers in volatile or hostile areas decreases (or it becomes easier for the nation to switch at will to more stable suppliers or to U.S. sources), there will not be much national security benefit to the United States. Reductions in import purchases from major suppliers like Mexico could even hurt U.S. national security (for example, by increasing poverty in Mexico and hence political instability in and immigration from that country).

In the political debate about CAFE policy, some observers have argued that the Gulf War of 1991–1992 would not have been necessary if the United States had been less dependent on Middle East oil. Although this claim has some plausibility, one should also consider a larger array of foreign policy factors unrelated to CAFE. In addition to the oppression of Kuwait, Iraq's rising military power was a serious threat to the entire region, including the national security of Israel and Saudi Arabia, two of America's closest and most insecure allies. Moreover, many U.S. allies (for example, Europe and Japan) depend on Middle East oil. Further, the action to stop the militarization and expansion of Saddam Hussein's regime, which appeared close to gaining nuclear weapons capabilities, may have been a preemptive effort to stave off a larger Middle East war, and to deter other regional aggressors (such as North Korea).

Economic Risks. It is unclear how much economic benefit would result from new increases in CAFE standards. Even if the 1974 OPEC oil embargo contributed to the ensuing recession, to the higher U.S. inflation rate in the 1970s, and to the nation's balance-of-payments problems, as well as to the tight money policy that contributed to the severe recession in the early 1980s, it is not clear that in the future such supply or price disruptions could occur, or with as much impact. OPEC has been unable to command control of world oil prices over the last several years, as diversification of suppliers and slackening demand in the 1991 recession have undercut its cartel power. And it would take quite a long time for an increase in new-car CAFE—even a large increase from 27.5 to 40 mpg—to make a big dent in total U.S. oil dependence. Moreover,

CAFE reduces use of all oil (not just imported oil), at some ecenomic cost to consumers.

Environmental Risks. Petroleum production and combustion contribute to the environmental problems of urban smog, potential global warming, and oil spills. How much would raising CAFE standards affect these environmental threats?

Almost 100 million Americans live in cities that do not meet the nation's air quality standards for photochemical oxidants (smog, chiefly consisting of ground-level ozone) (EPA 1990). This mixture of pollutants causes respiratory irritation and degrades visibility in the city environment. New scientific evidence suggests that ozone produces adverse health effects at lower concentrations than previously thought, which means that some cities now considered "healthy" may be judged "unhealthy" should the EPA tighten the air quality standard for ozone.

Since 1970 the United States has relied primarily on vehicle engine controls to reduce tailpipe emissions of volatile organic compounds (VOCs), which were then believed to be the primary precursors (pollutant contributors) of urban ozone. The tailpipe emission standards are expressed on the basis of grams emitted per mile, not total pollutant emissions or emissions per gallon of fuel. Manufacturers therefore design engines and emission control systems to just meet the grams per mile standard, so improved fuel efficiency does not necessarily lead to fewer VOC emissions. More fuel efficiency is just as likely to result in less stringent emission control systems that still meet the same grams per mile standard.

Assuming nevertheless that greater fuel efficiency would not be accompanied by a fully offsetting relaxation in emission controls, fewer VOC emissions may contribute to less smog in the urban environment. But the atmospheric chemistry of smog is proving to be more complex than previously thought. Recent scientific research suggests that nitrogen oxides (rather than volatile organic compounds) are the primary limiting factor in the formation of smog in many regions of the United States. Since stationary pollution sources (such as electric utilities and factories) are the primary man-made source of nitrogen oxides, a vehicle-oriented policy, such as

CAFE, might not make a major difference in the urban smog problem without complementary control of nitrogen oxide emissions sources (NAS 1992).

In the case of global warming, petroleum combustion leads to emissions of carbon dioxide (CO_2), one of the greenhouse gases. The effects of global warming, if it occurs, are uncertain but may include significant changes in weather patterns and rising sea levels. Global warming will be examined in detail in Chapter 10; here it suffices to say that U.S. CAFE standards can play only a minor role in addressing any problem that is emerging. All the cars and trucks in the United States account for only about 3 percent of worldwide CO_2 emissions and thus about 1.5 percent of total greenhouse gas emissions (Crandall and Graham 1991). The U.S. share will be even smaller in future years because emissions from developing nations are growing at a faster rate than those from the United Sates. Because of the slow rate of the nation's vehicle fleet turnover and the perverse effects of CAFE on driver behavior, as discussed earlier, changes in new-car fuel efficiency would barely affect this small and declining contribution.

The Safety Risks of Stricter CAFE Legislation

If Congress chose to require automakers to increase average fuel efficiency from 27.5 mpg to 40 mpg by the year 2000, as contemplated in the Bryan bill, auto manufacturers would be induced to install some technological improvements but would also produce smaller vehicles that require less fuel per mile. Vehicle manufacturers can improve fuel efficiency in their fleets through several compliance strategies: making technological improvements in engines, transmissions, and tires; reducing vehicle performance by cutting back on engine horsepower; reducing vehicle weight by substituting lighter materials; downsizing vehicles in both exterior dimensions and weight; and shifting the mix of vehicles offered toward the smaller and lighter end of their offerings. Between 1974 and 1985, vehicle manufacturers used each of these strategies in their attainment of a doubling in new-car fuel economy. Since the late 1980s, consumers have been in-sisting on increases in engine horsepower. Lack of consumer interest in fuel economy reflects the fact that the real price of gasoline at the pump has remained roughly constant since 1980 (CEA 1994, table B-60), and the U.S. price is now one-fourth to one-half the price paid by European motorists (largely because of higher gasoline taxes in Europe) (OTA 1990).

Safety professionals are concerned that future improvements in fuel efficiency may be accomplished by significant reduction in vehicle shadow (length times width) and curb weight. From 1974 to 1991, the average new car sold in the United States lost 16 percent of its shadow and 20 percent of its curb weight (Graham 1992). In the meantime, however, consumers have become increasingly interested in light trucks and vans, which now account for about one-third of all new vehicle sales (OTA 1990). New CAFE policy is likely to impose stricter fuel efficiency requirements on these vehicles as well as on cars.

The downsizing of the new car fleet has been associated with increases in occupant injury and fatality risk, compared with what would have occurred if cars had not been downsized. Fortunately, the deterioration in occupant safety has not led to absolute increases in the number of highway injuries and fatalities because other favorable forces, such as safety belt use laws and the national campaign against drinking and driving, have improved highway safety. But highway death rates would most likely have fallen even further if CAFE increases had not been imposed from 1974 to 1985.

When assessing the impact of downsizing on vehicle safety, it is important to distinguish single-vehicle from multi-vehicle crashes. While people may envision themselves dying in violent two-car collisions, only a quarter of automobile fatalities occur in that manner. The vast majority of fatalities result from single-vehicle crashes into roadside objects or from car-truck collisions (NHTSA 1992). As Figure 5.1 indicates, occupants of smaller vehicles face elevated risks of injury and death in both single-vehicle and multi-vehicle crashes.

In a single-vehicle crash, both vehicle size (that is, exterior dimensions) and vehicle mass work to protect vehicle occupants. More vehicle size provides more space for deceleration of the vehicle occupants, which reduces the severity of occupant impacts within the vehicle. Vehicle mass per se has no protective effect if the roadside barrier is absolutely immovable and impenetrable, because under these conditions speed at impact will determine the severity of occupant injury. Since most roadside objects, such as fences and trees, are somewhat penetrable, bendable, or breakable, extra vehicle mass results in occupants' experiencing less injurious crash forces (Evans 1991).

In a multi-car crash, vehicle weight per se is a mixed blessing

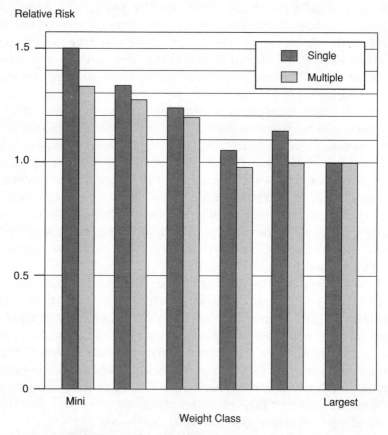

Figure 5.1 Relative probability of driver injury in a tow-away crash, by vehicle size. *Source:* Graham 1992, fig. 3.

for fleet safety, while vehicle size is unequivocally protective. Consider the case where vehicles 1 and 2, originally of equal weight and structural integrity, collide. Some extra vehicle weight in vehicle 1 would enhance the protection of the occupants of vehicle 1. Unfortunately, that extra weight would be hostile to the occupants of vehicle 2, the so-called "aggressivity effect." Holding constant the exterior dimensions and structural integrity of the two vehicles, it is not known whether extra weight in vehicle 1 would produce any significant change in the total number of injuries and fatalities in the two vehicles. If, however, the extra weight of vehicle 1 is provided by enhancing the crashworthiness of that vehicle (for example, by increasing exterior dimensions or adding stronger yet more flexible materials), then the net effect on safety is likely to be positive. The occupants of vehicle 1 and vehicle 2 will both benefit from the enhanced crashworthiness of vehicle 1, since the forces on the occupants of both vehicles will be attenuated. The aggressivity effect will still inflict some extra harm on the occupants of vehicle 2, but the empirical evidence indicates that reductions in vehicle size and weight tend to have a net harmful influence on occupant safety in two-car crashes (Graham 1992).

One might expect that smaller cars would be involved in fewer collisions than large cars, but the data on this point are very murky. Smaller cars are in fact involved in more collisions than large cars, but this difference is reduced or eliminated when driver age is controlled. Driver behavior is such a powerful determinant of collision frequency that it is very difficult to identify vehicle attributes that play a significant role. There is some evidence that small car drivers respond to their relative danger by traveling with more caution and fastening their safety belts more regularly (Evans 1985a).

The only type of crash whose frequency has been demonstrated to change with vehicle size is the rollover crash. Small cars exhibit less rollover stability than large cars, which is important because the rollover crash is likely to result in serious injuries or death to occupants. The studies of rollover crashes are unable to identify which vehicle attribute (vehicle weight, height, or shadow) is related to rollover propensity, although first principles emphasize the importance of the vehicle's center of gravity (Kahane 1991).

All told, the downward impact of CAFE on the size and weight of the automobile fleet is likely to increase traffic deaths. The most likely estimate from a recent study is that the Bryan bill (raising CAFE from 27.5 to 40 mpg by the year 2000) would cause 1,650 additional fatalities, and 8,000 additional serious injuries, per year in highway crashes than would occur in the absence of the bill, assuming full penetration of new vehicles into the fleet (Graham 1992).

Neglecting the Safety Risks of CAFE

The evidence that CAFE standards pose significant countervailing risks to motorists was not well recognized by Congress, the regulatory agency, or the public. Congress first authorized the Department of Transportation's National Highway Traffic Safety Administration (NHTSA) to implement CAFE standards in 1975. Since NHTSA is also the primary federal agency responsible for the safety of motor vehicles, one might have expected NHTSA to take a proactive role in identifying any adverse safety consequences of the CAFE program. NHTSA researchers did identify and publicize the safety problems associated with smaller, lighter vehicles available in the marketplace, but the policymakers in the agency never explicitly associated this stream of research findings with the CAFE program itself.

The impact of CAFE policy on vehicle safety was highlighted not by NHTSA but by risk analysts at the Brookings Institution and the Harvard School of Public Health (Graham 1983; Crandall and Graham 1989). Using data provided by researchers at NHTSA and General Motors Research Laboratories, Crandall and Graham (1989) estimated that each 500 pound reduction in vehicle size and weight was associated with a 14 to 27 percent increase in the risk of serious injury and fatality to occupants (given a crash). Since 1989 models were estimated to be 500 pounds smaller as a result of CAFE policy, the authors projected that the occupants of these vehicles would, over the lifetime of the vehicles, experience 2,000 more fatalities and 20,000 more serious injuries than would have occurred if CAFE standards have not been in place.

When President Reagan's appointees at NHTSA were presented with this information, they refused to change the agency's official policy on CAFE and safety. Indeed, in 1988 NHTSA was sued by the Competitive Enterprise Institute, a nonprofit "free-market" group, for ignoring adverse safety consequences when setting the CAFE standards for 1989 models. In this early litigation, NHTSA denied any link between CAFE and safety and persuaded a federal court that the nation's overall progress in reducing the traffic fatality rate indicated that CAFE policy was not compromising safety.

The major domestic vehicle manufacturers were also reluctant to be candid about the safety risks of CAFE. Although GM and Ford were steadfastly opposing tighter CAFE standards, their public speeches assiduously avoided the suggestion that downsized vehicles were less safe than larger vehicles. This reluctance may have reflected marketing or liability concerns.

In 1987 NHTSA's Office of Research and Development launched a series of in-house studies aimed at disproving the alleged relationship between CAFE policy and safety. As the Bush administration assumed office in 1989, the results of these studies began to be released at technical meetings. To the surprise of some NHTSA officials and CAFE advocates, the studies indicated that vehicle size and weight offered significant protection to motorists in both single-vehicle and multi-vehicle crashes (NHTSA 1990; NHTSA 1991). Once again, however, the published NHTSA reports were carefully written to avoid any direct link between CAFE and occupant safety.

Safety Concerns Go Public

While NHTSA remained silent on the safety issue, the Insurance Institute for Highway Safety (IIHS)—the trade association representing insurers who pay the claims for people injured in auto accidents—began to air concerns about Senator Bryan's proposal to raise CAFE to 40 mpg by the year 2000. Evidence submitted by IIHS suggested that such ambitious standards could not be achieved without more vehicle downsizing, which would lead to more occupant fatalities and injuries. IIHS also produced data indicating that GM's downsized vehicles were exhibiting higher occupant fatality rates than the same models prior to downsizing (IIHS 1991).

As the Bryan bill gained popularity during the Persian Gulf crisis of 1991–1992, the motor vehicle manufacturers began to reassess their strategy in the public policy debate. The Coalition for Vehicle Choice was formed under the leadership of Diane Steed, former NHTSA administrator in the Reagan administration, to provide information on the adverse impacts of the Bryan bill on consumer choice. With support from GM and other auto interests, the Coalition began to raise the safety issue explicitly in a concerted mass media campaign. With a powerful television advertisement aired throughout the country, the Coalition highlighted the danger to small car occupants when a big car and a small car collide.

Energy conservation advocates forged a powerful alliance with environmentalists to promote the Bryan bill, but they were concerned about the growing attention to the safety issue. In response to safety concerns, Joan Claybrook, president of Public Citizen and former NHTSA administrator under President Carter, came to the defense of the conservation advocates. She publicly accused Diane Steed of misleading the public about the safety risks of small cars. Claybrook insisted that vehicle manufacturers could build smaller and lighter cars without compromising highway safety, pointing to research by NHTSA showing that innovative crashworthiness designs could provide excellent crash protection to vehicle occupants.

Faced with this open debate, the key Bush administration appointees, Secretary of Transportation Samuel Skinner and NHTSA head General Jerry Curry, reversed the position of the Reagan administration and began to speak forcefully about the safety risks of the Bryan bill. When the administration threatened a presidential veto of the Bryan bill, safety was cited as one of the key motivating factors.

In public testimony, however, NHTSA officials drew a curious distinction between the current CAFE program and new legislative proposals. NHTSA said on the one hand that current

CAFE policy was not hurting safety, while stating publicly that overly stringent new CAFE standards could harm safety in the future. Under further litigation brought by the Competitive Enterprise Institute, NHTSA attempted to draw this distinction before a federal appeals court. In a stinging opinion decrying bureaucratic attempts to dodge the issue, the federal court ordered NHTSA to rethink its current CAFE standards in light of safety concerns (*CEI v. NHTSA* 1992).

Conclusion

Even when a countervailing risk threatens the lives of thousands of people, it may not gain currency in policy debates. The American political system does have some built-in checks to prevent omission of countervailing risks from the public policy debate. The potential victims of the countervailing risks, if they can organize themselves at reasonable cost, may advocate serious consideration of the countervailing risks. Here the insurers of crash victims (IIHS) ultimately stepped forward to highlight the safety issue, after years of willful neglect by the very agency charged with protecting motorist safety. And when administrative decisions are reviewed in the courts, federal judges may insist, depending upon factors such as the case law, the statute, and the evidence at hand, that regulators consider the countervailing risks (as well as the target risks) before issuing final rules.

Forcing *consideration* of countervailing risks does not, however, necessarily imply that policies to reduce the target risk will or should be abandoned. In the short term, considering safety in making automobile policy will simply require weighing risk versus risk—as described in Chapter 1 and as ultimately required by the court in *CEI v. NHTSA*. While the outcome of the fuel economy debate is far from clear, the countervailing risk of vehicle safety has added a new dimension to public policy discussions. Recent reports by both the Office of Technology Assessment (1991) and the National Academy of Sciences (1992) concur that the safety risks of fuel economy legislation need to be weighed against the anticipated benefits of energy conservation. Comparing safety risks with risks to national security, the economy, and the environment is by no means straightforward, but the application of risk tradeoff analysis can facilitate such comparison.

In the longer term, highlighting the countervailing risks *can* stimulate policymakers and scientists to consider innovative alternatives that reduce overall risk or that reduce target risks without increasing countervailing risks. In this case, it is worth considering both refinements of and alternatives to CAFE standards. For example, to diminish the adverse safety impacts of CAFE standards, Congress might consider applying separate CAFE standards to each size class of vehicles. This regulatory refinement might guide manufacturers to focus on technological advances rather than vehicle downsizing as a primary compliance strategy. The OTA (1991) study indicates the potential to increase fuel efficiency through innovative engine technologies that do not involve downsizing.

It may also be useful to consider refined CAFE standards in conjunction with fees on cars sold with powerful engines (a horsepower tax). This policy would make sense if engines with high horsepower ratings are associated with both high gas consumption and high safety risks, for example from excessive acceleration (Robertson 1991).

A logical but more publicly contentious policy alternative to tighter CAFE regulation is higher gasoline taxes. Stricter CAFE standards increase safety risks and place car makers in a predicament when consumers and regulators demand vehicles of different sizes. Gasoline taxes might help achieve CAFE's conservation goals through market-based incentives. From the consumer's point of view, replacing CAFE with gasoline taxes might not add costs: this switch would increase the variable cost of driving, but reduce the capital cost of purchasing a new car.

But wouldn't higher gasoline taxes induce consumers to switch to smaller, more fuel-efficient and hence less safe vehicles? Perhaps, but fuel taxes would also reduce traffic injuries and fatalities by discouraging the additional vehicle miles traveled (Leigh and Frank 1987; Leigh and Wilkinson 1991) that CAFE promotes. And gasoline taxes would not encourage motorists, as CAFE does, to keep their older, higher-emission vehicles in use longer. By shifting costs from initial capital cost to variable driving costs, fuel taxes would discourage extra driving and older cars, and thus reduce the concomitant extra fuel consumption, emissions, and accident risks that CAFE exacerbates. Thus, from the perspective of both target risks (energy consumption, emissions) and the countervailing risk (safety), higher gasoline taxes might prove to be superior to tighter CAFE standards.

6

Eating Fish

PAUL D. ANDERSON
JONATHAN BAERT WIENER

Decisions aimed at reducing target risks would be paralyzed if any suggestion of a countervailing risk were used to halt the decisionmaking process. Not all countervailing risks are equally serious. The key challenge is to distinguish the important countervailing risks and weigh their seriousness *relative* to the target risk.

This chapter illustrates how quantitative risk tradeoff analysis (RTA), described in Chapter 1, can be used to help gauge the seriousness of a countervailing risk. The target risk in this case, heart disease that results from eating foods such as beef with a high saturated fat content, can be reduced by substituting fish as a protein source, and national health institutions have therefore encouraged Americans to make this switch (NRC 1989). But eating more fish also entails a countervailing risk of cancer when the fish is contaminated with various carcinogenic pollutants. On this basis, agencies in nearly every state have warned consumers not to eat certain fish (Johnson 1992). Consumers are thus faced with conflicting recommendations and a risk tradeoff dilemma.

In this chapter, basic methods of RTA are used to weigh the risks. The analysis reveals that the elevation of cancer risk from eating fish with even high levels of contaminants is tiny compared to the expected protection against coronary heart disease provided by eating that fish instead of beef. This is so even for populations consuming large quantities of fish. Thus families should not ordinarily be deterred from replacing meat with fish in their diets. To put it another way, a consumer would have to dread dying of cancer over ten times more—and perhaps hundreds of times more—than dying of heart disease in order for the extra cancer risk from eating fish to begin to offset the reduced risk of heart disease from eating fish. And this estimate is based on several assumptions that tend to overstate the actual cancer risk from eating fish.

Recommendations about Eating Fish

A diet high in fat content is associated with an increased risk of a variety of diseases, including coronary heart disease (CHD) and certain types of cancers (NRC 1989). As a result, dietary experts assembled by the National Academy of Sciences (NRC 1989), the U.S. Senate (1977), and many national and international public health organizations recommend reducing intake of fat by substituting low-fat foods such as fish (NRC 1989). Specifically, the first dietary recommendation of the National Academy report reads as follows:

> Reduce total fat intake to 30% or less of calories. Reduce saturated fatty acid intake to less than 10% of calories, and the intake of cholesterol to less than 300 mg daily. The intake of fat and cholesterol can be reduced by substituting fish, poultry without skin, lean meats, and low- or nonfat dairy products for fatty meats and whole-milk dairy products; by choosing more vegetables, fruits, cereals, and legumes; and by limiting oils, fats, egg yolks, and fried and other fatty foods. (NRC 1989, p. 13)

Of the recommended foodstuffs, fish are unique because, in addition to being a low-fat source of protein, some of the components of fish oil have the potential added benefit of decreasing the risk of CHD directly by suppressing some CHD risk factors.

In contrast to these health benefits are some potentially countervailing risks associated with eating fish. The health risks can be grouped according to their causes: naturally occurring toxins, microbial contamination linked with pollution and improper handling after harvest, and environmental chemical pollutants (IOM 1991). Although public health officials have been cognizant of these potential risks for many years, several recent publications have focused on quantifying these risks (CU 1992; Fora and Glenn 1992; IOM 1991; Reinert et al. 1991) while acknowledging the beneficial aspects of eating fish. Although several of these authors recommend ways to reduce some of the countervailing risks, such as those associated with microbes (CU 1992; IOM 1991), none of the authors quantify the benefits of eating fish and compare them to the risks, such as the increased cancer risk associated with ingestion of carcinogenic pollutants. Similarly, the NRC report (1989) on diet and health recognized that pollutants in fish may pose a risk but did not quantify that risk. Meanwhile, states and the U.S. Environmental Protection Agency (EPA) have initiated programs to warn consumers against eating fish when pollutant contaminant levels are high (Tyson 1992; Johnson 1992), and more than 4,000 such bans or warnings have been issued by nearly fifty states (Wheeler 1992).

To help resolve this dilemma, this chapter quantifies the potential CHD risk of not eating fish and the potential cancer risks of eating fish, and compares them in order to explore whether the dietary recommendations should be changed to account for the risks associated with consumption of fish and, if so, under what conditions. In particular, for some lower-income communities, catching fish is an inexpensive, readily available, and potentially substantial portion of their diet, as well as being a source of low-fat protein. Because polluted waters and people with lower income can be collocated, at least a portion of the fish these people eat may have relatively high levels of carcinogenic chemicals. We also apply RTA to this subpopulation of high fish consumers.

The Health Benefits of Eating Fish

Benefits from consumption of fish can be realized in two distinct ways. The first, and the primary basis for the dietary recommendation to eat more fish, is the indirect effect that substituting fish for fatty sources of protein has on reducing dietary intake of fat and saturated fatty acids. High intake of fat and saturated fatty acids has been associated with an increase in CHD (and possibly certain cancers):

> There is clear evidence that the total amounts and types of fats and other lipids in the diet influence the risk of athero-sclerotic cardiovascular diseases and, to a less well-established extent, certain forms of cancer and possibly obesity. The evidence that the intake of saturated fatty acids and cholesterol are causally related to atherosclerotic cardiovascular diseases is especially strong and convincing. (NRC 1989, p. 7)

Second, consumption of fish may also directly reduce the risk of CHD through the specific effect of fish oils on CHD risk factors. Extensive studies, some with people who are genetically predisposed to greater CHD risk, have demonstrated a decrease in CHD risk factors when diets are high in fish oils (Simopoulos 1991). Several biological mechanisms have been hypothesized for this relationship (Cad 1985), all of which rely on the relatively high concentrations of a particular class of oils in fish, the "omega-3" polyunsaturated fatty acids. Diets high in omega-3 fatty acids have been shown to markedly decrease plasma cholesterol and triglyceride levels, to decrease the presence of very-low-density lipoprotein (Phillipson et al. 1985), and to affect the metabolism and function of platelets (Lee et al. 1985). All of these biological effects have been associated with, or hypothesized to cause, a decrease in the risk of CHD. (In addition, recent evidence suggests that omega-3 oils in fish help reduce chronic bronchitis and emphysema; Shahar et al. 1994.)

Limited epidemiological evidence lends some support to the hypothesis that people with diets high in fish content have a decreased risk of CHD. Several statistical studies have suggested that the consumption of fish may decrease the risk of CHD (Bang et al. 1980; Bang and Dyerberg 1972; Kagawa et al. 1982; Hirai et al. 1980; Kromhout et al. 1985). Although many of these studies focused on particular ethnic groups such as Greenland Eskimos (Bang et al. 1980; Bang and Dyerberg 1972) and Japanese (Hirai et al. 1980; Kagawa et al. 1982), they still provide evidence of relevance to residents of the United States. Other studies, however, have not found a relationship between increased fish consumption and decreased CHD risk (Curb and Reed 1985; Snowdon 1981; Vollset et al. 1985). Moreover, the studies that do show a decrease in CHD risk with increasing fish consumption are not able to discern whether that effect derives directly from omega-3 fatty acids or indirectly because diets rich in fish have lower levels of fat, saturated fatty acids, and cholesterol (NRC 1989, p. 8).

Estimating the CHD Benefits of Eating Fish. Kromhout and colleagues (1985) selected 1,088 Danish men, ages 40 to 59, living in Zutphen, a town that participated in the Seven Countries Study (Keys 1980), and investigated the relationship between their fish consumption rates and mortality from CHD. The composition of the diet of these men was recorded, as were other CHD risk factors including serum cholesterol, blood pressure, smoking habits, anthropometric measures, physical activity, and occupation. The vital status of these men was followed for twenty years, during which time 390 died (132 from cancer, 110 from CHD, 33 from cerebrovascular causes, and the remainder from other causes). The men were divided into five categories depending upon the amount of fish they ate: 0 grams per day, 1–14, 15–29, 30–44, and 45 or more grams per day. For each of these categories, both crude and adjusted risk ratios, and 95% confidence intervals, for death from CHD were calculated (see Table 6.1, Figure 6.1). Ratios were calculated for a twenty-year follow-up period, and were adjusted for the contribution of numerous other risk factors.

Both the crude and adjusted ratios show a marked decrease in the risk of CHD as fish consumption increases (Table 6.1). The largest decrease in risk ratio occurs between individuals eating 0 grams of fish per day (a ratio of 1.00) and those individuals eating 1 to 14 grams of fish per day (an adjusted ratio of 0.64; see Table 6.1, second row, and Figure 6.1). For example, increasing fish consumption from 0 grams per day to about 20 grams per day (equivalent to about one meal of fish every ten days) is estimated to result in a 44 percent decrease in the adjusted relative risk of CHD (from 1.00 to 0.56). The converse is also true: a person who decreased fish consumption from 20 to 0 grams per day would increase the adjusted relative risk of dying from CHD by about 75 percent (from 0.56 to 1.00).

The average American in fact eats about 15 grams of fish per day (EPA 1989), which places him or her on the cusp between Kromhout's categories of 1–14 grams per day and 15–29 grams per day. And the average American's risk of dying of heart disease is about 35 percent (Bureau of the Census 1990). Kromhout's results indicate that if the average American ate zero fish instead of 15 grams per day (and ate beef instead), that person's adjusted relative risk of dying from CHD would increase by about 66 percent (from 0.56–0.64 to 1.00; see Table 6.1), and the average total risk of mortality from CHD in this

Table 6.1　Heart disease and fish consumption

Fish consumption rate (in grams per person per day)		Risk ratio[a] (with 95% confidence bounds)	
Range	Midpoint	Crude	Adjusted
—	0	1.00	1.00
1–14	8	0.60 (0.33–1.10)	0.64 (0.32–1.26)
15–29	22	0.57 (0.30–1.09)	0.56 (0.27–1.15)
30–44	37.5	0.46 (0.20–1.06)	0.36 (0.14–0.93)
>45	45	0.42 (0.16–1.13)	0.39 (0.13–1.15)

Source: Adapted from Kromhout et al. 1985.

a. Risk of mortality from coronary heart disease, relative to the risk faced by a person consuming 0 grams of fish per day.

country would be not 35 percent but a staggering 58 percent. To put it another way, the current average fish consumption of 15 grams per day, rather than zero fish and more beef, is already reducing the national average risk of dying of CHD by an estimated 40 percent (reducing the adjusted relative risk from 1.00 to 0.56–0.64), or about 23 percentage points below what it otherwise would be. (Ideally this calculation would be expressed in terms of years of life expectancy added or lost, rather than the fraction of total deaths attributable to CHD.)

Increasing fish consumption above 15 grams per day would offer further benefits in decreased CHD risk. If the average American increased fish consumption from, say, 20 grams per day (a meal every ten days) to 40 grams per day (a meal every five days), that would reduce the adjusted relative risk of dying of CHD from about 0.56 to 0.36, a drop of about 36 percent (substantial but not quite as large as the 44 percent decrease in relative risk obtained by the first 20-gram increment, from zero to 20 grams per day, noted above). That would reduce the average American's total CHD mortality risk from its current 35 percent to about 23 percent, an additional 12 percentage points (Figure 6.1).

The relevance to the U.S. population of the results reported by Kromhout and colleagues (1985) can be questioned, but three reasons suggest that these findings are applicable to the United States. First, the phenomenon of reduced CHD mortality in people who eat large amounts of fish has been observed in three diverse populations: Dutch men, Greenland Eskimos, and Japanese. Although the relationship has not yet been confirmed in the U.S. population, there is little reason to believe that Americans would be unaffected.

Second, because the men studied by Kromhout and colleagues lived in Zutphen, the Netherlands city that participated in the Seven Countries Study, key risk factors between Dutch and U.S. citizens can be compared. Such a comparison shows that the only notable differences between the two populations were in the death rates from CHD and smoking habits. The death rates from CHD are 574 per 100,000 in the United States and 420 in Zutphen, a difference that is not statistically significant ($p > 0.05$). In the Netherlands, the majority of men (65 percent) smoked between 1 and 19 cigarettes a day, while in the United States the majority of men either never smoked (21 percent) or smoked 10 or more cigarettes a day (52 percent). The remaining key characteristics (systolic blood pressure, serum cholesterol, body mass index, resting pulse rate, percentage of diet calories consisting of total fats and saturated fat) were similar. Thus, with respect to at least two key CHD risk factors, serum cholesterol and percentage of diet consisting of saturated fats, the two populations are virtually identical.

Third, clinical experiments in the United States involving fish oils have led to several hypotheses about the potential biological mechanism. Although these experiments have been limited to observing changes in some of the risk factors for

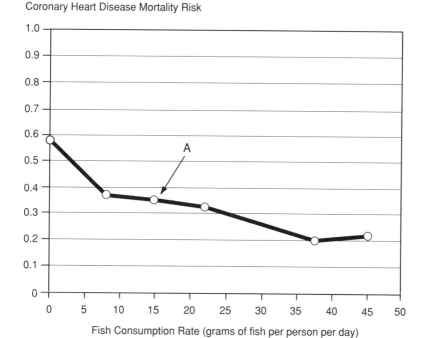

Figure 6.1 Fish consumption and risk of death from CHD. Note that in 1989 the average American ate 15 grams of fish per day and had a CHD mortality risk of 0.35 (denoted as point A).

CHD rather than the incidence of CHD itself, they have provided evidence that the risk factors decrease in Americans who have diets high in fish oils (Phillipson et al. 1985; Lee et al. 1985).

It is important to keep in mind, however, that some epidemiological studies have not found a relationship between CHD mortality and fish consumption, and the biological mechanisms for protection have often not been proved. This leaves open the possibility that the CHD benefits of eating fish are less than estimated here.

The Countervailing Risks of Eating Fish

A recent report by the Institute of Medicine (IOM) on seafood safety has summarized the different types and magnitude of risk associated with consumption of both seafood and freshwater fish (IOM 1991). The types of risk can be divided into three categories according to their causes: natural toxins and microbes; microbial contamination due to waters polluted by sewage or improper handling between the time of harvest and sale to the consumer; and contamination with environmental pollutants (IOM 1991).

The potential magnitude of these risks is governed by the severity of the hazard and the consumer's ability to reduce or eliminate the hazard. Thus, even though microbial contamination of processed or store-bought fish and shellfish has been shown to be disturbingly widespread and to pose anywhere from a mild to a severe hazard, consumers can greatly reduce, if not eliminate, this hazard by cooking the fish or shellfish (CU 1992; IOM 1991). Once cooked, store-bought fish poses little microbial risk. It is also noteworthy that the microbial hazards associated with improper handling or processing of fish are much smaller for anglers who eat fish soon after harvest, thereby reducing the amount of time available for fish to spoil.

The hazard associated with naturally occurring toxins may be severe, and in many cases there is little or nothing consumers can do, aside from not eating the affected fish, to reduce or eliminate this risk (IOM 1991). Fortunately, species with naturally occurring toxins tend to be localized, in both time and space, and tend to be the potential hazard recognized most easily by the public. As a result, the potential risks are also localized and can be further reduced through education and harvest restrictions (IOM 1991).

The hazards associated with anthropogenic environmental pollutants in fish range from mild to severe, and the occurrence of at least some chemical pollutants appears to be widespread (IOM 1991). Consumers can reduce the hazard by avoiding certain species of fish and by not eating selected portions of a fish, but unless they stop eating fish altogether, most people will likely be exposed to some level of pollutants through consumption of fish (IOM 1991; CU 1992; Fora and Glenn 1991; Reinert et al. 1991). The magnitude of risk varies, but if the commonly used methods to estimate risks are accurate, most people who eat fish incur some increased risk of getting cancer. For sport and subsistence fishing populations and their families who eat a great deal of fish containing relatively high levels of pollutants, the increased cancer risks, and possibly risks of other health effects, may be substantial.

Estimating Excess Lifetime Cancer Risks from Eating Fish. To estimate the potential excess lifetime cancer risk associated with a person's consumption of fish, we examined the six specific compounds with an "allowable concentration limit" set by the Food and Drug Administration (FDA) that are also assumed to be carcinogenic by the Environmental Protection Agency (EPA). This analysis assumes that every fish that a person eats contains all such compounds at a concentration equal to the limit derived by the FDA. We use a quantitative estimate of carcinogenic potential, derived by the EPA, called a Cancer Slope Factor (CSF) to estimate increased lifetime cancer risk. Given these assumptions, the relationship between a person's increased lifetime cancer risk and the amount of fish eaten is estimated using the following formula:

Potential Increased Lifetime Cancer Risk = Cancer Slope Factor (CSF) (milligrams of chemical per kilogram of bodyweight per day)$^{-1}$ × Fish Consumption Rate (kilograms of fish per person per day) × Concentration of Chemical in Fish (milligrams of chemical per kilogram of fish) / Bodyweight (kilograms per person).

The CSFs employed in the analysis are shown in Table 6.2. In accordance with EPA guidelines, we assumed that all people weigh 70 kilograms and that all consume fish contaminated with all six compounds at the FDA limits over their entire 70-year lifetime.

The increased lifetime cancer risk associated with eating 1 gram of fish containing the FDA limit of any one chemical is shown in Table 6.2, along with the cancer risk associated with eating 1 gram of fish containing all of the chemicals at their FDA limits. The relationship between the amount of fish eaten and increased lifetime cancer risk is assumed to be linear (Figure 6.2)—that is, doubling the rate of fish consumption doubles the potential cancer risk.

The increase in lifetime cancer risk associated with eating these contaminated fish is substantial, though small when compared to the existing background rate of mortality from cancer in the United States (see Figure 6.2). The lifetime risk of getting cancer for someone eating 1 gram per day (for a lifetime) of fish contaminated with all six compounds at their FDA

Table 6.2 Cancer risk from consumption of contaminated fish

Compound	FDA limit[a]	CSF[b]	PELCR[c]
DDT	5.0 ppm[d]	0.34	2.4×10^{-5}
PCB	2.0 ppm	7.4	2.1×10^{-4}
Chlordane	0.3 ppm	1.61	6.9×10^{-6}
Dieldrin	0.3 ppm	30.4	1.3×10^{-4}
Heptachlor	0.3 ppm	3.37	1.4×10^{-5}
Dioxin[e]	50 ppt[f]	156,000.	1.1×10^{-4}
All compounds			5.0×10^{-4}

a. Concentration limit set by FDA.

b. Cancer Slope Factor, in (milligrams of intake per kilogram of body weight per day)$^{-1}$, calculated by EPA as the 95% upper bound of the CSF distribution for the compound.

c. Potential Excess Lifetime Cancer Risk, for consumption of 1 gram of fish containing the FDA limit for the indicated compound, per day, for a 70-year lifetime.

d. Parts per million.

e. Dioxin refers to the 2, 3, 7, 8 tetrachlorodibenzo-p-dioxin isomer.

f. Parts per trillion.

limits is estimated at 5.0×10^{-4} (five in 10,000), which is equal
to one chance in 2,000. Eating 20 grams per day of such contaminated fish (equivalent to about one full meal every ten
days) would thus be estimated to increase the risk by twenty
in 2,000, which is equal to one in one hundred. That one percentage point increase in the risk of getting cancer would increase the total cancer risk faced by the average American
from 25 percent to 26 percent (from 0.25 to 0.26 in Figure 6.2).
Increasing contaminated fish consumption from 20 to 40
grams per day would increase the cancer risk by another one
percentage point, from 26 percent to 27 percent (see Figure
6.2).

This approach to estimating increased lifetime cancer risk
resulting from eating contaminated fish contains several elements that tend to overstate the actual cancer risk associated

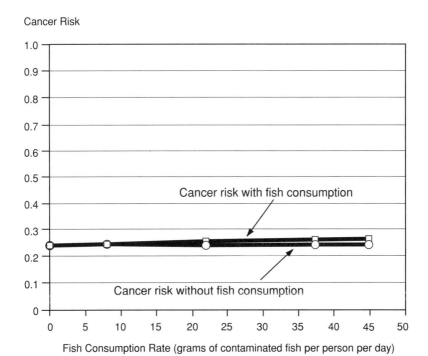

Figure 6.2 Contaminated fish consumption and risk of death from
cancer.

with consumption of fish. These elements are nonetheless typical of a "conservative" or protective risk assessment conducted by EPA.

First, the analysis uses several improbable exposure assumptions. A person is assumed to eat fish containing all six chemicals, at the FDA limits, for an entire lifetime. This analysis assumes that all fish contain all of these chemicals at their FDA allowed limits, even though the average concentrations of these chemicals in most fish in the United States are substantially below all of these limits (IOM 1991). It is possible that some fish are contaminated with significant amounts of a larger number of compounds, but this is unlikely.

Second, the cancer slope factors used in this analysis do not predict average increased lifetime cancer risk; rather, they are the 95 percent upper bound of a distribution of cancer slope factors. Thus 95 percent of the estimated cancer slope factors for these compounds are lower than that used in this analysis, and it is possible that the true cancer risk is zero. In addition, the distribution of cancer slope factors is derived in a manner designed to intentionally overestimate a chemical's cancer-causing potential. For example, in the case of dioxin, the cancer slope factor is based on those organs, and on the animal study, that gave the highest estimate of cancer-causing potential. Other animal studies showed that dioxin had a lower cancer-causing potential, and other organs showed a decrease in cancer incidence with increasing dose. Total cancer incidence was also lower in some laboratory animals exposed to dioxin than in animals not exposed. Dioxin's estimated cancer slope factor might be substantially lower if it explicitly incorporated these findings.

Third, this analysis assumes that all cancers caused by consumption of contaminated fish are fatal. The standard risk assessment methodology used here, however, only predicts cancer incidence. Some of the cancers predicted to be caused by consumption of fish may be curable and may not result in death. Thus the increase in an individual's risk of dying from cancer would be less than indicated by this analysis.

On the other hand, it is possible that various non-cancer

health effects could be caused by these same six contaminants. With the possible exception of dioxin (which is now suspected to cause immune system effects, and possibly developmental and reproductive effects, even at very low doses), the concentrations of contaminants in the fish are below the "safe" doses established by regulatory toxicologists. Cancer is the key issue because it is common to assume that any amount of exposure to a carcinogen increases risk.

Weighing the Risks

On the basis of the likely dependence of both decreased CHD risk and increased cancer risk on the fish consumption rate, it is possible to combine the two and develop a single relationship that predicts the net health risk (or benefit). Since both CHD and cancer are fatal chronic diseases, we use mortality risk as the yardstick for comparison. (This assumes that all cancers are fatal, as discussed above; and it assumes, perhaps incorrectly, that the reduction in quality of life for those suffering the two illnesses would be comparable.) Given the relatively small increase in excess lifetime cancer risk caused by consumption of contaminated fish (Figure 6.2) and the substantial reduction in CHD risk associated with consumption of fish (Figure 6.1), the benefits of eating fish appear to far outweigh the risks. The benefits, in fact, outweigh the countervailing risks to such a large degree that the relationship between net mortality risk and fish consumption is only marginally different from the relationship for CHD mortality alone (Figure 6.3). Indeed, as the analysis in this chapter indicates, going from zero to 20 grams of maximally contaminated fish per day would increase the average American's lifetime risk of dying from cancer by just one percentage point (from 25 percent to 26 percent), but is estimated to reduce that person's lifetime risk of dying from CHD by 23 percentage points (from 58 percent to 35 percent); and going from 20 to 40 grams per day of such fish would increase the cancer mortality risk another one percentage point, but would reduce the CHD mortality risk by 12 percentage points. The *net* effect in both cases is a substantial decrease in the overall risk of dying. (Of course, even a person saved from CHD by eating fish would eventually die of something else; ideally, therefore, the net effect of eating fish on life expectancy should be calculated in terms of the years of life saved rather than as a simple fraction of total mortality risk.)

It may be, however, that the two illnesses are subjectively different in ways that should be incorporated in this analysis. People may fear cancer more than CHD, perhaps because cancer is judged a more painful way to die. But even if cancer is considered two or three times more onerous than coronary heart disease, as suggested by Tolley, Kenkel, and Fabian (1994, pp. 339–344), its increased likelihood due to contaminated fish would still not overcome the estimated 12 to 23 times larger decrease in the risk of CHD mortality from eating those fish. Moreover, it should be remembered that this analysis includes all nonfatal cases of cancer (assuming them to

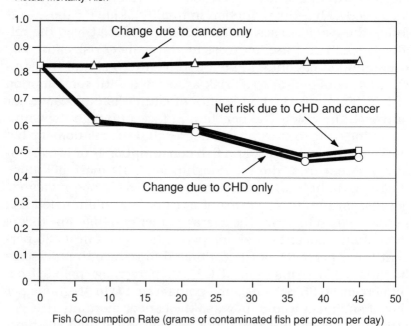

Figure 6.3 Contaminated fish consumption and combined risk of death from CHD and cancer.

be fatal), but excludes consideration of additional nonfatal cases of CHD, which are painful, debilitating, and expensive to treat.

Further, recall that for several reasons the cancer risk estimates used here are likely to overstate the true cancer risk. For example, the average level of these pollutants occurring in fish in the United States is less than that assumed by this analysis. The increased cancer risk associated with *actual* levels of chemicals in fish (at an average consumption rate of about 20 grams per person per day) in the United States is estimated to be about 7.5×10^{-5} (7.5 in one hundred thousand) (IOM 1991), or about one hundred times less than the increased risk of about 1×10^{-2} (one in one hundred) that was estimated in the analysis above. Thus the decrease in CHD mortality risk from eating realistically contaminated fish may be not 12 to 23 times larger but actually 1,200 to 2,300 times larger than the increase in cancer risk from eating those fish. Adjusting the cancer slope factors and accounting for the fraction of cancer cases that are not fatal would lower the cancer risk estimate further.

Prevention Strategies

One way to reduce the increased cancer risks would be to recommend that people eat less fish. This is the intended effect of the warnings issued by states. But the likely increases in CHD risk that would result from eating less fish suggest that such a recommendation, at least on a national scale, would not be wise public health policy.

Another way to reduce the increased cancer risks is to reduce the levels of pollution in fish eaten in the United States. Fortunately, numerous water quality regulations are accomplishing this either directly or indirectly. For example, water quality standards for dioxin have required many pulp and paper mills to curtail their discharges of dioxin into surface waters. (Still, if society could choose whether to put its marginal resources into further ratcheting down carcinogen pollution of waterways or into increasing the consumption of fish, on risk-reduction grounds it might choose the latter.)

Exposure to pollutants in fish can also be reduced on a national level by educating consumers to substitute fish having low levels of pollutants for those having high levels of pollutants in their diet (IOM 1991). In addition, the finding that most fish have relatively low levels of pollutants and that only a few have relatively high levels suggests that focusing environmental control efforts on those geographic areas and fish species with high levels of pollution provides the opportunity to bring about a significant decrease in national exposure to contaminated fish without a major nationwide expenditure of resources.

Thus, at least on a national level, a change in the long-standing recommendation to increase consumption of fish as a replacement for high-fat sources of dietary protein is not warranted. Indeed, although the direct evidence supporting a relationship between fish consumption and CHD is still limited, it is interesting to note that from 1970 to 1987 the risk of CHD decreased by 20 percent in the United States. During the same time period, fish consumption increased by 30 percent (Bureau of the Census 1990). Although this general association does not itself indicate a causal link, this dietary change may be working in conjunction with less smoking, more exercise, and better CHD treatment to reduce the risk factors for CHD mortality.

Special Populations at Risk and "Fish Advisories"

The increased cancer risk for people who fish recreationally, and for those who catch and eat a substantial amount of fish, depends upon the levels of pollutants in the fish from the local rivers, lakes, and estuaries that are heavily fished. Most areas and fish species with high levels of pollutants have been identified. These levels can vary greatly: some fish may have non-detectable levels of all pollutants, while others may have levels of one or more pollutants that approach or exceed the FDA allowable concentration limits. As a result, increased cancer risks can also vary from essentially zero to levels that may approach those predicted in this analysis.

The response of regulatory agencies has been to warn the

public of the increased cancer risks associated with eating fish from these areas through the use of "fish advisories." Depending upon the regulatory agency and the concentration of the pollutant(s) in fish, the advisory may range from a recommendation for some subsets of the general population to limit their intake of fish to a complete ban on consumption of fish for the entire population. A recent survey indicated that more than 4,000 advisories or bans had been imposed in nearly all fifty states, each covering certain types of fish from a specific location (Johnson 1992).

Given the large CHD benefits of eating fish, are these fish advisories a good idea? It seems clear that if an alternative source of "clean" fish is available, and if people affected by the advisory have access to this source at equal cost and will use it, then the advisory should be maintained. In theory, this holds true regardless of the level of cancer risk, because all fish are assumed to confer an equal CHD benefit. (If information on species-specific differences in CHD benefit becomes available, then cancer and heart disease risks for fish from different waters would, ideally, need to be considered in setting a fish advisory.) This theory should also be subjected to practical considerations and to the preferences of people who fish. Even with readily available "clean" fish species at equal cost, people may still want to catch and eat "contaminated" species if they provide more sport, offer a better fishing experience, or taste better.

Subsistence Fishing and Environmental Justice. When an alternative and accessible source of "clean" fish is not available or is more expensive, the results of this analysis suggest a change in how fish consumption advisories have typically been implemented. The potential excess lifetime cancer risk of subsistence fishing communities eating contaminated fish has been, and is, of particular interest and concern to public health officials. Because these populations, by definition, eat a large amount of fish, they often have the largest predicted excess lifetime cancer risk.

Moreover, there is an issue of "environmental justice" present in the risk of contamination faced by fish-dependent communities. Many of these subsistence fishing communities are relatively poor and disadvantaged, and some represent racial minorities such as Native Americans (Tyson 1992; Johnson 1992). Circumstances leading these populations to expose their families to carcinogenic contaminants, even if the net effect of the fish is still beneficial, may offend notions of fairness and may suggest the possibility of racial bias in the distribution of controllable environmental hazards.

Placing an advisory on waters that provide such communities with their source of fish may lead them to reduce the amount of fish in their diet. But as this analysis has shown, the likely result of such a change in their diet is probably to harm their overall health rather than to improve it. Interestingly, if the assumptions of this analysis are correct and the countervailing risks have been estimated accurately, then all other things equal, subsistence fishing populations eating "contaminated" fish are likely to have a lower risk of overall mortality (from cancer and CHD combined) than does a member of the general population who eats "clean" fish, but a lot less of it. Consequently, it may be that in exactly those instances where cancer risks appear to be the greatest, advisories should be implemented only after careful consideration of all risks combined.

To avoid misleading by omission, fish advisories could be continued but expanded to present audiences with the full set of consequences from eating or not eating fish, including both CHD and cancer risks. With more complete information about the countervailing risks of eating and not eating fish, families could then make their own decisions about how to resolve the risk tradeoff. In addition, measures such as reducing pollution discharges into the waterway could be (and are being) undertaken.

Conclusion

The suggestion that a public health measure might cause countervailing risk(s) should not paralyze decisionmakers. A risk tradeoff analysis, even a simple one based on "back-of-the-envelope" calculations, can provide insight into whether the countervailing risk is important enough to consider carefully. Although the cancer risk from eating contaminated fish may be plausible grounds for encouraging careful choice among fish types or pollution prevention, the RTA performed in this chapter indicates that it is not a large enough risk to discourage fish consumption generally.

Nor should decisionmakers shy away from RTA because of the need to consider subjective value judgments when comparing risks. Value judgments are sometimes crucial, and quantified RTA is designed to support, not displace, subjective factors in decisionmaking. Quantification of the objective elements of different risks (such as the mortality risks from CHD and cancer) can help clarify how substantial the subjective differences would need to be to change the decision. Some target and countervailing risks are so divergent in objective magnitude that subjective differences in outcome assessment are not likely to make an appreciable difference in choice. Thus, even if dying of cancer is felt to be more onerous than dying of CHD, it can still make good sense to replace meat with even somewhat contaminated fish in one's diet because the *net* reduction in mortality risk is so substantial. But for those for whom a given risk of cancer feels much worse than an equal risk of CHD, risk tradeoff analysis illuminates how much worse cancer must seem for those individuals to choose not to eat more fish.

7

Seeking Safe Drinking Water

SUSAN W. PUTNAM
JONATHAN BAERT WIENER

Americans have grown to expect a safe drinking water supply, but achieving safety is not simple. Aquatic pathogens, toxic chemicals, heavy metals, pesticides: the threats to our drinking water are myriad. As the list of chemical and biological risks expands, so do public concerns.

One of the most vexing issues in the effort to provide a safe water supply is that of risk tradeoffs. Efforts to reduce one risk in drinking water may introduce—either intentionally or unintentionally—a different risk to the population using the water supply. A primary example of this type of risk tradeoff involves the chlorination of drinking water. People have come to fear that chlorine in their drinking water may cause cancer. But chemical disinfectants like chlorine are used to combat serious waterborne microbial diseases. If we stopped adding these chemicals to drinking water in an effort to reduce the risk of long-term cancer, would we thereby increase the risk of waterborne microbial disease? Would we just trade one form of risk for another? This dilemma is at the core of modern drinking water policy (Craun 1993; EPA 1994a, 1994b).

The quandary of chlorination in drinking water is largely an issue of risk substitution. In general, the target population remains the same: everyone must drink water to survive. The disease outcomes posed by the target and countervailing risks, however, are very different. The concern about chemical disinfectants such as chlorine focuses on their chronic effects, most notably cancer. The health effects from waterborne pathogens, by contrast, involve acute diarrheal and gastrointestinal disease. (Because carcinogens and microbial disease may affect different sensitive subpopulations—in particular, waterborne disease can be especially devastating to the elderly and those with immune system deficiencies such as AIDS—issues of risk transfer and transformation are also present here.) Whereas cancer is now one of the major causes of death in the United States (accounting for about one of every four deaths each year), acute microbial diseases used to be among the primary killers in this country (causing one in every five deaths in 1900) but have since been largely controlled (CDC 1991). Still, microbial diseases remain the cause of millions of deaths worldwide, especially in poorer countries where clean water systems have not been constructed (World Bank 1992), and are again increasing in the United States in part because of AIDS. The incidence of acute disease from waterborne microbes is well documented; the relationship between chemical disinfection and cancer is far less certain.

In this chapter we explore the countervailing risks of waterborne microorganisms and the major chemical disinfectants used to control them. We focus on the health effects associated with these risks and examine some of the tradeoffs that must be considered in trying to compare and weigh these risks in the policy arena. Although the scientific data do not often provide certainty, it is essential for policymakers to consider the kinds of tradeoffs involved if they are to make sensible policy decisions for the protection of public health.

The Imperative of Safe Drinking Water

Safe drinking water has long been a key public health and environmental issue. Recognition of the importance of water quality to health dates back to ancient times: Sanskrit writings advocated heating and filtering of water as early as 2000 B.C.

(EPA 1986). Throughout history, water was known to be an essential element for survival and was hailed as the "scarce elixir of life" (Carpenter 1991).

With the advent of germ theory and greater understanding of the role of water in spreading infectious disease in the nineteenth century (NRC 1977), attention increasingly focused on the protection and purification of the drinking water supply. In the nineteenth century health-minded American communities began to separate drinking water, delivered to users from reservoirs and wells, from household and industrial wastes, discharged by users into sewage water systems. (Today many people in developing countries still do not have separate drinking water and sewer systems.) As early as the 1890s, U.S. municipal water companies began to establish filtration systems to remove bacterial microorganisms from the water supply. Chemical disinfection followed in the next decade with the introduction of chlorination technology in water treatment plants (EPA 1986).

The first health standard for drinking water was established in 1914 by the U.S. Public Health Service to protect against acute bacterial diseases. Standards have since been added to include water source protection as well as regulation of radioactivity and a host of chemicals (Walker 1989). With the congressional enactment of the Safe Drinking Water Act in 1974, "drinkable" water joined "fishable and swimmable" water—the latter delineated by the Clean Water Act of 1972—on the national agenda. The goal of the drinking water legislation was to protect the nation's groundwater system from contamination by organic and inorganic chemicals, radionuclides, and microorganisms. The Act was amended in 1986 to reinforce the federal government's commitment to protecting the water supply from toxic contaminants both in the distribution system and at the source.

Despite the scientific and technological advances made in water treatment processes over the last century, concern persists about drinking water contamination. Few areas of the country are without some form of current water quality problems or apprehension about safe sources for the future. Potentially toxic substances are continually being detected in both surface and groundwater supplies, in residential water pipes, and in agricultural runoff, underground storage and septic tank leakage, and toxic waste site leachate. Most recent concern has focused on toxic substances such as lead and chlorine. But microbes have not vanished: in 1993, a protozoan called cryptosporidium infiltrated public water systems, causing 400,000 cases of diarrhea and numerous deaths in Milwaukee. Residents of Washington, D.C. were forced to boil all their water for several days (EPA 1994b; Terry 1993).

Today Americans consume over three and a half billion gallons of treated water every day. There are nearly 250,000 public water supply systems in the United States, serving everything from the smallest towns to major metropolitan centers (AWWA 1984). Ninety percent of the population receives its water through these community water systems, with the rest using private wells or other individual sources. The Environmental Protection Agency (EPA) ranks drinking water pollution as one of the top four environmental threats to health (Carpenter 1991). At the state level, drinking water contamination ranked first among twenty-seven environmental health concerns of state public health officials in 1987 (Galbraith 1989), and the issue has also been included on the platforms of several recent major gubernatorial campaigns (Carpenter 1991). Internationally, where over a billion people lack clean drinking water and almost two billion lack sewage systems, waterborne microbial disease presents perhaps the world's single largest environmental health risk, afflicting more than a billion people and killing millions each year (World Bank 1992).

Worried by reports of chemical and biological hazards in the water supply, consumers are increasingly lured to the promise of "pure spring" water for their drinking water needs. Much of the tremendous growth in the bottled water and home filtration industries over the last two decades may be due to consumer anxiety about possible contaminants in the water supply.

The Risks of Chlorination

Chlorine is an element widely used in modern chemistry because it readily reacts with so many substances. The vast majority of public water systems in this country use chlorine to disinfect their drinking water. But the widespread application of chlorine as a drinking water disinfecting agent has raised concerns about the risk of human exposure to chlorine and its by-products. Past experience with chlorine-based compounds such as DDT, PCBs, and CFCs, which were later found to pose risks to health and the environment, have encouraged some environmental groups to call for a total ban on all uses of chlorine, rather than waiting to study each use of chlorine and its potential alternatives (Amato 1993).

Chlorine is toxic not just to microbes but to humans as well. Chlorine gas escaping at the treatment plant can cause acute health effects in workers, since the chemical is highly irritant to the eyes, nasal passages, and respiratory system. Inhalation of the gas can prove fatal at concentrations as low as 0.1% by volume (1,000 ppm) (AWWA 1984). At the minute amounts used in drinking water, however, the acute toxicity of chlorine is quite low. It is rather the potential long-term risk of cancer from chronic exposure to moderate amounts of chlorine that is the major concern with the chemical in the drinking water supply. Much of the cancer risk from chlorine stems from the class of complex chloroorganic compounds, known as trihalomethanes (THMs), that are formed as one of the major by-products of the chlorination process. Trihalomethanes are formed when chlorine is added to water containing organic materials, such as the humic and fulvic acids emitted from decomposing plant and animal materials in the water supply (Rook 1974; Bellar et al. 1974). Although THMs occur with chlorination of both surface and ground waters, their concentration is much greater with surface water because of its higher levels of naturally occurring organic materials.

Of particular concern among the THMs is chloroform, the most prevalent and thoroughly studied member of the THM group. Ingestion of chloroform has been associated with an increased incidence of cancerous tumors in multiple laboratory animal bioassays. These tumors occurred at several sites, most notably in the kidney and liver, as well as across several different species and strains of animals (National Cancer Institute 1976; Roe et al. 1979) (see Table 7.1). Although many of the animal studies focused on chloroform administered in corn oil or toothpaste, others also found increased evidence of tumors when the chloroform was administered in drinking water (Jorgenson et al. 1985).

Table 7.1   Summary of animal bioassay data for chloroform

Author	Animal	Route of Exposure	Dose[a]	Results[b]
NCI 1976	Osborne-Mendal rats	Oral-gavage, corn oil	M: 0/90/180 mg/kg/day F: 0/100/200 mg/kg/day	Stat. sig. increase in male kidney tumors
NCI 1976	B6C3F1 mice	Oral-gavage, corn oil	M: 0/138/277 mg/kg/day F: 0/238/477 mg/kg/day	Stat. sig. increase in male and female liver tumors
Palmer et al. 1979	Sprague-Dawley rats	Oral-gavage, toothpaste	15/60/75/165 mg/kg/day	No. stat. sig. increase in tumors
Roe et al. 1979	Multiple strains of mice	Oral-gavage, toothpaste, arachis oil	0/60 mg/kg/day	Stat. sig. increase in male kidney tumors
Heywood et al. 1978	Beagle dogs	Oral-capsules, toothpaste	0/15/30 mg/kg/day	No stat. sig. increase in tumors
Jorgenson et al. 1985	Male Osborne-Mendal rats	Oral, drinking water	0/19/38/81/160 mg/kg/day	Stat. sig. increase in male kidney tumors
Jorgenson et al. 1985	Female B6C3F1 mice	Oral, drinking water	0/34/65/130/263 mg/kg/day	No stat. sig. increase in tumors

Source: U.S. Environmental Protection Agency. 1985. *Health Assessment Document for Chloroform.* Washington, D.C.

a. Dose level(s) in milligrams of dose per kilogram of body weight per day (mg/kg/day). M and F denote sex of test animal.

b. "Stat. sig." = statistically significant.

Using the mouse liver tumor data (NCI 1976), the EPA originally estimated an upper-bound cancer risk—that is, a worst-case analysis—that indicated that the lifetime risk from exposure to chloroform could reach as high as one cancer per 2,500 members of the population exposed (EPA 1977). On the basis of this analysis, the agency began to regulate chloroform and other THMs in 1979, setting a "maximum contaminant level" of 0.10 milligrams per liter (or 100 parts per billion) for total trihalomethanes in the drinking water supply. The incremental lifetime cancer risk from ingesting chloroform in household water at this level has been estimated to be about two in 100,000 (Maxwell et al. 1991). In other words, if 200 million people drank household water at EPA's maximum chloroform level for their entire lives, about 4,000 would die of chloroform-induced cancer.

Chloroform is not the only by-product formed in the chlorination process that has been subjected to animal toxicity testing. Other major trihalomethanes, as well as trichloroacetic acid, dichloroacetic acid, various haloacetonitriles, and chlorophenols have been reported to show carcinogenicity, mutagenicity, or other toxic properties (Cotruvo and Regelski 1989; Simmon and Tardiff 1978; Herren-Freund et al. 1987; Bull 1982). For other by-products, however, such as various chlorinated acids, alcohols, aldehydes, and ketones, there is limited information on their potential toxic effects (Cotruvo and Regelski 1989). There is also a plethora of nonvolatile by-products formed in the chlorination process for which there are limited data on toxicity and other effects (NAS 1987). Identifying and testing these substances has been a relatively slow process, and much work is continuing in this area (Bull 1982).

In humans, chlorinated water has been associated with an increased risk of bladder, colon, and rectal cancer in multiple epidemiological studies (Crump and Guess 1982; Williamson 1981). These studies, in general, have found the risks of bladder, colon, and rectal cancer associated with drinking chlorinated water to be about 1.1 to 2.0 times higher than the risk for drinking the same quantity of unchlorinated water (Crump and Guess 1982). The aggregate cancer risk from drinking chlorinated water over a lifetime, however, remains modest.

One of the studies finding a significant positive association, the large case-control work by Cantor and colleagues (1987), suggests that lifetime consumption of chlorinated water increases the risk of bladder cancer by a factor of about two. The study compared those residing for more than forty years in communities where drinking water was chlorinated with those who drink unchlorinated water. This association may result in about 1,000 to 3,000 excess bladder cancers per year in the United States and could explain as much as 25 to 30 percent of the occurrence of bladder cancer in adults residing in chlorinated communities (Cantor et al. 1987).

As with many epidemiological studies, however, there are numerous problems with the studies of chlorinated water. Multiple uncontrolled confounding factors (for example, smoking, diet, occupation, lifestyle) could also explain part or all of the observed cancer rates. Inexactness in measuring the chlorine level, water consumption, population migration, and other variables detracts from the definitiveness of the estimated association. Also, because much of the nation's water is chlorinated, the number of individuals who can serve as study controls—those who drink unchlorinated water—is limited. Taken together, however, these studies have been interpreted as suggesting a significant association of bladder, colon, and rectal cancer with chlorinated drinking water (EPA 1985). This risk is highest in drinking water contaminated with organic material, but, given the myriad by-products formed in the chlorination process, any of a number of substances or combination of substances could be involved.

Additional health effects from chlorine have also been revealed in human studies. Of particular interest is a suggested relationship between consumption of chlorinated water and an increase in the total serum cholesterol levels of populations suffering from a diet deficient in calcium. While the increase in cholesterol levels was found to be small, it suggests that consumption of chlorinated water could be a possible risk factor for cardiovascular disease as well as for cancer (Wones et al. 1989; Zeighami et al. 1990).

Ingestion is not the only route of exposure to these substances in drinking water. There may also be adverse effects from inhalation or dermal exposure during showering, bathing, or swimming. It has been postulated, for example, that exposure to volatile chemicals in drinking water through inhalation may be as large or even larger than exposure from ingestion alone (Maxwell et al. 1991; McKone 1987).

As with most suspected carcinogens, the adverse health effects associated with chlorine by-products are largely chronic, cumulative, and may involve a long latency period before they appear. The health risks are estimated assuming a constant exposure of many years or often many decades. It may also be several decades before any adverse effects, such as excess cases of cancer, become apparent.

The Risk of Not Chlorinating: Microbial Disease

> Our drinking water is living. It is composed of one third green fine moss, one third polliwogs, and one third embryo mosquitoes. (George W. B. Evans, quoted in Carpenter 1991)

When this account was written one hundred and fifty years ago, much of the nation's water supply was teeming with various forms of aquatic organisms. Waterborne diseases, led by cholera, typhoid, and dysentery, were a top health problem in this country in 1900 (CDC 1991). They remain leading concerns abroad; the World Bank (1992) rated drinking water atop its list of preventable environmental hazards worldwide. For example, since 1991 the largest cholera epidemic in recent history has infected over 800,000 people from Peru to Mexico (Brooke 1991; Glass et al. 1992; Food Chemical News 1993).

With the introduction of filtration and disinfection systems during the last century, the risk of disease from drinking water in wealthier countries has been substantially reduced. Despite the enormous progress that has been made, however, there are still significant numbers of disease cases resulting from contaminated drinking water in the United States. Health risks from aquatic pathogens range from mild gastrointestinal distress to systemic disease and, in severe cases, death (Fowle and Kopfler 1986).

From 1971 to 1988, there were nearly 137,000 cases of waterborne disease—or an average of 7,600 cases per year—reported in this country (Levine and Craun 1990). It is suspected that there were numerous undocumented cases as well, because many cases of gastrointestinal illness are not recognized as part of a pattern of waterborne disease. It has been estimated that only half of waterborne disease outbreaks in community water systems and about one-third of those in non-community systems are detected, investigated, and reported (Craun 1986). Microbes in tap water may be responsible for as much as one in three cases of gastrointestinal illness in the United States (Carpenter 1991). Rates of waterborne illness as high as 900,000 cases and 900 deaths per year have been estimated by the Natural Resources Defense Council (Lee 1993).

Waterborne microorganisms encompass a broad range of pathogens, including coliform and heterotrophic bacteria, viruses, and protozoa. These organisms range in size over nearly three orders of magnitude, from extremely small viruses to relatively large protozoan cysts. They also vary greatly in the nature of their surface, living, and replication characteristics (Hoff and Akin 1986). These pathogenic microorganisms are naturally ubiquitous in lakes, streams, reservoirs, and most surface water sources. Groundwater supplies are also a subject of increasing concern, because enteric viruses and other organisms can leach into the groundwater system from the land application or burial of sewage sludge and other treatment wastes (Gerba and Haas 1988).

Although the "traditional" bacterial diseases of cholera and typhoid have largely been brought under control in this country, other microorganisms are constantly being identified and connected to waterborne illness. For example, the *Legionella hemophile* bacteria—the cause of legionnaires' disease—has recently been found in community water supplies (Stout et al. 1992), while tiny waterborne rotaviruses have been shown to be a major cause of acute gastroenteritis in infants and young children (Craun 1986).

The microbial agent most commonly identified and implicated in outbreaks of waterborne disease in recent years is the protozoan cyst *Giardia lamblia* (Levine and Craun 1990). Found in water as a result of deposition of fecal material from both humans and animals, *Giardia* is the most common pathogenic parasite in the United States. Surveys of various water supplies, for example, indicate that 26 to 43 percent of surface water is contaminated with *Giardia* cysts ranging in concentrations from 0.3 to 100 cysts per one hundred liters. *Giardia* strains are known to cause infection even at low doses, and outbreaks of disease have been associated with *Giardia* levels of 0.6 to 21 cysts per 100 liters (Rose, Haas, and Regli 1991).

The health risks associated with these types of microorganisms have been well established. The primary risks involve intestinal and gastroenteric diseases, such as diarrheal infections and dysentery. *Giardia*, for example, causes symptoms that are flu-like in appearance but are usually more severe, such as diarrhea, nausea, and dehydration that can last for months in some cases. The bacteria *Legionella* invokes severe pneumonia-like symptoms, especially in a less resilient population such as the elderly. Other health risks are present as well, such as hepatitis A or poliomyelitis from waterborne viral infections. In most instances, the adverse effects are acute, immediate, and readily apparent. Table 7.2 provides a summary of the diseases caused by waterborne microorganisms.

While many cases of waterborne disease are short-term and relatively minor, some are fatal and others drag on for months and can be chronically debilitating. The effects are particularly serious for the more vulnerable groups of the population, such as the very young, the very old, and those already weakened from other health problems. People with suppressed immune systems, such as those undergoing therapy for cancer or AIDS, for example, can be burdened with waterborne illnesses for many months, with often devastating fluid loss.

The infectious dose for waterborne microorganisms varies tremendously (see Table 7.3). The risk of infection for some of the viruses and protozoa is estimated to be 10 to 1000 times greater than for the bacterial organisms at a similar level of exposure (Rose and Gerba 1991). In general, viral and protozoan pathogens, such as *Giardia*, appear to be highly potent, with small numbers of the organism being capable of causing infection and disease in susceptible human hosts (Gerba and Haas 1988). Moreover, many of the protozoa and viral agents are more resistant to disinfection than pathogenic bacteria,

Table 7.2 Waterborne diseases

Waterborne disease	Causative organism	Source of organism in water	Symptom
Gastroenteritis	*Salmonella* (bacteria)	Animal or human feces	Acute diarrhea and vomiting
Typhoid	*Salmonella typhosa* (bacteria)	Human feces	Inflamed intestine, enlarged spleen, high temperature; can be fatal
Dysentery	*Shigella* (bateria)	Human feces	Diarrhea; rarely fatal
Cholera	*Vibrio cholerae* (bacteria)	Human feces	Vomiting, severe diarrhea, rapid dehydration, mineral loss; often fatal
Infectious hepatitis	Virus	Human feces, shellfish grown in polluted waters	Yellowed skin, enlarged liver, abdominal pain; lasts up to 4 months, seldom fatal
Amebic dysentery	*Entamoeba histolytica* (protozoa)	Human feces	Mild diarrhea, chronic dysentery
Giardiasis	*Giardia lamblia* (protozoa)	Animal or human feces	Diarrhea, cramps, nausea and general weakness; lasts 1 week to 30 weeks, not fatal

Source: Reprinted by permission from *Introduction to Water Treatment: Principles and Practices of Water Supply Operations,* vol. 2, p. 284. Copyright © 1984, American Water Works Association.

requiring larger quantities of chlorine and other disinfecting agents to successfully reduce their numbers in the water supply (Hoff and Akin 1986).

In addition to primary infection from direct ingestion of water laden with microbial contaminants, there is also the inherent risk with these pathogens of secondary or tertiary infection. Disease may be spread by person-to-person contact from infected individuals or by contamination of other materials, such as food, which can then expose previously noninfected members of the population.

Reducing Microbial Risk through Chlorine Disinfection

Chemical disinfecting agents, most commonly chlorine, have been used successfully to combat waterborne microorganisms since the early 1900s. The chlorination process proved so effective and easy to administer that by 1914 most of the drinking water supplied to cities in the United States was chlorinated in some manner (Fowle and Kopfler 1986).

Table 7.3 Probability of infection from waterborne microorganisms

Microorganism	Probability of infection from exposure to 1 organism	Number of organisms for 1% likelihood of infection
Salmonella (bacteria)	2.3×10^{-3}	4.3
Salmonella typhi (bacteria)	3.8×10^{-5}	263
Shigella (bacteria)	1.0×10^{-3}	10
Vibrio cholerae classical (bacteria)	7.0×10^{-6}	1428
Poliovirus 1 (virus)	1.5×10^{-2}	0.67
Entamoeba histolytica (protozoa)	2.8×10^{-1}	0.04
Giardia lamblia (protozoa)	2.0×10^{-2}	0.5

Source: Adapted from Joan B. Rose and Charles P. Gerba. 1991. "Use of Risk Assessment for Development of Microbial Standards." *Water Science Technology,* vol. 24, p. 31.

Chlorine is the most widely used disinfectant in the nation, with over half a million tons used annually by the water treatment industry (Manwaring 1985). It has become the predominant disinfecting agent for all types of potable water treatment operations in locations ranging from small rural communities to major municipal centers.

The addition of chlorine to the water supply is economical, convenient, and effective in virtually eliminating the transmission of bacterial and viral diseases from drinking water. Not only is it successful in destroying pathogenic microorganisms during the treatment process—the primary reason for using a disinfectant—but because it persists in the water distribution system, chlorine helps to prevent the regrowth of nuisance microorganisms (EPA 1981). It also is effective at reducing noxious odors and tastes in the water supply. The addition of chlorine has markedly expanded the drinkability of the nation's water resources by permitting the use of water not considered pristine and protected (Calabrese and Gilbert 1989).

The water treatment process involves a series of different steps. Some of the major steps include flocculation and coagulation (the joining of small particles of matter in the water into larger ones that can more readily be removed), sedimentation (the settling of suspended particles in the water to the bottom of basins from which they can be removed), and filtration (the filtering or straining of the water through various types of materials to remove much of the remaining suspended particles), as well as chemical disinfection. Chlorination is usually performed at several stages of the treatment process. Prechlorination may be performed in the initial stages to combat the algae and other aquatic life that may interfere with the treatment equipment and later steps. The major chlorination stage, however, occurs as the final treatment step after the completion of the other major processes, where the concentration and residual content of the chlorine can be closely monitored (AWWA 1984). In this postchlorination phase, the chemical is more effective in the filtered water, and less contact time is required for the chemical to disinfect the water supply (Clark et al. 1984–85).

Chlorination can deactivate microorganisms by a variety of mechanisms, such as damage to cell membranes, inhibition of specific enzymes, destruction of nucleic acids, and other lethal effects to vital functions (Hoff and Akin 1986). The effectiveness of the chlorination process depends upon a variety of factors, however, including chlorine concentration and contact time, water temperature, pH value, and level of turbidity (AWWA 1984). Disinfectant concentrations and contact times used by different water utilities vary widely, usually depending on the characteristics of the water being treated. Several states and advisory groups suggest minimum requirements or recommendations for these parameters, but there are no federal standards for them (Hoff and Akin 1986).

Alternatives to Chlorination?

The potential adverse health effects associated with the use of chlorine, the regulation of trihalomethanes (THMs) by the EPA, and the recent crusade to end chlorine uses (Amato 1993) have encouraged the water treatment industry to reexamine the disinfection process. The use of disinfectants other than chlorine is currently being explored to find ways of controlling pathogens in drinking water without forming halogenated by-products. Several alternative disinfectants are increasingly coming into use; three of the most common are chloramines, chlorine dioxide, and ozone. While other alternatives to chlorine are under focus as well, these three have received the greatest attention because they are effective, relatively inexpensive, and easy to use (Bull 1982).

One alternative to using straight chlorine in the disinfection process is to combine the chemical with another substance, such as ammonia. The mixing of ammonia with chlorine to form chloramines not only retards THM formation, but it also slows the reaction of chlorine with soluble organics and other compounds in the water supply (Moore et al. 1980). Chloramines have the advantage of being easy to generate and feed into the existing technology used for chlorination. They also produce a disinfectant residual that persists throughout the distribution system, preventing regrowth of microbes. In addition, they help to reduce unpleasant odors and tastes apparent with chlorine disinfection. The disadvantage of this alternative, however, is that chloramines are a weaker microbicide than chlorine, and their biocidal action becomes even weaker in water with high pH levels (EPA 1981). They must be used at higher concentrations and for longer periods of contact to achieve sufficient disinfection. Because of this, chloramines may not always be as successful as chlorine as the primary disinfectant in a treatment system, especially where more resilient viral or parasitic cyst contamination is potentially present (NAS 1987).

In contrast to chloramines, chlorine dioxide is a strong microbicide whose biocidal activity is consistent over the pH range usually occurring in water treatment and thus is useful in most systems. Chlorine dioxide is also easy to generate and feed into existing systems, but care is needed to monitor the chlorine concentration in generated chlorine dioxide. Like chlorination, it also produces a residual disinfectant that can persist throughout the water distribution system (EPA 1981).

Ozone is a powerful but unstable disinfectant, already in use in about 1 percent of U.S. drinking water systems (Amato 1993). It is an excellent microbicide whose biocidal activity is not affected by the pH of the water. Because of its instability, however, ozone does not produce a disinfectant residual to remain in the system after the water leaves the treatment plant, and there is thus a danger of biological regrowth as the water passes through the distribution system (Cotruvo and Regelski 1989). Moreover, the equipment that is required to generate ozone on-site is more elaborate and expensive than the technology required for either chlorine or the other two alternatives (EPA 1981; Amato 1993). The manufacturing of ozone requires a great deal of energy; rising energy costs make ozonation more expensive to use relative to the other alternatives, and high energy intensity potentially increases air and water pollution at the energy generating stations. In addition, because the ozone residual does not persist, the plant operator has no simple way to determine whether enough ozone has been added to the treatment process to destroy all the pathogens in the water (AWWA 1984).

The primary advantage to the use of chloramines, chlorine dioxide, or ozone as alternative disinfectants is that the THM concentration in drinking water is substantially reduced when these alternatives are used in place of chlorination. However, there are limited toxicological data on these chlorine alternatives. Currently there is no evidence to suggest that alternative disinfectants are any less (or more) toxic than chlorine (Bull 1982).

Although they do not produce THMs, the alternatives to chlorine do form their own organic by-products. Chlorine dioxide, for example, spawns the products chlorate and chlorite, which have been shown to cause consistent hematological (blood) effects—such as decreased red blood cell counts and glutathione levels—in multiple laboratory animals (Abdel-Rahman, Couri, and Bull; Bull 1982). In addition to similar hematological effects in rats (Abdel-Rahman, Suh, and Bull 1984), chloramines may also pose a danger for hemolytic anemia in kidney dialysis patients where the dialysate water was treated with chloramines (Kjellstrand et al. 1974; Moore and Calabrese 1980). Monochloramine has also been shown to be a weak mutagen (Moore and Calabrese 1980; Shih and Lederberg 1976). At present, little is known about the types of by-products produced by ozonation of natural organics (NAS 1987).

In general, then, less is known about the possible by-products formed by the alternative disinfectants and about their toxicological implications than is known about chloroform and the other chlorine by-products. Even though these alternatives are increasingly being used in disinfection processes, attention is only beginning to focus on their toxicology and possible health effects.

Moreover, as long as substantial quantities of background organic material are present in the source water, all chemical disinfecting agents will produce some type of by-product which, in all likelihood, will include certain chemicals that will be found to affect human biological activity (Bull 1982). Disinfectants are effective precisely because of their ability to kill or deactivate microbes and their ability to disrupt biological material (Fowle and Kopfler 1986). By their nature, they are reactive molecules capable of altering the chemical structure of organic substances present in the water supply (EPA 1981). The question then becomes whether their intended deadly effects on smaller life forms pose an unacceptable risk tradeoff for human health.

Weighing Risk vs. Risk

How do we compare the health risks of microbial disease and chemical disinfectants? The risks of microbial and chemical hazards differ substantially with respect to their outcomes, severity, certainty, timing, and distribution among population groups.

The adverse health effects of microbial disease are uncomfortable, debilitating, and potentially fatal. The diarrheal and other disabilities can last for only a few days, or they can drag on for many months. The effects occur promptly after exposure, often in a population already in a vulnerable state due to age (children and the elderly) or disability. For the most part in the United States, however, the disease effects are nonfatal and usually reversible. The issue is primarily one of morbidity, not mortality. (This is not true in developing countries, where diarrhea and dehydration due to poor water quality kill millions of children each year.) For example, mortality rates from enterovirus infections have been reported to range from less than 0.1 percent to 1.8 percent (Assaad and Borecka 1977). Since this may only reflect hospitalized cases, the actual mortality rate for all cases may be even lower.

Chlorine risks, on the other hand, present a very different picture. Disease occurs only after long-term, cumulative exposure of often many decades. The affected population is usually middle-aged or older; rarely are children afflicted with the types of cancer thought to be associated with chlorinated water. Here, as with most suspected carcinogens, the endpoints of interest include mortality as well as morbidity.

Microbial risks can be estimated and foreseen with a high

degree of certainty. Waterborne microbes can be isolated, identified, and studied to assess their risk level, and specific effects in humans can be shown to be caused by specific organisms. There is a wealth of historical data indicating the types of diseases that result from consumption of pathogen-infested water supplies. Although the dose-response relationship is not clearly defined for microbial disease, it is suspected that even a modest number of microorganisms can infect much of the population—particularly the most vulnerable groups—that drinks from the contaminated water supply. With the high prevalence of pathogens naturally occurring in water sources, the likelihood of disease resulting from untreated (or poorly treated) drinking water is high.

The certainty of cancer predictions from exposure to chlorinated drinking water, on the other hand, is much lower. With chlorine, as with many chemicals, it is more difficult to isolate the health effects and to prove a causal relationship between the chemical and human cancer. The data are far from conclusive. Risk assessments of chlorine's carcinogenic potential necessitate multiple extrapolations from animal bioassays (from high-dose experimental exposure to low-dose actual exposure, and across species from laboratory animals to humans) and various assumptions and choices made in the mathematical modeling processes. Similarly, the epidemiological data on human exposure are plagued by multiple confounding sources of cancer (such as smoking or diet), as well as by imprecise measurements of chlorine and chloroform levels, water consumption, and other elements. There are no dose-response data for humans, and the actual number of excess cancers seen in the studies is small. In addition, the data on other exposures to chlorine in drinking water, such as from swimming, showering, or washing fruits and vegetables, are very limited.

The issue remains how to weigh sensibly the target and countervailing risks. It is difficult to compare sudden, predictable episodes of diarrhea among children to latent, uncertain cases of cancer among adults. It is hard to balance an almost certain level of morbidity (and an uncertain level of mortality) in the present against a highly uncertain chance of cancer morbidity and mortality several decades in the future. Disease at hand demands action, but there is also strong support for protecting against future adverse outcomes; and the particular risk of cancer may provoke special public anxiety.

The challenge of trying to manage and reduce these diverse risks is further complicated by difficult economic, ethical, and attitudinal issues. For example, some say that a risk may be more acceptable to the public if it is naturally occurring (waterborne microorganisms) rather than technologically imposed (chemical disinfectants). But an immediate and present risk—the effects of which are readily apparent, unpleasant, and clearly consume resources in the form of medical treatment, work days lost, and so forth—may be less acceptable than the nebulous possibility of risk transpiring many decades down the road. The immediacy of disease raises the call for action—witness the recent clamor over microbial infections from fast-food hamburgers. Another factor is that some types of risk appear to be particularly dreaded, regardless of what the data show about likelihood and mortality rates (Slovic 1987). Many people in this country, for example, appear to have a deep-seated fear of cancer. Any time that the term "cancer" is even vaguely associated with a risk, no matter how uncertain the data may be, some people will demand that all possible steps be taken to eliminate that risk. The cancer risk associated with chlorine and its by-products triggers a demand from certain sectors of the population for removal of the chemical from public water supplies, even though such removal would increase the risk of immediate microbial disease.

An additional critical element in weighing these risks is the issue of who suffers each risk. Although risks in drinking water are borne by the same population in general—everyone must consume water to survive (though some can afford to purchase bottled water)—there is a difference in the subpopulations most vulnerable to each risk. Microbial disease would be injurious to many people, but especially to children, the frail elderly, and those with immune system deficiencies such as AIDS. The fatalities in the Milwaukee cryptosporidium outbreak in 1993 were concentrated among people with AIDS. Cancer from THMs, by contrast, is principally a threat to middle-aged adults who have consumed chlorinated water over many decades. As our society ages, cancers later in life may be of greater concern to a growing share of the electorate.

Similarly, the burden of risk alleviation may not be shared equally by different subgroups of the population. Were restrictions to be placed on the amount of chlorine that could be added to water supplies, lower-income and smaller communities and households, with more limited resources, would be less able to expend the necessary funds to switch to an alternative disinfection system or to purchase bottled water. These communities and households could be forced to lower the chlorine level to comply with the regulations without adequate protection against microbial disease. In addition, the solutions for the water systems of large communities may not be easily transferable to small systems. Given a choice, some communities might prefer to accept the long-term risk of chlorination rather than face the immediate risk of waterborne disease; others might decide differently.

Even in communities that could implement new alternatives to chlorine, the economic burden would not be easy to bear. Meeting federal requirements from the Safe Drinking Water Act and its amendments has been estimated to cost the nation's water suppliers more than $14 billion per year (Carpenter 1991), which is ultimately passed on to the consumer or taxpayer. Converting the nation from chlorination to ozonation might add another $6 billion per year (Amato 1993). Historically, Americans have enjoyed cheaper water than in many other countries, but many families will find their water bills rising as alternatives are sought to the present treatment technology. Water is not a commodity that consumers can do without, so a rise in price would most likely cause hardship for some American families. And increased regulations and restrictions placed on chlorination systems may induce the outlays of additional funds for drinking water that would otherwise have been spent for other public health activities or household purchases.

These dilemmas are not trivial in poorer communities. The devastating epidemic of cholera that began in Peru in 1991, for example, appears to have been unleashed (once cholera arrived in South America on ships from Asia) by a Peruvian government decision to stop chlorinating the urban water supply in response to fear of cancers from chlorination (Anderson 1991; Dowd 1994, p. 98). But in the absence of an affordable alternative disinfectant, the result was a dramatic increase in the risk of microbial infection. In short order more than 1,000 people died of cholera, and 150,000 were afflicted in Peru alone (Brooke 1991; ILSI 1991; *Nature* 1991). The epidemic then spread up the coast to Mexico; by 1993 it had killed more than 7,000 and afflicted over 800,000 people (Anderson 1991; Glass et al. 1992; Food Chemical News 1993).

Managing the Risks

Caught between the risks of cancer and microbial disease, the federal EPA has begun negotiated rulemakings, involving industry as well as community leaders, aimed at managing the risks of disinfection without undermining the control of microbial disease (EPA 1994a, 1994b). Many communities are beginning to search for "risk-superior" options for obtaining clean drinking water. At the technical level, there are currently various options available to Americans for managing the portfolio of drinking water risks. Chlorination as a disinfecting treatment has long been demonstrated as an effective system for achieving a substantially microbial-free drinking water supply. Many of the cases of waterborne disease that do occur every year can be attributed either to breakdowns or inadequacies in the treatment system or to areas where no disinfection has been implemented (Akin, Hoff, and Lippy 1982; NAS 1987)—though some, such as cryptosporidium, may be unaffected by chlorination (EPA 1994b).

Much of the risk associated with chlorine exposure may occur in extraordinary circumstances, not in routine situations. Most municipal drinking water supplies maintain chlorine levels such that the concentrations of chloroform in the systems range from 0.02 to 0.05 milligrams per liter (Wilson 1980), well below the standard of 0.10 milligrams per liter that the EPA has set as a safe level for ingestion of THMs. Trihalomethane levels can vary, however, particularly with seasonal or water quality changes. This is true especially in the summer months, when microorganisms grow more quickly and greater amounts of chlorine are added to the water supply to combat the increased microbial growth. In Washington, D.C., for example, THM levels can rise to 30 percent over the EPA limit, despite the $35 million water treatment plant that the city recently built (Carpenter 1991).

The concern over trihalomethane levels has spurred increasing use of alternative disinfectants. For example, both the state of Kansas and the Metropolitan Water District of Southern California now use chloramination for the maintenance of a disinfection residual in their distribution systems. Ozone disinfection processes, widely used in Europe, have also been on the increase in the United States. Recent improvements in the reliability and efficiency of ozonation technology, coupled with its high efficacy against resistant protozoan cysts and viruses, have strengthened the desirability of this chlorine alternative (NAS 1987).

New options include modifications to the chlorination process to reduce chlorine by-products. Particular attention has focused on reducing the level of organic precursors in the water to protect against trihalomethane production. Once THMs are formed, they are very difficult to remove, so the goal is to prevent their initial formation. One way to try to accomplish this is to pretreat the source water, with technologies such as granular activated carbon or other absorbants, to remove organic materials before the water enters the disinfection process. Another solution under investigation involves moving the chlorination step to a point in time after much of the organic material has been removed through the other treatment stages (AWWA 1984).

Again, however, these technological alternatives pose their own countervailing risks. For example, prechlorination of low-quality water is important to maintaining the efficacy of the other disinfection stages. This step is essential in removing algae and other growth from the treatment machinery and equipment and ensuring their optimum function and efficiency (White 1978). Without this step, the effectiveness of the disinfection process in preventing microbial diseases may be severely compromised.

Conclusion

Nothing known to science, including the content of drinking water, is one hundred percent "safe." Zero risk is a quixotic goal, whether in poorer societies or in our highly industrialized and chemical-dependent era.

But many people expect perfection—purity—in their drinking water. Not only is water an essential element of life, it is for many people an involuntary risk. Much of the population receives water from large community systems over which it has limited control. Many people believe that the government should be responsible for somehow eliminating all risks of drinking water contamination. The level of risk that society is willing to accept for drinking water may be lower than that for a more voluntary risk such as consuming alcohol or smoking cigarettes.

This case study illustrates the complex problems surrounding two different involuntary risks posed by modern drinking water: chemical versus microbial contamination. Concern over the potential carcinogenicity of chlorine and its by-products has pushed society to explore other disinfection alternatives. But would these options be worse than the process they replace? None of the chemical alternatives has both the biocidal and residual properties of chlorine, nor many of its secondary benefits. Even less is known about the toxicological properties of these alternatives and their by-products than is understood for chlorine. And reducing chlorination without effective alternatives may unleash deadly microbial diseases. Is the fear of cancer from chlorine pushing us to an inferior or even inappropriate solution for a safe drinking water supply? If we tinker with the present disinfection system, there is a distinct possibility that we may lose effectiveness in preventing microbial disease. One has only to look at many less developed countries to see the devastation that uncontrolled waterborne disease can cause—and recall that our country has only escaped these diseases relatively recently. It is not inconceivable that currently largely contained microbial pathogens in this country, such as the microbes that cause childhood diarrhea and cholera, could reappear with vigor if disinfection were not kept up to an adequate level.

It is interesting to observe that one era's target risk (waterborne disease) is now the modern era's countervailing risk, as target attention has shifted to the cancer risks of chlorination. In part this may reflect the perceived elimination of waterborne disease, in part increasing concern about cancer, and in part the aging of our society. But waterborne enteric pathogens are still responsible for much greater levels of illness in this country than are chemicals or other contaminants in drinking water (Gerba and Haas 1988). On the other hand, even a small excess risk of cancer or other adverse health effects from disinfecting agents could eventually account for a significant amount of latent illness (NAS 1987).

Policymakers need to consider and balance all the salient risks, target and non-target, in a coherent and comprehensive fashion. Given the countervailing risks of microbes and chemicals in drinking water, and the technologies available at present, there is no simple solution. The task for decision-makers is to manage the portfolio of risks intelligently and comprehensively. Because people's values and preferences for avoiding different risks and their abilities to afford alternatives to chlorination may vary considerably across communities, the choice of risk management strategies for drinking water may need to be made at the local rather than national level. In any case, we need to weigh all of the risks of drinking water in a thoughtful, sensible manner and search for solutions that reduce overall risk.

8

Recycling Lead

KATHERINE WALKER
JONATHAN BAERT WIENER

The U.S. Environmental Protection Agency (EPA) has come under increasing criticism for its fragmentary approach to managing the waste by-products of industrial activities (Hahn and Males 1990; Males 1989; Haigh and Irwin 1990; Dudek, Stewart, and Wiener 1992; National Commission on the Environment 1993). The agency's own Science Advisory Board has lamented the lack of a comprehensive, multimedia strategy for dealing with pollution (EPA 1990b). Critics charge that the current patchwork of environmental regulations for separate environmental media—air, drinking water, surface waters, and solid and hazardous wastes—fails to provide adequate mechanisms or incentives for managing risk tradeoffs such as the transfer of pollutants between environmental media. Policies intended to reduce, remove, and treat pollution in one medium often result in increased discharge or disposal of pollution into another. For example, sewage treatment plants, designed originally to reduce the threat to backyard water supplies from infectious and other pollutants, now generate sludges which have made their way to ocean dumpsites, landfills, and the air via incinerators. Air pollution rules requiring scrubbers to remove pollutants from smokestacks have generated new pollution in the form of "scrubber blow-down," which must then be disposed of in landfills where it may threaten ground or surface water supplies. Rules intended to reduce the contribution of air pollutants to local air quality problems have encouraged the construction of taller smokestacks, which essentially shift the impact to more distant geographic areas and populations.

The fragmentation in EPA programs and regulations largely reflects the narrow focus of the original statutes passed by Congress to protect the air, surface waters, drinking water, and food supply and to manage hazardous and solid wastes. Each of these media has its own statute—the Clean Air Act, the Clean Water Act (CWA), the Safe Drinking Water Act (SDWA), the Federal Insecticide, Fungicide, and Rodenticide Act (FIFRA), the Comprehensive Environmental Response, Compensation, and Liability Act (CERCLA or "Superfund"), and the Resources Conservation and Recovery Act (RCRA). While some statutes anticipated the potential for cross-media transfers and did not preclude their evaluation, they left the job of dealing with them to the agency (Hahn and Males 1990). But the fragmented statutory structure has spawned a similar fragmentation of responsibilities within EPA, and regulations issued by one EPA office have rarely (until recently) been designed to prevent pollution transfers to the media supervised by other EPA offices. As Table 8.1 indicates, EPA is beginning to analyze the phenomenon of cross-media risk tradeoffs, but in most cases before 1990 this analysis had still not been translated into regulatory provisions or adjustments to deal with the tradeoffs.

Why do these transfers of pollutants matter? At their worst, these transfers have been called a "toxics shell game" (Fortuna 1991) in which pollution is never reduced and no one really knows where the contaminants end up. The countervailing risks induced by cross-media pollutant transfers may in some cases outweigh the benefits of the reduction in risk to the target medium. More generally, the countervailing risk transfers may undermine the overall effectiveness of the regulation in protecting human health and the environment, and could mean that its *net* benefits do not exceed its costs (Dudek, Stewart, and Wiener 1992).

In this chapter we examine an EPA effort to take risk trade-offs seriously when evaluating an important proposed regulation, one that would require the recycling of 95 percent of the

Table 8.1   Evaluation of cross-media transfers in EPA[a] regulations

Regulatory program[b]	Regulatory status	*Federal Register* date	Multi-media analysis?	Evaluation of cross-media transfers?	Designed to mitigate cross-media transfers?
Used oil	proposed	11/29/85	yes	yes	yes[c]
Arsenic NESHAP	final	8/4/86	no	no	yes[d]
Chlorinated solvents	pre-proposal	10/17/85	yes	yes	yes
Superfund cleanups	ongoing	—	yes	sometimes	sometimes
Land disposal restrictions	final	11/7/86	yes	yes	no
Sewage sludge	proposed	2/6/89	yes	yes	no
Effluent guidelines (OCPSF)	final	11/5/87	yes	yes	no
Drinking water standard (8 VOCs)	final	7/8/87	yes	yes	no
Ocean incineration	proposed	2/28/85	yes	no	no
Municipal incinerators	pre-proposal	—	yes	no	no

Source: Adapted from Hahn and Males 1990.

a. Focusing on efforts between 1985 and 1989.

b. NESHAP = national emissions standard for hazardous air pollutants; OCPSF = organic chemicals, plastics, and synthetic fibers; VOCs = volatile organic compounds.

c. Cross-media shifts considered, but only as part of mitigating recycling impacts.

d. Cross-media provision in regulation has no practical effect.

lead acid storage batteries discarded into the municipal waste stream. Lead acid batteries, which are commonly used in automobile engines, account for more than three-quarters of all the lead used in the United States (EPA 1991c). Lead batteries that are not recycled may end up in landfills or may be incinerated by municipal solid waste combustors (MWCs) (EPA 1991c).

Lead (Pb) is an elemental metal found in the ground whose toxicity to humans has been known throughout the history of its extensive use. The Greek physician Hippocrates blamed lead poisoning for severe colic he observed in men engaged in extracting metals from ore (Ottoboni 1991). With scientific progress, the level or dose at which lead has been found to be associated with adverse effects has been steadily lowered. Most recently, the Centers for Disease Control (CDC) tightened its "level of concern" for lead in children's blood from 25 micrograms per deciliter (μg/dl) to 10 μg/dl, and suggested that there may be no safe level (CDC 1991).

In order to remove lead from incinerators that release it to the air and from landfills where it may threaten groundwater supplies, the Environmental Protection Agency's strategy for reducing lead exposures calls for environmentally sound recycling (EPA 1991e). Yet recycling of lead batteries is not risk-free. Secondary lead smelting, a key component of the recycling process, releases lead to ambient and workplace air, resulting in community and worker exposures to lead. The risks associated with these exposures must be weighed against the risks associated with population and worker exposures resulting both from primary lead smelting, necessary if new batteries are produced with new lead to replace discarded lead, and from incineration or landfilling of discarded lead acid batteries. These risks will depend not just on the quantity of lead put through each process, but on the likelihood of exposure and the size and sensitivity of the population exposed. Heightened demand for secondary smelting might increase the exposure of lower-income populations living near secondary smelters in the United States, or of populations in poorer countries where lead smelting processes are governed by fewer environmental or occupational controls.

The case of lead acid batteries provides an opportunity to explore some of the complexities involved in performing risk tradeoff analysis. It is also an unusual example of a situation in which an agency analyzed cross-media risk transfers and reached a different regulatory decision than might have been made if the decision had been based on consideration of the target risk alone: EPA decided *not* to require increased recycling of lead acid batteries, in part for fear of increasing the lead exposure of children living near secondary smelters where the lead recycling would take place.

EPA's Commitment to Recycling Lead

In the late 1980s, the conventional wisdom was that recycling lead acid batteries was obviously a good idea. EPA explained its "common sense" view and "expectation" that reductions in the amount of waste materials would reduce the amount of air emissions (EPA 1989b). The major policy disputes were about how best to accomplish recycling (for example, whether to mandate battery returns, or use a deposit-refund scheme). No one appeared to have contemplated the possibility of a problematic risk tradeoff.

EPA began to search for ways to require increased recycling of lead acid batteries. Although in 1987 the rate of lead recycling was already quite high (85 percent), it was largely driven by the high market price for lead (EPA 1991c). Had the market price for used lead softened, high rates of recycling would not have been maintained throughout the country. Only two-thirds of the states at that time had mandatory lead battery recycling laws. EPA wanted a federal rule to sustain high rates of recycling even if the market for used lead were to weaken.

EPA first tried to include mandatory lead battery recycling as part of new stationary source performance standards for municipal waste combustors (MWCs) under the Clean Air Act (EPA 1989b). In 1989 EPA proposed a mandatory materials separation requirement for MWCs, of which lead batteries were a part. This measure would have required MWC operators to reduce by 25 percent the weight of municipal solid waste incinerated by removing recoverable materials (glass, metals, yard waste, paper, and lead acid batteries) from the waste stream. EPA did not conduct a formal analysis of the cross-media consequences of the proposed Clean Air Act rule.

This proposal became the focal point of a contentious debate between the EPA and the White House Council on Competitiveness, headed at the time by Vice President Dan Quayle. The Council on Competitiveness had been established by President Bush to review major regulatory initiatives for their impact on the U.S. economy and to provide regulatory relief. The Council argued that the materials separation requirement only mandated separation, not actual recycling of the separated materials; since this was a rule proposed under the Clean Air Act, it could not address non-air disposal routes. Simply requiring separation might therefore just encourage landfilling instead of incineration, without increasing recycling. The Council also objected that the proposed rule removed decisionmaking authority from state and local governments, and more generally, that the rule was not supported by an adequate benefit-cost analysis (President's Council on Competitiveness 1990).

After this bureaucratic face-off, EPA dropped the materials separation requirement when issuing its final Clean Air Act rule in 1991 (EPA 1991d). The lead separation requirement, although not a specific target of criticism by the Council on Competitiveness, was dropped as part of this compromise (Barnett 1991).

Despite this defeat, EPA persevered in its "common sense" pursuit of increased recycling of lead acid batteries. A 1991 EPA strategy document identified recycling as the "Best Demonstrated Available Technology" (BDAT) for lead, making it the default or preferred treatment technology for lead wastes under the Resource Conservation and Recovery Act (RCRA). Under RCRA, technologies designated as BDAT did not need to be evaluated further for their public health or environmental impact. For most RCRA wastes, then, the question of whether or not there are other risks associated with the chosen technology has generally not been asked.

The lead acid battery initiative was also revived under a different regulatory authority, the Toxic Substances Control Act

(TSCA). This time, a proposed rulemaking was carried out in a formal Regulatory Negotiation ("reg-neg") in which representatives from the regulated industry, public interest groups, and state and local governments joined with the EPA in a federally chartered advisory committee to negotiate the text of the rule before it was proposed (EPA 1990a; EPA 1991b; EPA n.d.).

EPA's Risk Analysis

EPA's Office of Toxic Substances initiated a formal risk analysis of lead battery recycling as part of the TSCA regulatory negotiation. TSCA, unlike many other environmental statutes, charges EPA to prevent "unreasonable risk" based on a rigorous consideration of risks, costs, and benefits. EPA therefore conducted an extensive risk and economic analysis of increased recycling (EPA 1991a). Though simplistic in some respects and obscure in parts of its reasoning and calculations, this risk analysis was the basis on which EPA made its decisions, and we examine it for that purpose. It represents an unusual case in which the risk tradeoffs of a proposed regulation were explicitly evaluated.

EPA's analysis was limited to the risks associated with a marginal increase in the rate of lead acid battery recycling, from 85 percent to 95 percent. It did not address the question of the risks of lead acid battery recycling in general. In sum, EPA found that increasing the recycling rate from 85 to 95 percent would lead to a net reduction of the total lead emitted to the environment by 62,000 tons per year, but, surprisingly, that this reduction would at best not change the numbers of children with lead levels in their blood exceeding the CDC's 10 μg/dl level of concern and at worst might increase the number of children with such elevated lead levels. This unexpected result derived critically from EPA's analysis of projected changes in the specific routes of lead releases into the environment, and from its estimates of the populations exposed to each of those routes. EPA found that increased recycling would decrease releases of lead to land disposal (little affecting human exposure) and to air from primary smelters (reducing human exposure), but would also increase releases of lead to air from secondary smelters (increasing human exposure).

The Life Cycle of Lead Batteries. The life cycle of lead acid battery manufacture and disposal is illustrated in Figure 8.1. Lead begins its life in geologic deposits of lead ore. Metallic lead is removed from the ore in the primary smelting process and cast into metal grids. In the manufacture of batteries, the

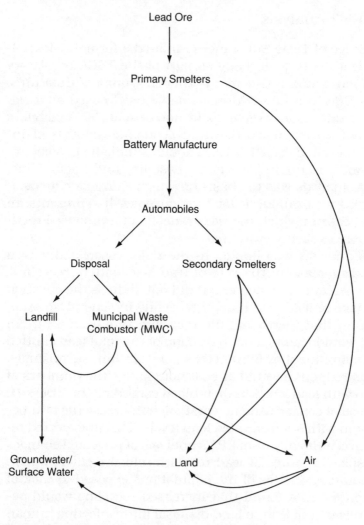

Figure 8.1 Life cycle of lead acid batteries.

metal grids are impregnated with a lead oxide paste and submerged in a sulfuric acid bath. The whole assembly is then enclosed in a plastic or metal box (EPA 1991c).

When the battery is spent, it may be disposed of in a municipal solid waste landfill, or in a municipal solid waste combustor (MWC) where not prohibited by state law (EPA 1991c). (Some batteries are improperly dumped in back yards or vacant lots.) The alternative to disposal is recycling, in which the lead metal/lead oxide grids are removed from the batteries, lead metal is recovered from the lead oxide paste, and lead is remelted in a secondary smelter. Some of the recovered lead is converted to lead oxide, and the rest is recast into metal grids. Since more than 90 percent of the lead from a battery is typically recovered, each recycled battery can essentially be transformed into a new one (EPA 1991c).

Only two primary lead smelters, in Missouri and Montana, refine virtually all the domestically mined lead in the United States. By contrast, as of 1991 approximately fifty secondary lead smelters were in operation in this country, with most located in the eastern United States and the states of California and Texas (EPA 1991a).

Lead may be released to the environment during primary smelting, secondary smelting, incineration in MWCs, or following disposal in landfills (see Figure 8.1). During smelting, lead is both emitted to the air and disposed of in land disposal sites. At MWCs, lead is released to the air in both stack and fugitive ash emissions. These fugitive emissions of ash are uncontrolled releases that typically occur during ash handling and disposal at ash landfills. Most of the lead remaining in incinerator ash ends up in municipal solid waste landfills. From landfills, small quantities of lead can dissolve in the groundwater percolating through the landfill, the leachate, and can migrate into groundwater or surface water supplies.

Routes of Exposure. The degree of risk associated with each of these releases depends on the extent of human or environmental exposure to the lead released. Lead has no known biological uses in the human body, and because it is an element, it cannot be broken down.

"Direct" exposures to lead occur when an individual inhales

lead in the form of the fine particulate released from smelter or incinerator stacks, or drinks water containing lead. "Indirect" exposures occur when lead released to the air settles into soil or water. Lead emitted from smelters and MWCs (and, until lead was phased out of gasoline, from automobile exhausts) is in the form of a fine particulate which can be distributed by the wind and can ultimately settle in soils. From the soils, the lead particulate may be re-entrained in air and further distributed, or it may follow myriad other pathways toward human exposure, turning up in household dust, in the soils adhering to garden vegetables, or in cow's milk, in which forms it may be ingested. Once deposited in soils, it becomes part of the general "background" level of lead in the environment, along with lead in the earth (EPA 1991c).

Both direct and indirect exposures contribute to the baseline level of lead in human tissues, typically indicated by the level of lead in blood or blood lead (PbB). Because of the difficulty of tracing lead concentrations back to their various sources, EPA assumed air emissions to be a surrogate measure of each source's contribution to background lead levels (EPA 1991c). A reduction in air emissions was assumed to result in a proportionate reduction in contribution to background lead levels and, consequently, the lead burden of the general population.

Reductions in Emissions. The agency's analysis, based on 1987 figures for lead consumption, emissions, and rates of recycling (then about 85 percent), found that increasing the rate of recycling from 85 to 95 percent would decrease the net release of lead to all media by 62,000 tons per year (EPA 1991c). Almost all (around 99 percent) of that net reduction would be reductions in land disposal, of which about 93 percent would be reductions in disposal at landfills and the remainder would be disposal on the premises of MWCs and primary smelters.

Because its analysis indicated that changes in land disposal would have little or no impact on human exposure and human health (as discussed in the following sections), EPA focused its attention on the 1 percent of the total reduction in lead emissions that would involve air emissions. EPA estimated that increased recycling would result in a net reduction of national emissions of lead to air of between 428 and 503 metric tons per year, or about 5 percent, depending on assumptions about changes in the amount of primary smelter activity after the policy change. This calculation is summarized in Table 8.2.

EPA's estimate assumed no compliance with state-mandated lead battery recycling programs. At the time of the study, approximately 68 percent of the states had mandatory recycling programs. The more compliance there was with existing state programs, the lower would be the additional impact of a federally mandated recycling program on national emissions. Under the assumption that all 68 percent of the state programs did achieve full compliance, the nationwide reduction in air emissions of lead attributable to a federally mandated program would only be about 1.5 percent instead of 5 percent. Thus EPA was estimating the maximum benefits of a federally mandated recycling plan (EPA 1991c).

Table 8.2 Effect of increased recycling on annual air lead emissions

Source	Annual lead emissions to air (metric tons)		
	85% Recycling[a]	95% Recycling	Change
Primary smelters	498	473 to 398[b]	−25 to −100[b]
Secondary smelters	509	560	+51
MWCs[c]	736	282[d]	−454
TOTAL	1743	1315 to 1240[b]	−428 to −503[b]

Source: EPA 1991c.

a. Based on baseline estimates by EPA Office of Air Quality Planning and Standards as cited in EPA 1991c.

b. Higher emissions (lesser change) reflects assumption that primary smelters will continue activity levels; lower emissions (greater change) reflects assumption that primary smelters will reduce activity levels.

c. MWC (municipal waste combustor) estimates do include both stack and fugitive emissions, but do not include impact of state laws with mandatory takeback and disposal ban provisions.

d. Assumes that batteries account for 65% of lead waste incinerated (Franklin Associates 1988).

More important than the net reduction in emissions was the location of each change in emissions. As shown in Table 8.2, air emission reductions occurred at primary smelters and MWCs, while air emissions from secondary smelters were projected to increase by 51 metric tons per year. One reason for this large increase is that, per pound of finished lead product produced, secondary smelters emit two to four times as much lead pollution as do primary smelters (EPA 1991c). This difference in emission rates reflects in part the presence of older, "dirtier" technologies at secondary smelters, and in part their history of lower compliance with the National Ambient Air Quality Standards (NAAQS) for lead.

The range of lead emissions projected for primary smelters in Table 8.2 (from 398 to 473 metric tons per year) reflects EPA's uncertainty about how primary smelters will respond when increased recycling boosts the use of secondary lead and in turn depresses demand for new lead. The larger reduction in emissions, a 100-ton drop to 398 tons per year, assumes that primary smelters will reduce operations commensurately when demand for primary lead falls. (EPA assumed that primary smelters would cut back by reducing the volume of lead they import.) The smaller reduction, a drop of 25 tons to 473 tons per year, assumes that primary smelters in the United States will find new markets for primary lead, and will therefore continue smelting (and importing lead ore) at nearly the same rate as before.

Reducing Human Exposure. Using its assessment of changes in air emissions resulting from increased recycling, EPA's Office of Toxic Substances, with help from its Office of Air Quality Planning and Standards, estimated the resulting changes in human exposure to lead. EPA's assessment of exposures to lead focused on children's exposures to airborne lead, but also projected adult worker exposures to lead at primary and secondary smelters, MWCs, and landfills, and exposures through land disposal of lead. Ecological impacts were not addressed in EPA's risk analysis.

The focus on childhood lead levels reflects EPA's strategy to evaluate impacts on the most sensitive segment of the exposed population (EPA 1991e). There is considerable evidence that lead exposure has the most severe impacts on children. EPA's rationale for focusing on the most sensitive subpopulation is that regulatory measures to minimize impacts on such sub-populations will provide adequate protection for the rest of the population.

For each emissions source, EPA estimated the change in the number of children aged from birth to 6 years whose blood lead (PbB) levels would exceed the CDC level of concern, 10 μg/dl, as a result of changes in lead emissions or exposures. The change in the number of children at risk was calculated by comparing the number of children exceeding the CDC level under the new rule to the number in the baseline year, 1987.

EPA (1991c) modeled the impact of lead air emissions on PbB levels using empirical measurements and estimates of lead concentrations in air surrounding lead emission sources, a statistical model of the relationship between air emissions and soil lead levels, assumptions about uptake (ingestion and inhalation) from air and soil, and a mathematical model of the relationship between lead uptake and blood lead levels. For each exposure, EPA projected the percentages of children who would have PbB levels greater than 10 μg/dl. The agency then multiplied this percentage by the total number of children aged 0–6 years who were estimated to be exposed to lead emissions from each source.

At each emissions source the EPA's analysis included conservative assumptions about the population's "background" level of exposure to lead in drinking water, soil, and air (EPA 1991c). Conservative assumptions were used so that the baseline levels of PbB in the exposed population, including the number of children with PbB levels already exceeding 10 μg/dl, would not be underestimated.

Results for Air Exposure to Children. The results of EPA's childhood exposure analysis contained a big surprise: even under optimistic assumptions, increased recycling would have *no impact* on the number of U.S. children with PbB levels exceeding 10 μg/dl; under pessimistic assumptions, it might *increase* the number of these children. These results are summarized in Table 8.3. The primary culprit was the increase in exposure to children living near secondary smelters; the impact of changes in MWC stack and fugitive emissions on PbB levels was estimated to be quite small.

The first two sections of Table 8.3 depict EPA's two scenarios for smelter emissions. In the first one, the "current NAAQS compliance" scenario, the agency assumed that smelters would continue their current rate of incomplete compliance with the National Ambient Air Quality Standard (NAAQS) for lead, which is now set at an ambient level of 1.5 µg/m³ (micrograms per cubic meter of air). EPA also assumed that no new smelters would be added to accommodate the increase in lead recycling. The changes in lead released from both primary

Table 8.3 Number of U.S. children at risk[a] from airborne lead emissions

	Number of children at risk[a]		
Source	85% Recycling	95% Recycling	Change
Current NAAQS compliance			
Primary smelters	226	198 to 219[b]	−28 to −7
Secondary smelters	525	525 to 563[c]	0 to +38
Improved NAAQS compliance			
Primary smelters	128	128	0
Secondary smelters	244	244 to 246[d]	0 to +2
MWCs			
Stack	0	0	0
Fugitive		−2	−2

Source: EPA 1991c.

a. "Children at risk" are U.S. children aged 0–6 years whose blood lead (PbB) level is greater than 10 µg/dl.

b. Higher number reflects assumption that primary smelters continue activity levels; lower number reflects assumption that primary smelters reduce activity levels.

c. Higher number reflects assumption of increased secondary smelting in the U.S.; lower number reflects assumption that increased secondary smelting occurs outside of the U.S.

d. Higher number reflects assumption of two new "greenfield" secondary smelters using cleaner technology.

and secondary smelters were therefore assumed to be proportional to changes in the volume of lead processed at each.

At primary smelters, the volume of lead processed was assumed to vary, as was the case in Table 8.2, depending on whether primary smelters reduced their activity after the increase in mandated recycling, or continued at prior levels by selling lead to other markets. If the activity of primary smelters remained constant, their emissions were estimated to decrease by only 5 percent; if their activity decreased, their emissions were estimated to decrease by 19 percent. EPA then translated these decreases in emissions into numbers of children in the United States aged 0 to 6 years with PbB levels greater than 10 μg/dl. These figures, shown in Table 8.3, suggest that the number of children with elevated PbB levels living near primary smelters would drop by 7 or by 28 relative to baseline numbers, depending on the assumption about the effect of increased recycling on the activity level at primary smelters.

At secondary smelters, the impact of increased recycling varied according to assumptions about where the lead was recycled. If all the lead were to be recycled through existing secondary smelters in the United States at their current rate of compliance with the NAAQS, EPA estimated that the number of children with PbB levels greater than 10 μg/dl would *increase* by 38. But if the capacity of existing smelters were exceeded, as the EPA's Office of Air Quality Planning and Standards expected it would be, then foreign secondary smelting operations were assumed to provide the additional recycling capacity (EPA 1991c). Under this assumption, EPA's estimate of the increase in the number of children *in the United States* with elevated blood levels was *zero*, as shown in the table. In this case, the emissions and risks would essentially be shifted to an unidentified population outside the United States. EPA's view was that such extraterritorial risks (or benefits if they existed) could not be considered under TSCA.

In the second scenario, the "improved NAAQS compliance" scenario shown in the second section of Table 8.3, EPA envisioned full industry compliance with the NAAQS of 1.5 μg/m³. At primary smelters, to be conservative, EPA assumed that even with a drop in the amount of lead processed and hence emissions, the number of children with PbB exceeding 10 μg/dl would not decrease. At secondary smelters, since compliance with the NAAQS would require limits on additional emissions, EPA assumed that any increase in demand for secondary smelting capacity generated by mandatory recycling would have to be met by foreign operations. Thus, as under the "current NAAQS compliance" scenario, *no* increase in the number of U.S. children with PbB levels greater than 10 μg/dl would be expected, but there could be increases in the numbers of foreign children with elevated PbB levels.

In a variation of this scenario, EPA estimated the impact of increased recycling if the additional demand for secondary smelting capacity were to be met by the construction in the United States of two new secondary smelters, known as "greenfield" smelters. EPA assumed that these new smelters would have the same lead emissions as those from "cleaner" examples of currently operating secondary smelters, and thus used emissions data from three cleaner secondary smelters to represent emissions from the new greenfield smelters. Population data for the "new" smelters were likewise taken from the populations living near the three existing smelters. As shown in Table 8.3, under this variation only *two* additional U.S. children were projected to have PbB levels greater than 10 μg/dl.

In addition to smelters, EPA estimated the impact on childhood PbB of reduced emissions from municipal waste combusters (MWCs), as shown in the third section of Table 8.3. Recalling that by far the largest reduction in airborne lead emissions caused by increased recycling—454 tons per year—was expected to occur at MWCs, as shown in Table 8.2, EPA expected to find a significant health benefit. EPA counted 186 MWCs in the United States that receive lead batteries, with approximately 2.5 million people living within 2 kilometers of these facilities, and additional workers who would otherwise handle lead in MWC ash.

EPA's analysis of the health impact of the reduction in air emissions from MWCs considered both community and worker exposures to lead. As in the study of smelters, EPA calculated the impact of exposures to the general population in terms of the effect on the blood lead (PbB) levels in children aged 0 to 6 years. EPA relied on estimates of airborne lead concentrations provided by the Office of Air Quality Planning and Standards (EPA 1989a). Concentrations of lead in air following mandatory recycling were assumed to be 65 percent lower, since lead batteries account for approximately 65 percent of the lead in the solid waste stream to MWCs. Thus, full compliance with the regulation was assumed in order to generate an estimate of the maximum benefit of mandatory increased recycling. The impact of MWC lead emissions on PbB levels was estimated for populations living near a sample of 41 facilities selected to represent the 186 MWCs in the United States.

Despite the large number of people potentially exposed to lead in stack emissions from MWCs, EPA's risk analysis projected that the impacts on blood lead levels would be very small. As shown in Table 8.3, *no* additional children were projected to exceed the 10 μg/dl PbB level. This result most likely stems from the facts that MWC emissions are lower than those for smelters, and that the populations living near MWCs already had quite low levels of PbB. Moreover, although the number of tons reduced (454) appears large, that reduction was spread over 186 facilities. The risk analysis projected that the reductions in lead emissions from MWC stacks due to increased recycling would merely reduce existing average PbB levels in exposed children from 3.02 μg/dl to 2.97 μg/dl—a difference of 0.05 μg/dl, and not across the crucial 10 μg/dl level of concern. (EPA [1991c] did not report whether these values were for the mean or the maximum child.) It is doubtful that even this difference could be demonstrated to be statistically meaningful given some of the broad assumptions used in the exposure analysis.

EPA's evaluation of the change in exposures to lead in fugitive MWC emissions was similar to its evaluation of MWC stack emissions. Using the highest concentration of lead in air estimated to result from fugitive emissions from MWCs with on-site ash disposal, EPA first calculated the corresponding blood lead levels in a population of potentially exposed children at current rates of recycling. Increased recycling was assumed to reduce the concentrations of lead in air by 65 percent (based on lead batteries constituting 65 percent of the MWC lead waste stream) and to result in lower blood lead levels as well. EPA then estimated the number of children whose blood levels would be likely to fall below 10 µg/dl as a result of mandatory recycling. Again, despite apparently generous assumptions about exposure to lead from fugitive emissions of MWC ash, the impacts on blood lead levels were relatively small. As shown in Table 8.3, EPA reported the upper bound number of children whose blood lead levels would fall below 10 µg/dl to be *two*. Blood lead levels for the mean (average) child were expected to fall from 4.71 µg/dl to 3.92 µg/dl for children in the 0 to 6 age group.

Results for Exposure to Workers. EPA's assessment of the impact of increased recycling on airborne exposures to workers at primary and secondary smelters was limited. However, citing limited data showing that exposures at both primary and secondary smelters can exceed Occupational Safety and Health Administration (OSHA) standards for lead, EPA concluded that recycling was unlikely to affect net occupational exposures at smelters (EPA 1991c).

Regarding workers at MWCs, who are potentially exposed to ash, EPA concluded that increased recycling might significantly decrease the prevalence of lead-induced disease among exposed workers at MWCs. Assuming that state-mandated battery return laws were not in effect, and therefore that the full impact of federally mandated recycling would be felt, EPA estimated that PbB levels would fall below 10 µg/dl for 3,300 of the 15,000 workers at MWCs. Approximately 3,000 workers whose PbB levels still exceeded 10 µg/dl could expect to see about a 32 percent decline in those levels. But these estimates are not necessarily meaningful, because the 10 µg/dl PbB level set by CDC was based on evidence of its health effects in young children (CDC 1991), and its applicability to adult workers is unclear. The focus of EPA's assessment of lead exposure in MWC workers was lead-induced hypertension (high blood pressure and its associated impact on the risk of cardiovascular disease and stroke), and although there is a well-documented association between PbB and hypertension at levels substantially higher than the CDC level of concern, the impact of PbB levels approaching or lower than 10 µg/dl on hypertension is quite uncertain (Davis 1991). By contrast, the standard for adult workers set by the Occupational Safety and Health Administration (OSHA) is an action level of 40 µg/dl PbB; at this level the frequency of PbB monitoring must be increased and efforts made to reduce exposure in the workplace, and removal from work is required when an individual's PbB level reaches 60 µg/dl.

Results for Land Exposure Routes. The other route of exposure to lead that EPA explored for the general population was the ingestion of lead in drinking water contaminated by leachate from municipal solid waste landfills. Here the agency was estimating the health benefits of a major reduction in total lead released—about 93 percent of the projected 62,000-ton reduction due to increased recycling would otherwise have gone to landfills. But despite making conservative assumptions about exposure, the agency's analysis suggested that lead in landfills is not currently posing any significant hazard to drinking water supplies. Thus EPA found that the impact of increased battery recycling would be small.

Using the maximum concentration of lead detected in recent studies of leachate (at landfills built before RCRA design requirements went into effect in 1980), and assuming a dilution factor of 100 (as employed by EPA's Office of Solid Waste; see EPA 1991c) for leachate migrating to a hypothetical residential well, EPA estimated the "worst case" PbB level in infants (less than 1 year old) to be 3.9 µg/dl. The contribution of lead from landfilled batteries to infant PbB accounted for 2.4 µg/dl of the total. For newer landfills (post-1980), the maximum concentration projected for a hypothetical nearby well was 10-fold lower than the estimate for worst-case landfills.

EPA's Decision

On the basis of its multimedia risk analysis, EPA ultimately decided not to move forward with a regulation to mandate recycling of lead acid batteries. In doing so, the agency acted contrary to its stated policy in favor of recycling, and changed course from its years of efforts under three different statutes (CAA, RCRA, and TSCA) to mandate increased recycling.

The decision not to push for federally mandated recycling of lead acid batteries was based on several factors. No doubt among them was the fact that many states—68 percent at the time of the risk analysis—had already instituted mandatory battery recycling programs, and more had plans to institute them, making an additional federal mandate less urgent. Moreover, at the time EPA abandoned its rulemaking, the current rate of lead recycling had already reached 95 percent (Battery Council International 1992). But that rate fluctuates with the market price for lead, and it could fall again in the future.

Certainly, TSCA's requirement to evaluate risks, costs, and benefits, and EPA's resulting risk analysis showing that the increase in recycling would yield little measurable benefit and might even increase net risks, was pivotal. EPA's analysis demonstrated that even though recycling was likely to reduce the net quantity of lead released to the environment by impressive amounts, these physical amounts alone were not the whole story. In the evaluation of human health risks, what mattered was where the lead went and to what degree populations were exposed to the lead released. Even though 99 percent of the reduction in lead release to the environment would come from diverting lead batteries from land disposal (93 percent at solid waste landfills and the rest on the premises of MWCs and smelters), the assessment could predict no substantial health benefit from this reduction. Although landfills have received batteries for years, the documented release of lead in leachate turned out to be low even from the older, less environmentally well-designed landfills. In the area of air emissions, EPA's study found that the net elimination of 400–500 tons per year emitted to air would not be an appreciable improvement, since some children would be less exposed but others (those living near secondary smelters) would be more exposed. Recycling had the effect of shifting some releases from one area to another and thus from one population to another: from primary smelters, MWCs, and landfills to secondary smelters (and, perhaps, to activities in other countries). At best, these shifts resulted in no apparent health benefit. At worst, the shifts in the point of release resulted in increasing net risks to the recipient population, because switching lead disposed of in landfills to secondary smelting facilities increased the estimated number of children with PbB levels greater than 10 μg/dl living near those facilities. Banning lead from incinerators and landfills essentially transformed small exposures to the large populations living around those facilities into larger exposures to the smaller populations living around secondary smelters. If EPA's study indicated that MWC workers might benefit from lower risk of lead-induced hypertension and heart disease, they would do so at the expense of higher risk to children living near the secondary smelters.

Even the scenarios in which recycling appeared to cause no increase in risk to populations living around secondary smelters were somewhat illusory, because in these cases recycling simply shifted the risks out of U.S. regulatory eyesight, to populations employed in or living around secondary recycling facilities in other countries. The actual impact on foreign health would depend on the size and age of the populations living near secondary smelters and their background blood lead levels, and on the emissions control restrictions placed on secondary smelters in those countries. The last item can be quite decisive: as shown in Table 8.3, moving from the equivalent of full compliance with the U.S. NAAQS (second section) to less than full compliance (first section) would expose many, perhaps hundreds, more children to elevated blood lead levels. Thus if mandatory increased recycling caused secondary smelting to shift from the United States to countries with more children living nearer to secondary smelters, or with less stringent air emission controls on lead, the net effect could be a substantial increase in risk.

Still, major questions remain about EPA's risk analysis and its decision. Chief among these is the difficulty of quantifying impacts that are clearly important. EPA's study only briefly touched on potential ecological impacts, concluding that they might be important, but that EPA was not able to quantify them. It is not clear whether the net ecological impacts of increased recycling (and secondary smelting) would be positive or negative, but the issue could conceivably be dispositive. Moreover, EPA worried that its inconclusive findings of health impacts from land disposal were themselves unsteady. EPA's risk analysis concluded, despite its quantitative analysis to the contrary, that "our most important conclusion is that increased recycling greatly reduces the total lead emissions and concomitant indirect lead exposure . . . Reducing these emissions would provide a public health benefit" (EPA 1991c). Perhaps limitations in current understanding of all the indirect pathways through which lead can result in human exposure and of the environmental and PbB levels at which lead ceases to have an impact, among others, prevented the public health benefit from being quantified.

Conclusion

As EPA's risk analysis revealed, with current technologies, recycling lead acid batteries reduces risks to some people but increases risks to others. This "risk transfer," when analyzed carefully, caused the agency to step back from its unqualified, "common sense" commitment to increasing the recycling of lead acid batteries. Although EPA's analysis leaves room for technical criticism, and several questions remain unanswered, it shows how an investment in risk tradeoff analysis can yield decisions that are superior to what uninformed conventional wisdom would dictate. Even if EPA had decided to go ahead with mandatory battery recycling—a decision which some could argue, perhaps on grounds of ecological effects or worker exposure, would be warranted even given EPA's risk analysis—then the analysis of risk tradeoffs that EPA performed would provide the key to modifying or complementing that policy to protect children who live near secondary smelters.

EPA's explicit use of risk tradeoff analysis is encouraging, and portends broader attention to multimedia risk tradeoffs in future decisionmaking. Perhaps in a few years it will be possible to recast Table 8.1 to reflect numerous cases of consideration and action based on comprehensive risk analyses. An accretion of multimedia analyses would also help to build institutional bridges within EPA, mirroring the interconnections among environmental systems, so that as EPA offices conduct such analyses, they may be increasingly drawn to work with each other rather than in isolation and to think ahead about the impacts of their decisions on other environmental media. In this case, for example, the Office of Toxic Substances collaborated with the Office of Air and the Office of Solid Waste in order to generate multimedia risk estimates.

The lead acid battery recycling analysis also suggests rethinking of the Best Demonstrated Available Technology (BDAT) specified for RCRA wastes in the current RCRA program. The application of BDAT to hazardous wastes under RCRA was intended to stop the "toxics shell game," to have one piece of environmental legislation take final responsibility for safe disposal or destruction of toxic materials (Fortuna 1990). Once BDAT is specified for a particular type of waste, no further analysis is typically required. Yet as the lead acid battery recycling case illustrates, BDAT does not necessarily mean that overall risks are reduced.

The case study raises other troubling questions. First, if it is not a good idea to mandate an increase in recycling from 85 percent to 95 percent, why are we sure that with current technology even the 85 percent rate is desirable? EPA did not address the countervailing risks induced by the current market rate of recycling, or by the 68 percent-plus states that are enacting recycling programs. Perhaps the ideal policy would actually be for the federal government to discourage lead battery recycling; EPA's risk analysis raises this question without investigating it. Or perhaps the ideal policy would be to find ways to reduce the adverse environmental consequences of the recycling process, such as by reducing air emissions from secondary smelters. EPA has recently embarked on that tack under the Clean Air Act, proposing to require technology-based limitations on lead emissions from secondary smelters (EPA 1994). For the longer term, perhaps the best policy, illuminated by risk tradeoff analysis, will be to explore less toxic alternatives to lead-based batteries.

A second troubling aspect of this case study is the subtle omission of people in foreign countries from the EPA's quantitative estimates of children at risk of elevated blood lead. This omission graphically demonstrates the risk transfers to which those without any voice in the decisionmaking process may fall victim. Under the method used by EPA (perhaps required by TSCA), the assumption that risky facilities would be relocated abroad generated a risk estimate of "zero" in the quantitative tables, even though it was clear that the true risk was positive and significant. Though explained in footnotes, such skewed bottom-line estimates can quickly feed the "tyranny of numbers" that generates bad policy. Although TSCA may not permit EPA to make a regulatory decision to protect foreigners, it is hard to imagine that the law requires willful blindness in analysis.

9

Regulating Pesticides

GEORGE M. GRAY
JOHN D. GRAHAM

One of the principal objectives of U.S. environmental policy is to protect human health and wildlife from excessive exposure to toxic chemicals. The birth of the modern environmental movement is often traced to the publication of Rachel Carson's *Silent Spring* (1962), which highlighted the injurious impacts of chemicals such as DDT on birds and fish.

Current policy operates on a chemical-by-chemical basis. Rules are promulgated to reduce or eliminate either the use of a suspect chemical or discharges of the chemical into the environment. In recent years, the wisdom of "one-at-a-time" chemical regulation has been questioned because that approach fails to take account of the risks and benefits of substitute chemicals (Whipple 1985). Nowhere is this conundrum more salient than in the field of pesticide regulation, where chemical producers, farmers, and regulatory agencies are all faced with the phenomenon of risk tradeoffs.

The history of DDT is instructive. Although DDT has relatively low toxicity compared to many pesticides, it was intensely criticized by Carson and others and ultimately banned by the Environmental Protection Agency in 1972 because of its persistence in the environment and threat to wildlife. In its place, farmers have turned to a number of organophosphate pesticides to control pests that damage crops. The organophosphates are less persistent yet more acutely toxic than DDT, and have caused incidents of serious poisoning among unsuspecting workers and farmers who had been accustomed to handling the relatively nontoxic DDT (Ottoboni 1991). Meanwhile, DDT was heavily used in the worldwide campaign to eradicate insect-borne malaria—once declared a success— and the decline in its use since 1972 may have contributed in part to the revived malaria epidemic that is now afflicting more than 200 million and killing over 2 million each year (though excessive use of DDT in earlier decades may also have contributed by fostering resistant strains of insects) (Brown 1994; Drogin 1992).

In this chapter we explore the risk tradeoffs inherent in U.S. pesticide regulation. We consider in particular detail EPA's dilemma in the re-registration of the fungicide "maneb" for use on lettuce. This case study illustrates how current regulatory strategies, by focusing on pesticides one at a time, lead to policies that may increase, not decrease, risk to public health and the environment. The current approach does not encourage decisionmakers seeking to regulate a particular pesticide to compare the risks of that chemical with the risks of substitute pesticides, or of alternative (potentially nonchemical) pest-control methods. The chapter concludes with suggestions for improvements in the methods of risk analysis that can better serve the public's goals for pesticide regulation.

U.S. Pesticide Regulation

Pesticides are agents used to control pests such as insects, weeds, fungi, and other pathogens; thus they are purposefully designed to be harmful to some organisms. The first U.S. laws regulating pesticides were passed early in this century and were designed to protect the farmer from unscrupulous peddlers of ineffective pest control agents (NRC 1980). Today pesticides are regulated primarily to protect workers and the public from toxic effects while ensuring the benefits of pesticides for farmers and food consumers.

The public's primary concern about pesticides is the risk of consumer exposure to pesticide residues remaining on produce or in processed foods. Even if the risk of illness to an individual consumer is slight, when the risk is applied to the entire U.S. population through the food supply, the incidence of adverse health outcomes can be significant. For example, if 200 million food consumers are each exposed to an incremental lifetime cancer risk of one chance in a million, then 200 excess cases of cancer can be expected to occur over a lifetime. Although such estimates of risk are often worst-case scenarios, the point is that the large size of the exposed population spurs regulatory concern.

Pesticide use on crops is regulated under two laws administered by different federal agencies. The Environmental Protection Agency (EPA) is responsible for pesticide registration under the Federal Insecticide, Fungicide, and Rodenticide Act (FIFRA), while both EPA and the Food and Drug Administration (FDA) are responsible for managing pesticide residues on food under the Federal Food, Drug, and Cosmetic Act (FFDCA) (NRC 1987).

The central function of pesticide regulation under FIFRA is registration, the granting of permission for manufacturers to market a pesticide for use on a particular crop against a particular pest. FIFRA requires the manufacturer of the active ingredient in the pesticide product to demonstrate efficacy against the target pest. In addition, FIFRA requires the manufacturer to supply health information on the compound, such as data on acute toxicity, developmental and reproductive toxicity, neurotoxicity, and potential carcinogenicity. Since human data are usually unavailable, EPA relies on information from animal studies.

Registration under FIFRA requires the setting of a "tolerance" under FFDCA for pesticide residues on food crops and products. A tolerance is the maximum level of pesticide residue allowed on food. Tolerances under FFDCA are set by EPA. The tolerance level is determined in two stages: first the manufacturer, using studies in test fields, determines how the pesticide must be applied to a crop to control the target pest; then the amount of pesticide remaining in or on the produce after this treatment, the residue level, is examined to determine if it is safe.

If a compound has *not* been found to cause tumors in laboratory animals, EPA makes the determination of "safe" by comparing the residue level to the Acceptable Daily Intake (ADI) for that pesticide. EPA calculates the ADI in such a way that even a lifetime of exposure at the ADI will cause no adverse consequences to a human being. The toxicological data are evaluated to find the most sensitive toxic response to the pesticide. From the dose-response relationship for this effect, a no-observed-effect level (NOEL) is determined. The NOEL is the highest dose at which no toxic effects were observed in animal tests. This dose is then divided by a safety factor, usually 100, to determine the ADI for humans. This ADI level is used by EPA in setting a tolerance for registration of the pesticide.

If the compound *has* been shown to cause a statistically significant increase in tumors in laboratory animals, then EPA uses quantitative risk assessment (QRA) to set the tolerance. QRA uses mathematical models and science-policy assumptions to estimate the potential cancer risk from exposure to carcinogenic compounds (EPA 1986). The risks calculated by QRA are expressed as probabilities of developing cancer with a lifetime exposure to the compound. Unlike the ADI for non-cancer toxicity, there are no statutorily designated levels of acceptable risk for pesticides that are animal carcinogens. However, a survey by a National Academy of Sciences panel found that EPA usually allows upper-bound lifetime cancer risk estimates of 1×10^{-6} (one in one million) or less, but rarely allows upper-bound lifetime cancer risk estimates of 1×10^{-4} (one in ten thousand) or higher (NRC 1987).

A pesticide must have a tolerance level for each crop on which it may be used. Some widely used pesticides have a hundred or more tolerances. At the farm, the levels of pesticide residue on crops can be controlled to some extent by adjusting application amounts and rates as well as the intervals between application and harvest of the crop. These adjustments will sometimes be made to bring residue levels below the ADI or the acceptable risk level.

A pesticide with FFDCA-approved tolerances can then be registered for use under FIFRA. The registration contains a legally binding requirement of a label on the pesticide, which gives details about the crops on which the pesticide may be used, application rates, the pre-harvest time interval, and special clothing to be worn or work practices to be followed when using the product.

Modern requirements for pesticide testing came into effect in the early 1970s. In order to register and obtain tolerances, the manufacturer of a pesticide is required by EPA to submit extensive data on toxicology, chemistry, and anticipated residue levels of the compound and its metabolites and degradation products. These data are evaluated by EPA and a preliminary tolerance is set. EPA then publishes the proposed tolerance in the *Federal Register* and invites public comment. After a full analysis of the data and comments, EPA chooses either to set a tolerance or to deny the request for registration.

A large number of pesticides currently in use that were registered prior to the development of current testing standards have an incomplete toxicological data base. For example, many of the older chemicals have not been tested for carcinogenic potential in long-term animal experiments. The incomplete data base raises concerns about the safety of tolerances set many years ago. In 1981 EPA instituted its new "data-call-in" program to increase its toxicological knowledge of these older compounds. This program requires older pesticides to be re-registered on the basis of scientific data that meet modern toxicological standards. Congress has mandated that re-registration decisions for these older compounds be completed by 1997, which is considered a very ambitious schedule.

Fungicides are the type of pesticide used to control damage to crops by fungi and to treat seeds and small grains that become infected with fungi during storage. They are also used in the cultivation of ornamental flowers, shrubs, and grasses. As with other pesticides, there is concern about potential adverse effects on human health and the environment from exposure to fungicides. When fungicides are tested for carcinogenic potential, they are typically tested at doses far greater than those experienced by humans in daily life. This testing at the so-called maximum tolerated dose (MTD), defined as the highest dose that does not cause weight losses in test rodents, is unrealistic but is intended to compensate for other weaknesses in the animal experiment such as the small number of rodents (typically 50) in each test. Serious questions have been raised about whether tumors in animals observed near the MTD are relevant to humans, since the tumors may result from secondary toxicity rather than from the compound itself (Ames and Gold 1990; Carr and Kolbye 1991; NRC 1993).

It has proved difficult to develop an effective fungicide that does not cause tumors in rodents at doses near the MTD. More than 90 percent of fungicides that have been tested in standard animal experiments have caused tumors when large doses are applied for the lifetime of the animal (NRC 1987). Some reports estimate that fungicides may account for 60 percent of the predicted cancer risk to humans from all pesticides in the diet (NRC 1987).

When information from the data-call-in program suggests that a pesticide may pose a significant cancer risk, EPA initiates a "special review" of the compound. Historically, in special review as in tolerance setting, EPA has informally considered a cancer risk to be negligible if lifetime exposure to the predicted residue level increases a consumer's probability of contracting cancer by less than one chance in a million. Risks greater than one in a million may induce special review, a process where risks and benefits are scrutinized to inform a judgment about whether continued registration of the compound poses an "unreasonable risk" to human health and the environment. This "unreasonable risk" standard requires EPA to weigh the benefits of the pesticide against its risks.

The Risks of Substitutes

When examining the risks and benefits of a pesticide, EPA typically assumes that revoking the registration of the pesticide will eliminate the associated risks to human health and the environment. However, this would be true only if no pesticide replaced the banned compound and the target pest spontaneously disappeared. In practice, either the pest flourishes, with associated damages to crops and potentially to humans; or a different pesticide or alternative pest-control method, with its own risks and benefits, is used in place of the banned product. Yet the current approach to pesticide regulation has not made it a practice to consider such countervailing risks or to weigh the relative risks of all likely pest control scenarios.

Substitution is the process of replacing a banned or restricted pesticide with other available alternatives. The substitution issue is most salient when EPA makes a decision, usually through "special review," to revoke the registration of an existing pesticide product. Substitution is a less obvious but still important issue when EPA makes a decision to grant or refuse registration of a new pesticide.

The use of substitute pesticides can cause countervailing risks in many ways. First, new health risks can occur if the substitute pesticide is itself potentially carcinogenic, or if it has the capacity to cause other adverse health effects such as birth defects or neurobehavioral damage in children. (As mentioned earlier, the substitutes for DDT proved to be less persistent in the environment but more acutely toxic to farm workers.) Second, the pests do not just disappear when a pesticide is banned. The pest itself, if not adequately suppressed by the substitute pesticide, may be responsible for direct risks to human health (for example, through the spread of infections diseases, such as malaria, or through ingestion of fungal carcinogens left by pests on food crops). Third, when a substitute pesticide is less effective at controlling the target pest, or acts against fewer pests at a time, farmers may respond by increasing the overall use of pesticidal products (or by selecting plant strains with higher levels of natural pesticides), with potentially adverse implications for human health and wildlife. Finally, restricting pesticides may generate indirect but important risks to the health of farm families and food consumers. If substitute pesticides are less effective or more expensive than the banned products, crop yields may be constrained and the prices of critical foods, especially fruits and vegetables, may rise significantly (Zilberman et al. 1991). By curtailing the essential nutritional intake of lower-income families, increased food prices can cause health risks that potentially outweigh the health benefits of avoided exposure to pesticide residues.

The Maneb Story

In July of 1987 the Environmental Protection Agency began a special review of the ethylene bisdithiocarbamate (EBDC) fungicides, primarily because of concerns about cancer risk from consumers' dietary exposure to residues (EPA 1987). The use of EBDCs in the United States began in the 1930s, and they are now the most widely used family of fungicides in the world. The EBDCs are easy to use, have little problem with pest resistance, are inexpensive, and are effective against a broad range of fungal pests. It is estimated that approximately one-third of all fruits and vegetables in the United States are treated with EBDCs (NRC 1987). EBDC tolerances have been set for a large variety of food crops, from casaba melons to turnips (EPA 1987).

Maneb, a member of the EBDC family of fungicides, has a tolerance for use on lettuce. Because of the dry climates in which lettuce is grown, irrigation is necessary, but irrigation and climatological factors bring the threat of downy mildew. Downy mildew is caused by the fungus *Bremia lactucae*, a fungal pathogen that, even with fungicide use, has a significant effect on lettuce yield in this country. Maneb is used to control downy mildew. In December of 1989 EPA proposed to ban the use of maneb on lettuce (EPA 1989b). The ban was based on EPA's estimate that dietary exposure to maneb residues on lettuce might increase a consumer's lifetime risk of cancer by 3.0 chances in a million. If every person in the United States consumed lettuce for seventy years with estimated levels of maneb residue, EPA estimated that about one additional case of cancer would occur, in addition to the background incidence of 900,000 cases of cancer per year due to all genetic and environmental causes (Rosenthal et al. 1992).

Several environmental groups applauded EPA's proposal because they believed that banning the use of maneb on lettuce would remove an unnecessary risk from the food supply. Lettuce growers, on the other hand, challenged the wisdom of the proposal. They questioned the scientific basis of EPA's cancer risk estimates, arguing that extreme assumptions had inflated the risk estimates. The growers also questioned EPA's estimate of small benefits resulting from maneb use, instead predicting that without maneb the $1 billion annual lettuce crop in California and Arizona would be jeopardized.

Maneb is currently the chief means of controlling downy mildew on lettuce. In evaluating the effects of the cancellation of maneb use on lettuce, EPA identified three alternative fungicides: captan, metalaxyl, and copper compounds, which are also registered for use on lettuce to control downy mildew. One additional alternative, aliette (Fosetyl-Al), is widely used in Europe but is not registered for use in the United States. When EPA proposed the ban of maneb, it granted aliette a special waiver for use on lettuce in California.

In March 1992 EPA reversed its position and decided to reregister maneb for use on lettuce (EPA 1992). While EPA's official position was that the cancer risks of maneb use were shown to be much smaller than the agency had originally thought, some of the risk tradeoffs described in the following sections may have contributed informally to the agency's decision.

Trading One Cancer Risk for Another?

Since it is very difficult to design an effective fungicide that will not cause tumors in laboratory animal experiments, the relative cancer risks of alternative fungicides should be analyzed carefully. EPA's predicament with maneb illustrates this point.

One of the principal alternatives to maneb, captan, had also recently been subjected to EPA's special review process (EPA 1985; EPA 1989a). In February 1989 EPA had decided that the use of captan on various crops might pose significant cancer risks to consumers. EPA proposed cancellation of 45 out of 69 previously allowed food uses of captan. Another 13 out of 69 uses were retained because benefits outweighed risks, but even these uses might be suspended in the future if the manufacturer did not submit further data requested by EPA. Lettuce fell into this category because EPA decided that the cancer risks from the use of captan were slight and were outweighed by the benefits of captan use on lettuce (EPA 1989a). Thus, when EPA proposed to ban maneb in December 1989, captain remained available as a substitute.

At the time of EPA's decision, captan was only used on an estimated 5 percent of the lettuce crop (EPA 1985; EPA 1989a). EPA permitted captan's use on lettuce in part because it was not expected to be widely used. If captan were to replace maneb as the chief means of controlling downy mildew, perhaps 65 percent of the lettuce crop would then be treated with captan (the 60 percent currently treated with maneb plus the 5 percent currently treated with captan). If captan had been in such widespread use on lettuce in 1989, EPA might have revoked its tolerance in the special review process.

Using EPA's standard risk assessment methods, it turns out that the estimated cancer risks of using maneb versus captan on lettuce are roughly comparable, which means that cancer risks would not necessarily decline if captan were substituted for maneb. Indeed, the actual cancer threat from captan use may be more serious than the threat from maneb use if the entire body of toxicological data is considered. For instance, captan's carcinogenicity appears to be of greater concern than maneb's because captan exhibits mutagenic (DNA-damaging) activity in the standard Ames test, and causes a rare form of intestinal tumors in rats that is unambiguously related to captan exposure (EPA 1985). In contrast, the evidence for maneb's mutagenicity is limited, and the rodent tumors caused by maneb may reflect biological mechanisms that are not relevant to the low doses experienced by humans. Maneb's carcinogenicity is primarily related to a breakdown product, ETU, which causes thyroid tumors in rats at high doses. The only other evidence of tumor formation from maneb exposure occurs in the rodent liver, which many scientists believe is a poor predictor of human cancer risk (Chambers et al. 1987).

Trading Cancer Risk for Other Health Risks?

Frequently it is a finding of tumors in rodents that leads EPA to question the re-registration of a pesticide. Tumor findings in laboratory animal tests can also doom new pesticides under development even before they reach the marketplace. Is this focus on carcinogenicity necessarily protecting public health? Insufficient attention is given to the possibility that slightly carcinogenic pesticides may be preferable to noncarcinogenic pesticides in cases where the latter cause other pernicious health effects such as neurotoxicity, birth defects, and damage to the body's immune system.

Cancer risks dominate EPA's registration process because of public concern over cancer and the technical assumptions that are made by EPA risk assessors. As discussed earlier, for all noncancer health effects, EPA assumes that safe levels of exposure (the ADI) can be established at roughly a factor of 100 below the highest dose that causes no observed adverse health effects in laboratory animals (the NOEL). For cancer, however, EPA assumes that there are no safe levels of exposure. Any nonzero level of pesticide residue is predicted to increase cancer risk, as long as the compound has been shown to cause cancer in laboratory animals. EPA's assumptions about the dose-response relationships for cancer and other health endpoints are not universally shared in the scientific community and are topics of considerable technical dispute (see Upton 1988; OMB 1991; Evans et al. 1992; Holland and Sielken 1991). Many experts argue that low doses of carcinogens can pose no cancer risk, and some (for example, Ames 1992; Calabrese 1994) claim that low doses may even help the body's immune system develop the ability to withstand higher doses.

As the choice between maneb and captan illustrates, EPA's assumptions may cause non-cancer effects such as reproductive abnormalities to be downplayed relative to cancer effects. In the initial review of captan, EPA noted that available data suggest that captan has the ability to cause fetal abnormalities in laboratory animals. The NOEL for reproductive effects, including reduced offspring size in rats, was set at 12.5 mg/kg/day (milligrams of captan per kilogram of body weight per day); when EPA applied its standard 100-fold safety factor to the NOEL, it generated an acceptable daily intake (ADI) of captan of 0.125 mg/kg/day (EPA 1985). In a contemporaneous study, the National Academy of Sciences estimated that the levels of captan residue on foods (predicted on the basis of worst-case exposure assumptions) might exceed this ADI (NRC 1987). This potential problem disappeared for two reasons: EPA determined that by measuring the actual residues of captan in food, rather than using worst-case assumptions of exposure, the actual dietary exposure to captan was likely to be *less than* the ADI; and EPA reconsidered the animal studies in 1989 and made a final determination that captan is not a teratogen (reproductive toxin) (EPA 1989a).

Needless to say, a reasonable person might disagree with EPA's assessment of the reproductive risks of captan. Since the cancer risks of maneb are highly speculative, some citizens might regard the reproductive dangers of captan exposure as more serious than the slight cancer risks of maneb exposure. Others, such as those past their childbearing age, might prefer to face higher risks of reproductive toxicity and less cancer risk. As important as this issue might be, the current regulatory process does not permit a rigorous comparison of the non-cancer and cancer effects of alternative pesticides.

Trading New Risks for Old Ones?

The more rigorous regulation to which new pesticides are subject, relative to older pesticides, often means that effective, less toxic compounds may be kept unavailable while less effective or more toxic older pesticides remain in use (Huber 1983). Under FIFRA and FFDCA, Congress has set in motion a process that makes it close to impossible for less dangerous new pesticides to replace more dangerous old ones. When EPA sets a tolerance for a new compound, it must consider only the risk of the new pesticide (as compared to the ADI or acceptable cancer risk) and implicitly ignore the risks associated with older pesticides already on the market. Yet older pesticides are often more toxic and less carefully tailored to pest-specific impact than are the new compounds that have been developed in accordance with modern toxicological testing protocols.

Under the FFDCA, which regulates substances added to foods, including pesticide residues, the tolerance-setting procedure is governed by two sections of the statute, sections 408 (administered by EPA) and 409 (handled by FDA). Section 408 concerns the levels of pesticides found on fresh commodities. This section allows the consideration of the risks and benefits of a pesticide in setting a tolerance, acknowledging that pesticide use is necessary for the maintenance of a "wholesome, adequate, and economical food supply." Section 409 is concerned with substances purposefully added to foods (food additives), including artificial colors, flavors, and sweeteners. Section 409 has been interpreted to include pesticide residues on food, but because under section 408 a commodity can have a legal amount of a pesticide present, a pesticide is not considered a food *additive* unless it becomes concentrated during the processing of the food product. The process of making a vegetable sauce or fruit juice, for example, may lead to the concentration of a pesticide in the processed food. In this section of the statute, Congress made the determination that substances added deliberately to food must never cause cancer, and so no risk/benefit balancing is allowed under section 409. This is because section 409 is subject to the Delaney Clause in the FFDCA, which states that "no additive shall be deemed safe if it is found to induce cancer when ingested by man or animal or, if it is found, after tests which are appropriate for the evaluation of the safety of food additives, to induce cancer in man or animals." This clause has been interpreted to mean that no pesticide can be granted a section 409 tolerance if it concentrates at all in processed food and has any evidence of carcinogenic potential in animals (*Les v. Reilly* 1992). Denial of a section 409 tolerance frequently dooms the use of a pesticide on a particular crop because it is impossible to determine and enforce which part of a crop will be used for raw consumption and which is used in processed foods.

In addition, the Delaney Clause applies to pesticide registrations after 1958 but not to pesticides registered before the 1958 amendment. Delaney may therefore rule out lower-risk substitutes for dangerous pre-1958 pesticides. A clear example occurs in the case of downy mildew control on lettuce. Aliette, the potential alternative to maneb, is a new organophosphate fungicide first registered in the United States in 1983. It is an effective fungicide with very low acute toxicity, and it has been subject to extensive toxicological studies. All of the evidence suggests it is an effective fungicide with fewer health risks than maneb, but aliette is not allowed for use on lettuce in the United States, primarily because of some evidence of carcinogenic effects in rodent bioassays. Tumors were found in male rats fed approximately 40,000 parts per million (ppm) aliette in their diet—equivalent to having an enormous 4 percent of their total diet made up of the pesticide. Meanwhile, aliette showed no evidence of carcinogenicity in either female rats or male or female mice; and aliette is not a mutagenic compound. EPA's Office of Pesticide Programs has placed aliette in category C—that is, it is considered a possible human carcinogen, but the carcinogenicity data are so weak that they do not support quantitative risk assessment (Quest et al. 1991).

Aliette, although widely used in Europe, is only registered for use on pineapples in the United States, a use where residues are not a serious problem. It seems that it is the finding of possible carcinogenicity, and the legal regime's narrow response to that finding, that has prevented its use on lettuce in the United States. Because the regulatory system does not allow the risks of old versus new pesticides to be weighed explicitly, it may be keeping an effective fungicide with much lower risks than those of the fungicides currently in use from even being considered as an alternative.

Trading Pesticide Risk for Pest Risk?

An important risk tradeoff that is frequently overlooked is the risk posed to the public health by the pest itself. Not only can some pests destroy crops and decrease farm yields, but some pests also pose a direct risk to human health.

For an example of this kind of tradeoff in the United States, consider the use of ethylene dibromide (EDB) to control fungus on corn and peanuts. EDB kills a fungus that produces a potent carcinogen, aflatoxin, as it grows on corn and peanuts in storage silos. Aflatoxin is one of the most potent animal carcinogens known, and it is believed to be responsible for many cancer cases worldwide, especially in developing countries with poor grain storage techniques (Yeh et al. 1989). When the fungicide EDB was found to be an animal carcinogen, its use was revoked by EPA because of concerns about cancer risk. When evaluating the risk of EDB, the EPA never considered formally that the actual public health risk could increase with the loss of EDB for the control of aflatoxin. In fact, in 1988 the U.S. corn crop had much higher than usual aflatoxin levels as a result of drought conditions, and it is quite possible that the public was exposed to a much higher cancer risk through aflatoxin than EDB would have presented (Kilman 1989).

Comparative Efficacy

An important property of alternative pesticides that must be considered is efficacy. Some pesticides will control pests, and thus crop losses, better than others. Some control the pests but have possible negative aspects, such as the potential for damaging the crop, or pest resistance. Since some pesticides are effective against many pests, a single application can take the place of several compounds effective against only one pest.

The alternative fungicides for control of downy mildew on lettuce illustrate these points. As a service to member farmers, the Iceberg Lettuce Research Program sponsored field trials of registered and unregistered downy mildew control agents (Kurtz 1990). The results of these trials were sent to the EPA. In these tests, which measured the ability of fungicides to control downy mildew when used alone, it was demonstrated that metalaxyl is the most effective agent when used alone. Maneb was slightly less effective than metalaxyl, and aliette was similar to maneb. The copper compounds were the least effective at controlling downy mildew, and captan was judged ineffective. However, this was a rather artificial comparison because under actual use conditions the fungicides are frequently applied together. For example, the most common combination used in California is maneb as a contact fungicide and metalaxyl acting systemically. Using the compounds together helps control downy mildew better and helps prevent resistance (EPA 1989b). From this comparison it appears that either metalaxyl, aliette, or maneb would be an adequate fungal control agent. A comparison of their risks and efficacy would then be useful to help choose among them.

Control of downy mildew is not the only aspect of efficacy that is important in analyzing control strategies. Metalaxyl and the copper compounds, both registered for lettuce, have serious problems that decrease their apparent efficacy. On crops treated with metalaxyl, fungi frequently develop resistance to its antifungal properties. Metalaxyl is currently used together with maneb in disease management, but its sole use may lead to resistance in downy mildew. In fact, it has been estimated that fungal resistance to metalaxyl is likely to develop within one year of the cancellation of maneb's tolerance and that within five years metalaxyl would be completely ineffective (EPA 1989b). Indeed, some lettuce fields in California are already resistant to the fungicidal action of metalaxyl (EPA 1989b; Kurtz 1990). The copper compounds cause leaf damage, often called "spotting" or "bronzing" when used in high moisture situations. The leaf damage makes the lettuce less cosmetically appealing to consumers and may also lead to decreased lettuce yield (EPA 1989b; Kurtz 1990). The copper compounds are currently used sparingly in an integrated pest management system with maneb and metalaxyl. If the use of copper compounds were to increase, as a result of the unavailability of maneb, the severe phytotoxic effects of the coppers would affect the quality of the lettuce crop. In fact, some manufacturers of copper-based fungicides have removed the use of the product on lettuce because of liability worries over crop damage and loss.

Trading One Pesticide for Many?

An additional aspect of efficacy that should be considered when weighing alterative pesticides is their specificity. For example, anthracnose is another fungal disease of lettuce that is controlled with pesticides. Controlled tests indicated that maneb and captan were effective in controlling anthracnose, while metalaxyl and aliette were not (Kurtz 1990). Restricting multiple-action compounds, which must then be replaced by several single-action pesticides, may increase the overall environmental burden of pesticides and the resulting human health risk. The current "one-at-a-time" focus of pesticide regulation can lead to a situation in which many pesticides, each with risks judged to be acceptable, are used on a single crop. The sum of these individually acceptable risks might be considered unacceptable. Current pesticide regulatory schemes do not address this problem.

Trading Off-Farm Risk for On-Farm Risk?

In some cases, efforts to reduce pesticide residues on foods can increase farm workers' exposure to pesticides. Pesticides that wash off foods more easily may also come off more readily on workers' hands. Pesticides that are less persistent in the environment may accumulate more quickly in the workplace or be more acutely toxic. As mentioned earlier, this has been the experience as DDT (moderately toxic but persistent) has been replaced by organophosphates (less persistent but acutely toxic to workers). Thus the beneficiaries of reduced residue and persistence—consumers and wildlife—may be enjoying the benefits of a risk transfer to farm workers. Farm workers are not fully protected by the EPA or the Occupational Safety and Health Administration (OSHA) (GAO 1992), and may be particularly vulnerable when they are migrant, low-income, minority workers who lack a political voice or the English skills to read labels.

Similarly, pesticides selected to reduce residue on foods may achieve that goal by evaporating prior to shipment, thus transferring risk from consumers to the atmosphere. For example, methyl bromide is widely used as a fumigant on crops, wood, and soils, in part because, although toxic, it leaves little or no residue to affect consumers (USDA 1992). But methyl bromide avoids leaving residue by evaporating, and in the upper atmosphere its bromine atoms contribute to depletion of the earth's stratospheric ozone layer, admitting increased ultraviolet radiation (UNEP 1992). (The risks of ozone depletion and ultraviolet radiation are discussed in Chapter 10.)

Trading Pesticide Risks for Nutrition Risks?

In addition to direct health risks from a pesticide and its replacements, an evaluation of overall risk should also consider the potential health effects due to changes in food consumption patterns that result from restriction of the pesticide use.

The use of pesticides has dramatically lowered the cost of food in the United States. Before 1950 the average family spent about 24 percent of its income on food, whereas today food occupies only about 12 percent of average family income. A part of this decrease in price may be attributed to pesticide use (Carpenter 1991). More to the point, economic studies indicate that restricting pesticides to reduce carcinogenic residues would likely raise the prices of foods significantly, in particular the prices of fruits and vegetables (Zilberman et al. 1991). For example, the price of "organically grown" broccoli in organic food stores is currently about four times the price of ordinary supermarket broccoli (Graham 1993). Although these price effects might be moderated in the longer term as alternative means of controlling pest losses were brought into use, the short-term price effect could be substantial.

If the prices of fruits and vegetables rose, the effect would be very regressive, with the largest impact on the poorest segment of the population. The risk tradeoff is that putting fresh fruits and vegetables out of the reach of poorer citizens may burden them with an even larger risk of disease than the pesticide residue presents. Consumption of fresh fruits and vegetables is associated with major reductions in the risk of heart disease and several types of cancer (Steinmetz and Potter 1991). Thus extremely stringent restrictions on pesticide residue may pose adverse countervailing risks, from both a net risk perspective and an environmental justice perspective.

Conclusion

The countervailing risks of regulating pesticides are so pervasive that a rigorous methodology of risk tradeoff analysis is required if EPA is to assure citizens a "safe, wholesome, and economic" food supply. The current one-at-a-time focus on the risks of individual pesticides may lead well-meaning decisions to cause perverse outcomes. The current system of pesticide regulation may be increasing rather than decreasing net risk. And it may be creating problems of environmental injustice, by shifting risk from the average consumer to disadvantaged segments of society such as farm workers and low-income families. In addition, EPA's one-chemical-at-a-time approach ensures that each chemical is replaced by another, instead of assessing the net risk of chemical and non-chemical options in a more coherent fashion (GAO 1991).

This tunnel vision can be corrected by a new form of risk tradeoff analysis that requires consideration of substitute risks and aggregates the overall risks of alternative methods of pest control for particular crops. Full consideration of all the risks posed by pest control options, through RTA, would highlight the need and opportunity for lower-risk methods of pest management. These may include better chemical pesticides as well as alternatives to chemical pesticides. For example, in some cases, biological methods (such as introducing bird-eating insects) or biotechnological methods (such as genetically engineering crop plants to erect their own defenses) may be as or more effective than chemical pesticides, especially when pest resistance is considered, and may pose lower risk to humans and the environment.

The methodology proposed here is in some ways a refinement of the improved analytic strategies being employed by EPA's Office of Pesticide Programs (Reinert et al. 1990). EPA analysts deserve credit for embarking on a more rigorous approach to risk-benefit analysis of pesticides in a political environment that appears to focus more on quick decisions than on decisions based on the use of good science. And recent initiatives by the current and preceding EPA Assistant Administrators for Pesticides, Lynn Goldman and Linda Fisher, have helped bring consideration of the relative risks of alternative pesticides into EPA's calculus. Goldman has considered the risk that would be posed by substitute pesticides in her decision whether to allow use of a candidate pesticide, and Fisher began a "safer pesticides" initiative to clarify the relative risks of different pest control options.

But EPA efforts are ultimately limited by the narrow, piecemeal approach taken in the pesticide statutes. Congress can
play a constructive role by reconciling the inconsistencies in
FIFRA and FFDCA in favor of a more comprehensive form of
risk analysis. The separate rules under FIFRA, FFDCA 408,
and FFDCA 409 (and its Delaney Clause) should be replaced
with a directive to EPA to license pest control methods to "reduce overall risk," entailing consideration of the several countervailing risks enumerated in this chapter. Non-chemical
methods (such as biotechnology) should be compared with
chemical pesticides on the basis of the overall risk of each
agent in each target environment, rather than put in a separate regulatory box erecting far higher hurdles simply based
on the technological process of production (NRC 1989; OSTP
1992). If Congress chooses instead (as it has recently been
urged) to mandate more simplistic approaches to pesticide
regulation, such as tolerances based on predetermined cancer
risk levels (for example, "one in a million") without regard to
the countervailing risks and benefits of alternative pesticides,
then the result may just as likely be an overall decrement
rather than an improvement in public health and environmental quality.

10

Protecting the Global Environment

JONATHAN BAERT WIENER

Protecting the global environment is now a major challenge of public policy and international diplomacy. An international agreement to phase out chemicals that may deplete the stratospheric ozone layer was signed in 1987 and beefed up in the 1990s. International agreements aimed at conserving biodiversity, avoiding adverse climate change, and reducing deforestation were signed at the "Earth Summit"—the U.N. Conference on Environment and Development held in Rio de Janeiro in June 1992.

But proclaiming a global environmental goal through an international agreement or a national law does not guarantee success in reducing overall risk to the global environment. The potential for unexpected risk tradeoffs, so evident in the preceding chapters regarding specific domestic policies, is exacerbated where policy must address multiple activities and effluents arising in virtually every sector of human endeavor in every country. The pathways through which risks may shift, plentiful enough at the micro level, only proliferate at the global level.

This chapter surveys several, but by no means all, of the risk tradeoffs associated with policy to protect the global environment. Each of these risk tradeoffs could make a full case study on its own, and experts familiar with each problem may find the presentation here too brief. The purpose of this chapter is not to settle the debate on any particular issue, but simply to show the ubiquity and complexity of the risk tradeoffs that face those seeking to safeguard the health of the earth, and to begin exploring how international institutions might weigh the most important target and countervailing global risks.

We examine here the two target risks to the global environment that have been of paramount recent concern: ozone depletion and potential global warming. It may turn out that the largest environmental risk facing the world is something else, such as the collision of an asteroid with the earth (Kerr 1992; Hoyle 1991), or disease due to poor local water quality (World Bank 1992), but ozone depletion and the "greenhouse effect" have dramatically captivated international and national policymaking attention. By applying the tools of risk tradeoff analysis, we seek to illuminate the array of countervailing risks confronting policymakers working to combat these two threats, and we suggest potential "risk-superior" moves that might address the target risk without unacceptably increasing countervailing risks.

The Threat of Ozone Depletion

If the theoretical predictions and empirical observations are correct, one of the most dire threats to the global environment is the potential depletion of the ozone layer high in the earth's stratosphere. This layer of ozone (O_3) molecules, 20 to 50 kilometers above the planet's surface, shields the earth from the sun's ultraviolet (UV) radiation (WMO 1991; Solomon and Albritton 1992). But in the mid-1980s scientists discovered a seasonal "hole" in the ozone layer around the South Pole (Farman et al. 1985). Recent observations and new understandings of middle-atmosphere chemistry suggest that ozone depletion has been occurring faster and more pervasively than previously thought, not only creating a springtime "hole" above Antarctica but also thinning the ozone shield significantly (perhaps 5 percent or more) over temperate latitudes in spring and summer months (WMO 1991).

If short wavelength UV-B or UV-C radiation increases at the earth's surface when the ozone layer is depleted, as evidence is beginning to confirm (Crutzen 1992; Kerr et al. 1993), that may entail damage to cell function and DNA in humans, plants, animals, phytoplankton, and other critical elements of the global food web (German Bundestag 1989, pp. 308–320; Smith et al. 1992). The sensitivity of organisms to UV varies enormously (Stevens 1992). If UV-B or UV-C radiation increases, there could be higher rates of skin cancer, immune system disorders, cataracts, and other illnesses among humans (Monasterksy 1992). For plants, one five-year study found that a simulated 25 percent reduction in the ozone layer was associated with roughly a 20 percent decline in soybean production (German Bundestag 1989, pp. 315–316), although that study showed increased growth during water stress, and other studies with other species have shown lesser effects (Stevens 1992). Researchers trying to solve the mysterious worldwide decline in populations of many frogs and other amphibians have recently discovered a possible link to ozone depletion, because amphibian eggs appear to be damaged by increased UV-B (Yoon 1994). Perhaps most disturbing is the evidence that the springtime "ozone hole" over Antarctica in 1990 (up to 50 percent reductions in the ozone layer) was correlated with a 6 to 12 percent decline in the primary productivity of marine phytoplankton inside the hole (Smith et al. 1992). Marine phytoplankton are the basic resource of the oceanic food web, producing about 60 billion tonnes of vegetable solids per year, or about twice the total annual production by terrestrial plants (German Bundestag 1989, p. 317).

Reducing Ozone Depletion

The primary culprit in this global risk appears to be the increased production of chlorofluorocarbons (CFCs) over the past several decades. In 1974 two chemists theorized that CFCs could rise to the stratosphere and be broken apart by the sun's UV radiation, freeing the CFCs' highly reactive chlorine atoms to destroy ozone molecules (Molina and Rowland 1974). In the 1980s, empirical observations of trends in upper-atmosphere chlorine levels supported this hypothesis, and the discovery of very rapid "heterogeneous" reactions between solid chlorine ions (frozen on stratospheric ice clouds) and gaseous ozone helped explain how ozone depletion could be occurring so quickly (WMO 1991).

The threat of global ozone depletion was soon identified as a target risk warranting international policy action, though negotiations progressed somewhat deliberately until the scientific evidence of the ozone "hole" spurred a decisive response. In the 1987 Montreal Protocol, the major CFC-producing and using nations agreed to phase out 50 percent of their use of CFCs by the year 2000; that has since been advanced to a 100 percent phaseout by 1995.

The Target Risk in Historical Perspective

Ironically, today's target risk—the problem of CFCs depleting the ozone layer—is itself a countervailing risk of steps taken in the 1930s to deal with a target risk of that era. CFCs were unveiled in 1930 by Thomas Midgely, a General Motors scientist and later president of the American Chemical Society, with the promise to be a wonder chemical: a nontoxic, nonflammable coolant that could replace the highly toxic ammonia compounds used in refrigeration (Weiner 1990, p. 45; Hallett 1993). Their inert nature soon lead to uses as fire extinguishers and later as cleaning fluids for silicon computer chips.

It was the same inert quality of CFCs that made them a solution to the target risk of toxicity that then created the countervailing risk of ozone depletion. Because CFCs do not react with other compounds, they leave humans unharmed by exposure and rise to the stratosphere intact. Only under the intense bombardment of solar UV radiation high in the stratosphere do CFCs break down, liberating chlorine ions, which attack the ozone. That risk transformation was not recognized until the 1970s.

Curiously and conversely, efforts to reduce concentrations

of ground-level ozone—the key component of urban smog—are now being reevaluated in light of findings that ground-level ozone, like its stratospheric counterpart, helps shield those underneath from elevated UV radiation (Bruhl and Crutzen 1989; Crutzen 1992, pp. 104–105). Researchers have observed 40 to 80 percent higher UV levels in New Zealand, with clean air, than in Germany, with smoggy air, even controlling for differences in latitude, stratospheric ozone density, and other factors (Seckmeyer 1992). Yet ground-level ozone may have deleterious effects on human health (Krupnick and Portney 1991, pp. 523–525), and it has been estimated that the currently elevated levels of tropospheric ozone in the United States are impairing crop productivity and damaging forests (Mooney et al. 1991, p. 96). At least some locales will need to face the question whether the protection from UV (and the attendant risks of cancer, immune disorders, and other maladies) that is afforded by ground-level ozone could make it worthwhile to tolerate the increased lung, crop, and forest ailments.

Countervailing Risks

Meanwhile, the phaseout of CFCs, aimed at the target risk of global ozone depletion, is turning out to pose its own countervailing risks. The substitutes for CFCs in refrigeration, cleaning silicon chips, and other applications will in most cases be compounds with similar properties: hydrochlorofluorocarbons (HCFCs), which contain much less chlorine than CFCs and deplete ozone at roughly a tenth the potency of CFCs (WMO 1991; Solomon and Albritton 1992) and hydrofluorocarbons (HFCs), which contain no chlorine and pose no ozone depletion risk.

But HCFCs and HFCs pose other problems. First, some of these compounds are toxic, at least to laboratory animals (Naj 1991), renewing the original concern that led CFCs to replace ammonia. Second, using HCFCs for refrigeration can be significantly more costly than using CFCs, up to five times the price (Weisskopf 1992). This may be a small issue in industrialized countries, but it is a critical issue of public health risk in poorer countries. Unless other steps are taken, a great deal of new CFC use is forecast to occur in China, India, and other developing countries as they make refrigeration available to their two-billion-plus populations. From the perspective of those countries, the target risk of most vital concern is food spoilage, which afflicts millions of people annually through hunger, malnutrition, and food-borne disease (World Bank 1992). As they see it, switching from CFCs to HCFCs at the behest of industrialized countries could slow their campaigns for widespread refrigeration, and CFC-induced ozone depletion is a risk transformation—a different issue largely affecting other countries' populations. From the perspective of many in industrialized nations and environmental groups, the target risk is global ozone depletion, and increased CFC use in developing countries would pose a risk offset—the same risk imposed globally—thus providing these wealthier countries strong incentives to assist the developing countries to make the transition to refrigeration without increasing the use of CFCs.

Third, switching to HCFCs and HFCs to reduce ozone depletion may pose an increased risk of a different environmental threat: global warming. Scientists at first believed that CFCs themselves, for reasons distinct from their effect on the stratospheric ozone layer, were a potent greenhouse gas (Ramanathan 1975). The direct "radiative forcing" effect of CFCs (the ability to trap heat in the atmosphere) is extremely powerful—several thousand times that of carbon dioxide (CO_2), the most abundant "greenhouse gas," per unit of emissions—and CFCs tend to reside in the atmosphere for many decades, giving them a very high direct "global warming potential" (IPCC 1990a; see Table 10.1). Global warming potential or GWP is an integrated measure of a compound's radiative forcing and its expected residence time in the atmosphere. Thus, despite their small volume in the atmosphere, CFCs were estimated to account for as much as 25 percent of the human contribution to radiative forcing over the period 1980–1990 (see Table 10.2).

HCFCs and HFCs also have significant GWP. The direct GWP of HCFCs and HFCs is, very roughly, about a fifth of that of the CFCs they would replace (IPCC 1990a, table 2.8). The twist is that it now appears that CFCs, in addition to their direct GWP, also produce surprisingly powerful indirect cooling effects, by depleting ozone in the lower as well as the upper stratosphere. Because the lower stratosphere ozone is itself a significant greenhouse gas, its depletion by CFCs exerts a negative influence on potential warming. Globally averaged, the cooling from CFCs' depletion of lower stratosphere ozone appears to roughly offset the warming effect from CFCs' direct radiative forcing (WMO 1991; Ramaswamy 1992). This new finding suggests that CFCs in the global aggregate may have no net global warming potential (IPCC 1992) (though the indirect cooling effect, and hence the net GWP of CFCs, varies with latitude [Kiehl 1992]).

Thus if CFCs are close to a wash in terms of GWP, and HCFCs and HFCs still pose significant GWP (since they do not deplete lower stratosphere ozone to a comparable degree), it appears that replacing CFCs with HCFCs and HFCs could

Table 10.1 IPCC "global warming potential" (GWP) indices[a] for selected greenhouse gases

Gas	Relative instantaneous radiative forcing (per kg)	Typical atmospheric residence time (estimated years)	GWP: relative radiative forcing potential over years		
			20	100	500
CO_2	1	120	1	1	1
CH_4[a,b]	58	10	63	21	9
N_2O	206	150	270	290	190
CFC-11[a]	3,970	60	4,500	3,500	1,500
CFC-12[a]	5,750	130	7,100	7,300	4,500

Source: Adapted from IPCC Scientific Assessment, 1990, tables 2.3, 2.8.

a. In light of new scientific information acquired since the 1990 IPCC Assessment, IPCC science panels have revised the GWPs for CFCs downward (toward zero), and have revised the GWP for CH_4 upward (above 21 toward 30, for a 100-year time horizon). The 1994 Interim IPCC Report and 1995 IPCC Second Assessment Report will further clarify the state of knowledge.

b. Including indirect effects of CH_4 on tropospheric O_3, CO_2, and stratospheric H_2O.

pose an unexpected risk substitution: greatly reducing ozone depletion but somewhat increasing contributions to potential global warming.

Weighing the Risks

The various risk tradeoffs involved in the use of CFCs are illustrated in Table 10.3. These results do not necessarily counsel changes in plans to phase out CFCs. Evaluating the risk tradeoffs requires weighing the various risks according to the factors enumerated in Chapter 1, such as their severity, imminence, and certainty. If it is correct that the depletion of stratospheric ozone due to CFCs is a well-documented and highly hazardous phenomenon occurring now, while any greenhouse warming due to HCFCs and HFCs is more distant and uncertain, it may make sense to continue phasing out CFCs despite the potential increase in warming from CFC-substitutes. The prospect of continued mortality and morbidity due to food spoilage in developing countries may be a more grave concern, and warrants further study.

Table 10.2   Radiative forcing in the 1980s

Gas	Share (%)
Carbon dioxide	55
CFCs (11 and 12)[a]	17
CFCs (other)[a]	7
Methane[b]	15
Nitrous oxide	6

Source: Adapted from IPCC Scientific Assessment, 1990, Policymakers' Summary, p. xx. (The contribution from ozone and its precursors may also be significant, but was not quantified by the IPCC.)

a. These estimates were based on the direct warming effect of CFCs only, and did not account for later findings of an offsetting cooling effect due to CFCs. In light of new scientific information acquired since the 1990 IPCC Assessment, IPCC science panels have revised the net GWPs for CFCs downward (toward zero).

b. Estimated using a 100-year GWP for methane (CH_4) of 21 relative to carbon dioxide (CO_2). In light of new scientific information acquired since the 1990 IPCC Assessment, IPCC science panels have revised the GWP for CH_4 upward (above 21 toward 30, for a 100-year time horizon).

The Environmental Protection Agency is recognizing the need to weigh these risk tradeoffs in its policy to replace CFCs with substitute HCFCs and HFCS. Under a congressional directive to give preference to substitutes that "reduce overall risk" (Clean Air Act, section 612(c)), EPA is proposing to evaluate alternative substances within a "comparative risk framework," taking account of their ozone depletion potential, toxicity, contribution to global warming, effects on water and air quality, and effects on workplace health and safety (EPA 1993). Although EPA proposes to weigh these factors qualitatively, rather than calculating a quantitative index of net risk, this proposal comes very close to employing a method of risk tradeoff analysis that we are suggesting in this volume.

Toward Risk-Superior Moves

There may also be ways to phase out CFCs without incurring unacceptable countervailing risks. Risk tradeoff analysis highlights the possibilities for such risk-superior moves. For example, under the Montreal Protocol, an assistance fund has already been created to help developing countries meet the costs of refrigerating while avoiding increased use of CFCs.

Table 10.3 Risk tradeoffs in use of CFCs and substitutes

Technology	Toxicity	Cost	Approximate[a] ODP	Approximate[a] GWP 1990 est.	1992 est.
Ammonia (to 1930s)	high	low	—	—	—
CFCs (1930–2000)	none	med.	1.0	5,000	0
HCFCs (1990–)	some?	high	0.1	1,200	900
HFCs (1995–)	?	high	0.0	1,000	1,000

Sources: See text.

a. Figures for ODP and GWP are *illustrative approximations* of the median estimate for each class of compounds, and do *not* represent precise estimates for specific substances.

This fund is modest in size, but it may help jump-start the diffusion of non-CFC technologies to developing countries before they refrigerate extensively. Or it may need to be supplemented with additional arrangements, such as some form of market-based incentive to spur private-sector cooperative arrangements to transfer non-CFC technologies.

New technologies might also be developed that operate without using CFCs at all, such as aqueous cleaning solutions and desiccant cooling systems. Or equipment might be designed that does not leak HCFCs and HFCs to the atmosphere. Although these technologies could help replace CFCs without posing a global warming risk from increased HCFC and HFC releases, they are likely to be even more costly, thus exacerbating the dilemma of refrigeration in poorer countries.

The Threat of Global Warming

The other global atmospheric risk of greatest concern has been the threat of global warming or the "greenhouse effect." After three decades of cooling global temperatures, measurements began rising in the mid-1970s, with particularly rapid warming in the 1980s (Jones and Wigley 1990). Evidence from ice cores indicates that "greenhouse gas" concentrations in the atmosphere and surface temperature have been closely correlated over the last 160,000 years (Schneider 1989b, p. 40). Enormous computer models constructed to forecast the effect of increasing levels of greenhouse gases such as carbon dioxide (CO_2) on the earth's climate predict that if the amount of CO_2 in the atmosphere doubled from its preindustrial level (about 275 parts per million [ppm]), global temperature would rise about 1.5 to 4.5 degrees centigrade—a larger change than recorded in the last 10,000 years (Schneider 1989). However, numerous uncertainties and gaps in the computer models have made these forecasts subject to challenge and periodic recalculation, and debate has raged over the likelihood that global warming will occur (for example, see Balling 1992). There has also been controversy over the potential consequences of global warming, with some fearing a "runaway greenhouse" that would turn the earth into an uninhabitable

Venus (Chandler 1992) and others seeing potential benefit in the longer growing seasons that a warmer world might bring (Gribbin 1982).

Political Salience and Scientific Uncertainties

Public attention to the long-run potential mega-risks of a greenhouse planet seems to have been driven less by important changes in scientific understanding of the global climate than by very short-run, transient, local temperature events. Public anxiety about global warming peaked during the hot summer of 1988, when droughts hit the midwestern United States and Congress held hearings on whether the heat might be a result of global warming under way (Schneider 1988, p. 35; Hirsh 1988). Yet these short-term trends are within the range of natural climate variation (IPCC 1990a) and say little to nothing about the potential for sustained future changes in global climate that would be of real importance. (When Mt. Pinatubo's eruption yielded a bout of temporary cooling in the 1990s, public fears of a greenhouse effect waned, even though the underlying risk of long-term global warming was not affected.)

Partly in order to surmount such short-term politics, nations organized the Intergovernmental Panel on Climate Change (IPCC) in 1989 to produce a consensus scientific report on the issue. The mainstream scientific view coalesced on a fair degree of confidence that global warming would be promoted by continuing increases in atmospheric greenhouse gas concentrations (IPCC 1990a). But the IPCC noted that the slight warming observed in this century (about 0.5 degrees C) might just be natural variation; that when run on historical data, the computer models tended to overpredict warming by about a factor of 2; and that the computer models did not do a good job of representing the dynamics of major climate parameters such as the oceans and clouds. Thus the IPCC cautioned that any actual greenhouse effect might be at the low end of the forecast 1.5 to 4.5-degree range for a doubling of atmospheric CO_2, and that the temperature change might be lagged several decades after the doubling of CO_2 levels. In addition, the IPCC envisioned a wide variety of impacts of global warming on human and non-human communities, many adverse but some beneficial (IPCC 1990b). The debate about impacts turned from the level of ultimate temperature change to the rate of warming, which some thought the oceans would moderate (Balling 1992, p. 44), but which others feared might be so rapid that it could cause wrenching dislocations and outstrip the ability of ecosystems to adapt (IPCC 1990b; NAS 1991b; Peters and Lovejoy 1992).

Since the late 1980s and the first IPCC report, several new findings have suggested a more complex, and possibly less pessimistic, outlook. While climatologists' models continue to forecast a 1.5 to 4.5-degree C rise in average surface temperature for a doubling of preindustrial greenhouse gas concentrations, the fundamental questions of the rate, timing, and magnitude of potential warming remain highly uncertain (IPCC 1992). Model calculations of the sea-level rise resulting from a given level of warming have successively declined as the models have incorporated more realistic ocean-atmosphere couplings. There is now empirical evidence that the modest 0.5-degree C warming of the last century is occurring mostly at night and in the winter, hence softening rather than worsening climate variations (Karl 1991; Rensberger 1993). It is now well recognized that in addition to CO_2, several other greenhouse gases—among them methane (CH_4) and nitrous oxides (N_2O)—are also important contributors (Ramanathan 1985; see Tables 10.1 and 10.2). And further study has indicated that particulates (such as sulfur pollution) are helping to reflect heat away from the earth, suggesting that continued emissions of these pollutants may be offsetting a substantial share of the warming effect of greenhouse gas pollution (IPCC 1992; Wigley 1991). Moreover, since the chlorofluorocarbons (CFCs), formerly the most potent greenhouse gases, are now believed to be greenhouse-neutral (as discussed earlier), the estimate of total greenhouse forcing contributed by human activities has been cut by about 25 percent (IPCC 1992; WMO 1991). The last decade's debate over the physics of climate models, including ocean-atmosphere heat transfer, cloud formation, and solar variations (Stone 1992), is now being followed by a new era of uncertainties in the staggeringly complicated atmospheric chemistry of greenhouse gases (Kiehl 1992).

Action to Prevent Global Warming

Policymakers cannot wait endlessly for "all the evidence to come in," since the evidence is never all in: we are always learning more and always making decisions in the face of some uncertainty. The combination of complex and uncertain scientific information with political and economic pressures on all sides helped shape governments' negotiation of the Framework Convention on Climate Change, which was signed at the 1992 U.N. Earth Summit in Rio de Janeiro.

The convention cites global warming as its target risk and, in somewhat contorted language, calls on industrialized countries to aim to return their emissions of greenhouse gases to their 1990 level by the year 2000. Developing countries are not bound to limit their emissions, but they are encouraged to move to lower-emissions paths of economic growth, and are offered financial resources and technology transfer to assist in that transition.

Countervailing Risks of Preventing Global Warming

There are some countervailing risks of reducing global warming, irrespective of the type of policy that is used to achieve that goal.

Impacts of Warming. An enhanced global greenhouse effect would likely bring adverse impacts for various communities, but it could also bring benefits to some. Global warming could lead to myriad environmental changes, including altered precipitation patterns, sea level rise, and shifting agricultural and forest zones (IPCC 1990a; IPCC 1990b; IPCC 1992). Ecosystems might have great difficulty adapting to rapid changes in temperature, rainfall, wind, and habitat zones (Peters and Lovejoy 1992; WWF 1992). Some of the effects, such as sea level rise in low-lying developing countries, could have important distributional impacts even if their aggregate damage is comparatively low (Glantz 1991). At the upper bound, few experts fear a "runaway" greenhouse effect spurred by positive feedbacks (Schneider 1989b, pp. 37–38), but there is concern about unpleasant "surprises" (such as reversals of ocean currents) which could entail abrupt increases in the damage to societies and ecosystems (Schneider 1989a, pp. 78–79; Schelling 1991, p. 204).

The impacts of warming on agriculture are worth examining because of the importance of farming to human survival and its sensitivity to climatic change. Greenhouse warming would be likely to alter both the total amount and the distribution of food production. It could harm farmers and food consumers in some parts of the world, and benefit others.

Historically, the warm "Medieval Optimum" around 900–1000 A.D., when average temperatures were about 1 degree C warmer than the present, was especially generous for world agriculture, while the "Little Ice Age" of 1650–1850, when average temperatures in the northern hemisphere were 1–2 degrees C cooler than today, was decidedly uncongenial (Schneider 1989b, pp. 61–62; Bernard 1980, p. 127).

Looking to the future, the computerized "general circulation models" (GCMs) used to forecast the climate indicate that some areas (such as southern Europe and central North America) might experience declining crop yields as global warming raises temperature and reduces precipitation, while other areas (such as northern Europe, Russia, Australia, and China) could enjoy significant crop yield increases (IPCC 1990b, pp. 2.7–2.17; Kane et al. 1992a, 1992b). For the United States, tests with two GCMs indicate that a 3 to 4-degree C warming could bring yield declines of about 24–54 percent for dry corn, 26 percent for irrigated corn, 35–60 percent for dry soybeans, and 16–31 percent for dry winter wheat (Kane et al. 1992a, p. 120, citing Smith and Tirpak 1989); but other studies have predicted smaller yield declines in this country (for example, Dudek 1987), or even some increases (Brookes 1990, citing IPCC/Coolfont report). Meanwhile, comparable increases in crop yields could occur in areas around the globe favored by changing climate (Adams, Rosenzweig, et al. 1990; Kane et al. 1992a, pp. 121–122; Brookes 1990, citing IPCC/Coolfont report).

Several factors make these crop yield predictions uncertain. These modeling exercises try to depict the effect of warming resulting from a doubling of preindustrial greenhouse gas concentrations by the mid-twenty-first century, but if there were further warming as concentrations kept rising, that might generate larger crop yield declines (Cline 1992, pp. 100–101; Pearce 1992). On the other hand, even the most negative yield changes noted above are more optimistic than previous estimates (for example, the older studies relied on by Cline 1992, p. 98). More importantly, the GCM-based estimates do not account for any farmer adaptation to warming, or for increases in farm productivity over time, both of which have been enormously important over the past 100 years and could well moderate predicted crop yield declines (Kane et al. 1992a, p. 129). Model runs that incorporate farmer adaptation to changing relative crop prices during warming (Dudek 1987; Adams, Rosenzweig, et al. 1990) and an empirical study of the warming that occurred in the 1930s (Rosenberg et al. 1991) all show much smaller crop yield declines in the United States than do the simple GCM runs. In addition, the GCM-based forecasts do not fully account for the recent finding that essentially all of the observed 0.3 to 0.6-degree C warming of the last fifty years has been an increase in minimum (nighttime and winter) temperature and not in maximum temperature (Karl et al. 1991), suggesting that gradual warming may smooth out temperature extremes, reduce crop freezes, and perhaps facilitate agricultural productivity (Rensberger 1993).

Changes in crop yields, however, do not translate directly into changes in overall agricultural output value or overall social well-being. Simply multiplying predicted yield changes by the value of output in the base year, without accounting for attendant price changes, readjustments via international trade in agricultural products, and the gain to producers as well as the loss to consumers that would occur if yields fell and prices rose, can exaggerate the real damages to farming under global warming. Analysts accounting for these factors have found that, assuming a hypothetical yield decline of even 50 percent in the United States, Canada, and the European Community (EC), no change in yields in Russia, northern Europe, China, Japan, Australia, Brazil, and Argentina, and a 25 percent decline in yields in the rest of the world (that is, the remaining developing countries), the net effect on world gross domestic product (GDP) would be a loss of only 0.40 percent (Kane et al. 1992a, p. 127). Using the smaller yield changes estimated by more recent models to occur under gradual global warming (that is, yield declines of perhaps 0–20 percent in the U.S./Canada/EC and gains in the other major crop exporters), the effects on world GDP are essentially zero: from a 0.07 percent loss to a 0.06 percent gain (Kane et al. 1992a).

Thus global warming might have no adverse impact on world agriculture in the aggregate, although it could cause significant risk transfers from some farming areas to others (Adams, Rosenzweig, et al. 1990). It bears repeating that these estimates of the impacts of warming relate only to its effects on agriculture, not on other sectors such as coasts, forests, and ocean ecosystems.

Global Cooling. In addition to the direct benefits of warming that would be foregone, concern has been expressed that preventing global warming might accelerate global cooling toward the next ice age. Not long ago, the global environmental risk enjoying the most attention was not global warming but global cooling. Most climatologists agree that over the next thousand years or more, the earth is headed toward a cooler period, perhaps an ice age; the climate of the present millennium is warmer than it has been since the last major ice age receded about 15,000 years ago, and long-term cycles in the earth's tilt, rotation, and revolution suggest that the planet may again be approaching a glacial period (Schneider 1989b, pp. 38–40). The transient cooling in the middle of this century made many observers worry that the next ice age might be upon us (Ponte 1976; Hoyle 1981; Gribbin 1982, p. 51; Schneider 1989b, p. 64; Will 1992), disrupting weather and food-growing areas and perhaps decimating much of the planet's life-supporting areas (Budyko 1982, pp. 278–285; Ponte 1976, p. 237). As noted, the Little Ice Age in the 1800s was particularly hard on world food output. Some therefore fear that action to curtail potential greenhouse warming could trigger more rapid onset of an ice age (Gribbin 1982), while others argue that global warming in the nearer term (the next 100 years) would not affect ice ages that move on the scale of thousands of years (Bernard 1980, p. 23). With the hot spell of the 1980s, popular attention began to shift away from the ice age risk to focus on warming; but the underlying tradeoff—a potential risk substitution of planetary proportions—may remain important over the longer term.

Countervailing Risks of Narrow Policies to Prevent Global Warming

Putting aside the pros and cons of preventing global warming and assuming that such action is in the world's best interests, countervailing risks may still arise from the narrow policy prescriptions that nations have put forward in the rush to act. Some of these policies pose other risks (risk substitutions or transformations), while some could cause as much or more global warming than they prevent (risk offsets).

Cross-Gas Shifts. Policies to reduce CO_2 emissions could inadvertently cause risk-offsetting increases in emissions of other greenhouse gases. Before the Framework Convention on Climate Change signed at the Earth Summit committed its signatories to address all greenhouse gases, most proposals by national governments to curb potential global warming focused specifically on limiting emissions of carbon dioxide (CO_2) from fossil fuel combustion (MacNeill 1991, pp. 75–77, 97; Dower and Zimmerman 1992). CO_2 is the most abundant anthropogenic greenhouse gas, so it is an obvious first target for greenhouse policies. For example, in 1990 Germany declared a goal of reducing its CO_2 emissions 30 percent from 1990 levels by 2005 (MacNeill et al. 1991, p. 97), and in late 1991 the environment and energy ministers of the European Community proposed a plan to impose a CO_2 tax on all EC energy consumption (Lascelles 1992; BNA 1991).

Policies singling out CO_2 for control would likely induce some electric power producers to switch from burning high-

CO_2 coal to burning low-CO_2 natural gas. Some observers have expressly urged that coal "be replaced by [natural gas] whenever possible" (Levenson 1989, p. 205), and several countries have proposed requiring a switch from coal to natural gas as key parts of their domestic plans to limit CO_2 emissions (Netherlands 1990, sec. 3.2.1., p. 6; German Bundestag 1990). More generally, imposition of a constraint or tax on CO_2 emissions would likely lead energy markets to undertake considerable fuel-switching from coal toward natural gas (DOE 1990, pp. 26, 29; CBO 1990, pp. 27–30, 44; EC 1991a; Dudek and LeBlanc 1990, pp. 38–39). In Europe, natural gas supplies would come primarily from the former Soviet Republics (EC 1991, pp. 35–38).

But CO_2 is only one of several greenhouse gases, which also include methane (CH_4) and nitrous oxides (N_2O). Per unit of emissions, CO_2 is the least potent of these gases in causing global warming (see Table 10.1). The difficulty with policies spurring a switch from coal to natural gas is that natural gas is about 90 percent methane, and in some places leakage of CH_4 from natural gas wells, pipelines, and other systems is substantial. The CO_2/CH_4 risk offset can be quantified. With current combustion techniques, burning coal generally produces almost twice as much CO_2 per BTU (unit of energy) than burning natural gas (Rodhe 1990, p. 1218). CH_4 is a much more potent greenhouse gas per unit than CO_2, with a global warming potential (GWP) of about 20 relative to CO_2, over a 100-year period (see Table 10.1). And the 1995 IPCC Second Assessment, when published, is likely to raise the GWP of methane relative to CO_2 even higher, toward 30. Thus seemingly low CH_4 leakage rates can offset large CO_2 reductions. If CH_4 has twenty times the GWP of CO_2, then about a 6 percent rate of CH_4 leakage from natural gas systems would negate all of the CO_2-related savings in GWP accomplished by switching from coal to natural gas (Rodhe 1990, p. 1217.) If CH_4 has a GWP higher than 20, the break-even leakage rate would be lower than 6 percent.

As depicted in Figure 10.1, a policy to restrict CO_2 alone (such as an EC tax on CO_2), by encouraging a switch from high-CO_2 coal to lower-CO_2 natural gas, could actually boost

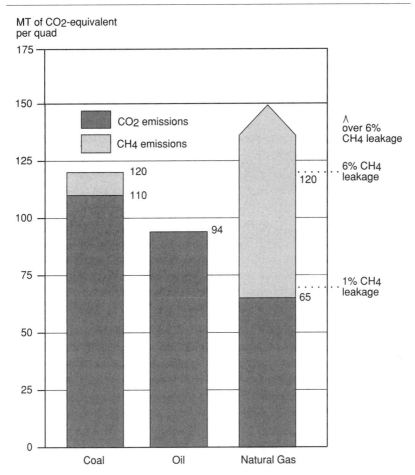

Figure 10.1 Net global warming potential (GWP) from fuel switching, expressed in megatonnes (MT) of CO_2-equivalent emissions generated per quad (quadrillion BTUs of energy produced). This depiction assumes conservatively (see text) that the GWP (100-year warming potential per tonne of emissions) for CH_4 is only 20 (relative to CO_2 = 1). See IPCC Scientific Assessment 1990, table 2.8. The calculations are based on Rodhe 1990.

a net *increase* in potential global warming where CH_4 leakage rates exceed the 6 percent break-even point. Actual CH_4 leakage from natural gas systems can often exceed 6 percent. Unless remedial action is taken to reduce leaks, EC imports of natural gas from Russia would entail CH_4 leaks of 4 to 10 percent (Rabchuk and Ilkevich 1991; Arbatov 1990), quite possibly averaging 6 percent or higher (Hogan et al. 1991, p. 182). Worldwide (including developing countries), CH_4 leakage from gas systems could be as high as 6 to 9 percent (Crutzen 1991). Even in industrialized countries, CH_4 leakage rates can be high: in the U.K. the range is a surprising 1 to 11 percent (Wallis 1991, p. 428), with a conservative best estimate of the national average falling somewhere between 5.3 and 10.8 percent (Mitchell et al. 1990, pp. 809–818). In Australia, leaks are said to average 3 percent (Falk and Brownlow 1989, p. 270). The CH_4 leakage rate in the U.S. natural gas system is estimated at only about 1 to 2 percent (Hoffman 1991).

Reducing CO_2 by switching from coal to other fuels could also pose a second risk offset, not reflected in Figure 10.1, because sulfur particulates emitted in coal combustion exert a cooling influence on the earth by reflecting solar radiation (IPCC 1992, pp. 20–21; Wigley 1991). Burning natural gas emits a much smaller quantity of these particulates than burning coal, and of course nuclear power, hydropower, and solar/wind power emit no sulfur particulates. Thus, wholly apart from the tradeoff between reduced CO_2 and increased CH_4 from natural gas, switching from coal use to other fuels could yield a net increase in relative warming influence in the short term because of the declining emissions of reflective sulfur particulates (Wigley 1991, p. 505). Indeed, recent analysis under the central emissions scenario used by the IPCC indicates that the sulfur effect alone is so important that replacing coal with no-sulfur energy technologies would actually cause a net increase in average global temperature through the year 2050 (though a net decrease after 2050, when long-lasting CO_2 begins to outweigh the more transient effects of sulfur) (Edmonds et al. 1994). Of course, controlling sulfur emissions can have important regional benefits in risk reduction, such as reducing acid precipitation (NAPAP 1991) and reducing the human health effects of particulate air pollution (Dockery et al. 1993). Thus, from the perspective of sulfur emission control, important risk substitutions and transformations need to be weighed.

From the perspective of global warming prevention, high CH_4 leaks and declining sulfur particulate emissions could mean that policies to restrict CO_2 by inducing switching from coal to natural gas would cause a global risk offset by increasing net global warming, at least in the short term. Although the effect of decreased CO_2 would likely dominate over the long term (given the long residence time of CO_2 in the atmosphere), the increased *rate* of global warming in the short term could be more important to sensitive ecological systems.

Cross-Border Shifts. The greenhouse gases mix globally in the atmosphere, so emissions anywhere on the planet contribute to an aggregate global effect. A wide variety of sources and sinks (removal mechanisms) of greenhouse gases is susceptible to human influence. These sources and sinks occur in every sector, from industry to agriculture to forestry, and they are widely distributed around the globe (IPCC 1990c). Limits on emissions imposed on one group of emitters will only be effective if they translate into reductions in overall global emissions.

Yet the major proposals to limit greenhouse gas emissions generally provide that such action shall be taken first, or only, by the industrialized countries—typically the members of the Organization for Economic Cooperation and Development (OECD). Even without additional policy restrictions, the emissions of the OECD members are fast becoming a minority of global CO_2 and CH_4 emissions. If current trends continue, the OECD members will account for less than 30 percent of global emissions by 2025 (Leggett 1992). Stabilizing OECD member country emissions of CO_2 at 1990 levels after 2000—the most common proposal—would reduce global CO_2 emissions by only a few percent from baseline forecast emissions in 2020 (DOE 1990, pp. 19–21); by 2025 the OECD countries could not keep global emissions from growing even if they eliminated 100 percent of their own emissions (Bradley et al. 1991, p. II-10.7).

Against this backdrop, limitations on emissions in the OECD countries could be frustrated by cross-border "leakage" of emitting activities to other locales where no restrictions apply. The first type of leakage is short-term: if the industrialized nations reduced their consumption of fossil fuels, world prices of those fuels would fall, leading to increased quantities consumed in other nations where limits on emissions were not in place (DOE 1990, p. 27). One econometric simulation of unilateral action to reduce U.S. CO_2 emissions by about 15 percent indicates that this short-term price effect would offset about 20 percent of the planned savings in the United States (Bradley et al. 1991, pp. II-10.7–10.8). A model of an oil tax ($10/barrel in 2000, rising to $23/barrel in 2007) imposed in all OECD member countries found a 33 percent offset through increased oil consumption elsewhere (Reinsch and Considine 1992). A model of stabilizing EC country CO_2 emissions by 2000 found an 11 percent offset in the total CO_2 emission reduction; in that estimate, part of the increase in emissions from cheaper oil consumption outside the EC was itself offset by a slower transition away from oil to higher-CO_2 coal supplies in areas like China (Burniaux et al. 1992, p. 15).

Over the longer term, the immediate price-driven offset would be magnified by a second type of leakage: emissions-intensive activities would increasingly relocate in unregulated areas and export their products back to the regulated areas. Taken together, the price effect and the capital mobility effect could substantially undercut efforts by a subgroup of emitters to affect global emission trends. If the OECD members attempted to impose significant reductions in emissions, some models indicate that the short- and long-term effects in combination could drive the marginal rate of offsetting geographic leakage to nearly 100 percent (Rutherford 1992).

Countervailing Risks from Non-Warming Impacts

Each of the greenhouse gases has other impacts on the environment besides its impact on global temperature. In addition to its potential impact on the planet's heat balance, CO_2 stimulates the growth and water use efficiency of plants. Thus, policies to reduce levels of CO_2 in the atmosphere may pose a risk transformation by limiting the atmospheric carbon available to plants.

Doubling the CO_2 concentration of the atmosphere from its recent level of 300 parts per million (ppm) to 600 ppm is estimated in laboratory studies to boost average plant growth and crop yield by about 33 percent in "C3" plants, and about 14 percent in "C4" plants (Rosenberg et al. 1990, p. 157). C3 plants, so named for the type of photosynthetic process they perform, include wheat, rice, barley, legumes—in total, 80 percent of the world's food supply—and virtually all trees. C4 plants, which include maize, sorghum, millet, and sugarcane plants, employ a photosynthetic process that already uses carbon efficiently, and therefore they derive less aid from increased CO_2 concentrations (IPCC 1990b, p 2.5).

This finding should be no surprise, since carbon is the grist of photosynthesis. Commercial greenhouse operators typically keep their facilities in the range of 600–2000 ppm CO_2—two to six times the level in the normal atmosphere today—precisely in order to stimulate plant growth (Grodzinski 1992, p. 517). There are questions, however, whether increasing CO_2 concentrations will exhibit similar effects outside laboratories and nurseries: lab conditions may be superior to field conditions, the latter constrained by the availability of water and nutrients; rising global temperature due to CO_2 might inhibit the gains from carbon fertilization; the carbon fertilization effect may decline over time as plants return to original growing conditions; competing weeds may also benefit from elevated CO_2; and the benefits of CO_2 fertilization may peak after about 600–800 ppm (Cline 1992, pp. 90–91; Bazzaz and Fajer 1992).

Recent research tends to confirm the CO_2 fertilization hypothesis in more realistic situations. Several experiments in the field have shown significant fertilization effects, in some cases even larger changes in yield and growth than predicted by lab studies, on the order of 25 to 50 percent increases for C3 plants (Drake and Leadley 1991, pp. 858–859). A study of grasses in the Chesapeake Bay exposed to 800 ppm CO_2 has shown increased photosynthetic carbon assimilation (a mea-

sure of overall plant matter growth) of 88 percent in C3 grasses
and 40 percent in C4 grasses, and no decline in this response
rate over the four years of the study (Drake and Leadley 1991,
p. 858). Because of internal positive feedback mechanisms,
sour orange trees turn out to respond to a doubling of the CO_2
concentration by tripling their growth rate and total biomass
(Idso and Kimball 1991). Meanwhile, field studies suggest that
one reason for lesser response in some lab studies may be that
labs use potted plants whose root growth is constrained and
which therefore cannot respond fully to the rising availability
of carbon; in field trials where roots can expand, robust CO_2
enrichment is consistently observed (Drake and Leadley 1991,
p. 858).

Rather than fading under stressed growing conditions, the
positive effects of elevated CO_2 appear to be comparatively
larger in the face of stresses—limited nutrients or water, sa-
linity, cool temperatures, or pollution—than in already optimal conditions (IPCC 1990b, p. 2.5). Increasing CO_2 concentrations spurs plants to close their stomata (small openings in
leaf tissues) and thereby to reduce transpiration (water loss to
the air through the stomata) per unit of photosynthesis, increasing their water use efficiency and their resistance to
drought by about 30 percent (Rosenberg 1990, 1991; IPCC
1990b, pp. 2.4–2.5). CO_2 fertilization could therefore be especially valuable in arid areas and areas that might lose precipitation under global warming. And doubling CO_2 concentrations actually raises the optimum temperature for
photosynthesis in C3 plants by about 4 to 6 degrees C, so
global warming itself is not likely to inhibit the carbon fertilization effect (IPCC 1990b, pp. 2.4–2.5). As for weed competition, the IPCC noted that fourteen of the world's seventeen
worst weeds are C4 plants amid C3 crops, so that CO_2 enrichment might in fact help crops outperform these weeds (IPCC
1990b, p. 2.5).

Of course, important uncertainties remain regarding the impact of elevated CO_2. Like the computer-generated forecasts of
the effects of global warming, the predictions of enhanced CO_2
fertilization have not yet been tested on complete ecosystems.
But at least in the case of CO_2 fertilization there is already

some corroboratory evidence at the macro level: as atmospheric CO_2 has risen from 275 ppm in the 1800s to about 350 ppm today, the amplitude (annual variation) of the earth's historical CO_2 record has increased, implying an increase in the total biomass of the world's carbon sinks (Rosenberg 1991, p. 333). Still, the detailed effects on unmanaged ecosystems, such as rainforests, have not yet been fully studied (see Peters and Lovejoy 1992). There are also important questions about the nutrient needs and nutritional value of CO_2-fertilized larger plants (IPCC 1990b, p. 2.6; Cline 1992, p. 90). Researchers are currently studying the effect of elevated CO_2 on successive generations of plants, and are attempting to test increased CO_2 without changing other variables, such as light, that may have varied in previous field tests when CO_2 chambers were attached to plants (Oren 1994).

As CO_2 levels increase, the fertilization effect may not continue with equal vigor. The incremental impact of elevated CO_2 levels appears to drop off after 550 ppm for maize and 850 ppm for wheat (Cline 1992, p. 91). But since present CO_2 levels are about 350 ppm, increasing concentrations over the next century would continue to make a sizable difference. And the incremental impact of CO_2 on global temperature will also drop off: by 350 ppm, the part of the thermal radiation spectrum that CO_2 blocks is already mostly occluded, so additional inputs of CO_2 in the atmosphere will have a steadily declining marginal effect (Rowland 1989, p. 40; IPCC 1992, p. 21).

Ideally, one could estimate the combined effect of warming and carbon fertilization due to each increment of CO_2 in the atmosphere. Some analysis has been conducted of the net effect of both influences on agricultural yields. An early effort found that although warming alone would imply substantial reductions in yields of several crops in the United States, warming and CO_2 fertilization together would impose only mild to insignificant reductions in yields (Dudek 1987). More recent studies examining the two effects in concert, using a variety of general circulation models of the earth's climate (GCMs), have predicted a 17 percent *increase* in yields in subarctic Russia and Siberia (Parry et al. 1988, cited in Kane et al. 1992b, p. 25), and from no change to large crop yield increases in the

United States (Adams 1989; Smith and Tirpak 1989, cited in Kane et al. 1992b, p. 25) and in other countries (Brookes 1990, citing IPCC/Coolfont report). These estimates do not fully incorporate the findings described earlier about night-time-wintertime warming and farmer adaptation, which tend to brighten the prospects for world agriculture further. Yet the analysis of adjustments by international food markets (Kane et al. 1992a), as discussed earlier, suggests that modest in-creases in world crop output, like modest decreases, would not appreciably affect world economic well-being.

Forests and Global Warming

Another set of risk tradeoffs may be posed by suggestions made by some researchers to plant trees to sequester CO_2 from the atmosphere. Already terrestrial biota (chiefly forests, but also including grasses and soils) remove one-half to two-thirds of the CO_2 added to the atmosphere each year (Quay et al. 1992; Tans et al. 1990). Because young growing trees store carbon more rapidly than mature forests, some have sug-gested growing large tree plantations as a greenhouse miti-gation strategy. The question remains where to put those trees: some suggest planting them on unused land, while others propose clearing currently mature forest stands and re-placing them with new, growing stands.

The latter strategy could pose a risk substitution: fore-stalling global warming at the expense of global biodiversity. Tropical forests, for example, cover less than a tenth of the earth's surface but harbor about half of the earth's several mil-lion species (Peters and Lovejoy 1992). The diversity of species is already under stress from land conversion and other causes, and clearing older forests to erect new, single-species planta-tion forests would further compromise that diversity. The rich-ness of forest life forms is critical to the viability of ecosystems. Forest biodiversity also provides important genetic resources for human purposes, such as life-saving medicines and har-dier agricultural strains.

In addition, replacing old forests with new plantations could constitute a risk offset, by inadvertently emitting more carbon to the atmosphere than is sequestered. Young trees store carbon rapidly as they grow, while mature trees do not; hence the proposal to replace the old with the new. Of course it matters what is done with the harvested trees—if they are burned, their carbon is returned to the atmosphere, for no net sequestration. But even if the old trees are stored in solid form (for example, as furniture), the exercise can be a net carbon loss, because forests store significant carbon in the soils as well as in trees, and the disruptive effects of clearing old forests would liberate that soil carbon (Harmon et al. 1990). In temperate and boreal forests, it could take many years, perhaps over a century, for the new plantation trees to recoup the carbon lost from the soil in just the first few years after the mature forest was cleared (Dudek and LeBlanc 1993).

Weighing the Risks

Recognizing that risk tradeoffs could be occasioned by preventing global warming, or by specific policies intended to do so, does not, by itself, mean that these goals and policies are unwarranted. Sound risk tradeoff analysis can help decisionmakers weigh the risks carefully.

In terms of the total output of agriculture, initial RTA suggests that the fertilization benefits of CO_2 molecules added to the atmosphere are sufficiently significant and near-term that these benefits at least counsel caution before imposing restrictions on CO_2 emissions as a way to prevent global warming. Moreover, policies to control CO_2 alone could be ineffective at reducing global warming because of CH_4 and sulfur shifts. Depending on the relative magnitude and timing of these countervailing risks, it may make sense to shift priority from controlling CO_2 to controlling non-CO_2 greenhouse gases, such as methane, in steps to begin preventing global warming.

When weighing these risks, the uncertainties surrounding the predictions of both the CO_2 fertilization effect and the greenhouse warming forecast should be compared. Neither has been fully tested on real ecosystems, but there is empirical evidence from present-day field trials showing observable CO_2 enrichment in real plants, whereas the warming predictions are based on incomplete computerized general circulation models (GCMs) that have difficulty representing oceans and clouds and that overpredict current temperature when fed historical emissions data (Stone 1992). Moreover, the plant fertilization effect would occur promptly with rising atmospheric concentrations of CO_2, whereas any global warming as a result of those added CO_2 molecules would occur decades or more later.

The bottom line for agricultural impacts is not the net change in crop yields resulting from warming and CO_2 fertilization, but the effect on human well-being. If even large changes in the total output of crops have little impact on aggregate world GDP (Kane et al. 1992a), as discussed earlier, it may be that the effects of warming on the distribution of food are more important than on total output levels. Studies should therefore focus on the combined impacts of warming and CO_2 fertilization on the regional distribution of food supply and prices: the critical parameters will likely be the influence of warming on regional precipitation and soil moisture, the rate of warming, and the role of CO_2 in increasing the drought-resilience of plants. And weighing the risks of warming and CO_2 fertilization should pay increased attention to impacts on resources and ecosystems other than agriculture, such as forests, marine life, and insects and microbes.

Under the Climate Convention signed at the 1992 Earth Summit, countries are obligated to take some actions to limit greenhouse gas emissions, with a long-term objective of avoiding dangerous climate change. The questions for policymakers from a risk tradeoff perspective therefore include the following: Do our climate policy measures actually achieve reduced risk of global warming, or are their intended effects undercut (or even reversed) by risk offsets such as cross-gas or cross-border shifts? If warming is to be prevented at some level of effort under the Convention, then how shall we prevent it in the way that best minimizes all the other risks that such policies could entail? Or, more generally, what is the optimal set of policies that will minimize the overall risks, considering warming, plant fertilization, loss of biodiversity, ozone depletion, toxicity, and so forth? To date these crucial questions have not generally been asked by governments seeking to protect the global environment.

Some form of "global change index" incorporating all of these multiple effects—warming potential, carbon fertilization, biodiversity loss, UV radiation, and other impacts—would offer policymakers an understandable estimate of the relative overall risk reduction benefits to be realized from avoiding an incremental unit of each of the gases (Stewart and Wiener 1990, p. 77; DOJ 1991, pp. 24–27; Stewart and Wiener 1992, pp. 88–89; see initial calculations of a two-impact index in Reilly 1992). Such an index, or a reliable approximation, would help policymakers devise strategies that maximize the overall risk reduction per unit of social cost. The index need not be framed in single-number point estimates, but could be a set of ranges, or equations, or a simple PC-based program. The index should reflect both "coincident" reductions in risk and increases in countervailing risks that would result from various strategies to limit emissions, such as coal-to-gas switching or conserving forests.

Risk-Superior Options

Risk tradeoff analysis demonstrates the bewildering array of countervailing risks that face efforts to prevent global warming, but it is not purely a predicate for pessimism. It helps reveal opportunities as well. For example, RTA indicates that, at least as far as the two global risks of climate change and biodiversity loss are concerned, a strategy of conserving existing forests rather than clearing older forests to create new tree plantations would be a risk-superior way to limit net greenhouse gas emissions (Gray 1992). The Food and Agriculture Organization of the United Nations estimates that tropical forests were being cleared at over 17 million hectares per year in 1990 (up 35 percent since 1980); this rapid destruction was contributing an impressive 10 to 30 percent of global net CO_2 emissions (IPCC 1990c). Pressures on boreal forests are mounting as well, especially in Siberia, from both logging and fires.

Or instead of reducing CO_2 and just tolerating CH_4 leaks, one could work to reduce CH_4 leakage from natural gas systems, which account for about 75 of the 500 teragrams of methane emitted annually from human activities (Crutzen 1991). Reducing CH_4 leakage may be a particularly cost-effective means of reducing contributions to potential warming (Rabchuk and Ilkevich 1991, p. 12), because CH_4 is itself the product being transported and sold in natural gas systems, so there is an economic incentive to capture fugitive CH_4 emissions (Hogan et al. 1991, p. 1981). Leakage will persist where the cost of capture exceeds the revenue that the capturer can gain from the recovered CH_4. This discrepancy is especially likely where energy is not traded in a competitive marketplace, but even in competitive energy markets private CH_4 recapture is still likely to fall short of social goals because some of the social benefits of CH_4 recapture (for example, reducing its potential to cause global warming, smog, and explosions) are not incorporated in the market price for recovered CH_4. A policy aimed only at reducing CO_2 emissions provides no incentive to correct such market failures, but a "comprehensive approach" would fully account for both CH_4 and CO_2 emissions (as well as other gases) and thereby achieve cost-effective attention to overall warming risk (Stewart and Wiener 1992; Stewart and Wiener 1990). The Framework Convention on Climate Change signed in 1992 embodies such a comprehensive approach, but it remains to be seen how countries will implement it.

As for the choice between a warmer world and a colder world, RTA suggests that the goal should not be framed in terms of a "stable climate" (see, for example, Zimmerman 1992). We know that the earth's climate varies perpetually and considerably, even on human time scales (Schneider 1989b, pp. 36–65), mostly for reasons that humanity appears powerless to control. A goal of "stability" could encourage humans, with the clumsy tools we possess, to try to intervene to fine-tune the earth's climate toward an illusory "stable" course. Perhaps a better formulation would be to manage our own emissions of trace gases toward an "optimal anthropogenic contribution" or an "optimal atmospheric composition." Then, given the constant dynamism of the climate and the importance of short-term as well as longer-term climate variations to human welfare, a key goal should be increasing the ability of societies to adapt to changing climate. Although reducing greenhouse gas emissions may help forestall long-term warming, it would not address many more immediate climatological threats such as regional hurricanes and droughts.

A strategy of adaptation could, however, pose its own countervailing risks. Some argue that human society could adapt to global warming at less expense than it would cost to limit emissions to prevent that warming (NAS 1991b). For example, protecting coastal development from a sea-level rise of 65 cm through 2100 is estimated to cost on the order of 0.04 percent of world GNP (undiscounted) over 110 years (IPCC 1990c). But ecological systems may be more vulnerable to climate stress and less able to adapt quickly (NAS 1991b; Peters and Lovejoy 1992). Protecting coastal ecosystems (such as wetlands and river deltas) from sea-level rise, for example, might be much more costly than protecting human installations, or impossible, and coastal biota might even be injured by efforts to protect human development (for example, dikes built to protect coastal development may obstruct needed salt exchange between sea and coastal wetlands). In that sense, allowing warming to occur while humans adapt could mean not so much an increase in global risk but a risk transfer from human societies to ecological systems. Even if one takes a purely anthropocentric and utilitarian perspective, the risk of warming to human society would need to include the impact on human society of these ecological damages; and since ecosystems ultimately sustain life on the planet and provide many of the resources needed for economic growth, some positive level of investment in their conservation—in this case, measures to prevent or soften global warming—would likely be worthwhile to humans, even in present-value monetary terms.

Conclusion

Attempting to care for the health of the planet is no small task, and it is not surprising that the degree and complexity of risk tradeoffs confronted in that arena are so great. What is trou-

bling is that the tunnel vision exhibited in domestic environmental policy appears unabated in global environmental
policy: dogged focus on one target risk with little attention paid
to potential side effects, or even to the efficacy of the chosen
policy measures.

Neglect of risk tradeoffs at the global level may arise from
several causes. First, mental heuristics, such as the salience
of recent events, may distort decisionmaking about more complex underlying risks (Noll and Krier 1990); thus the politics
of climate change seem to have been driven less by long-term
forecasts than by short-term trends (cooling from the 1940s
through the 1970s, warming in the 1980s, and cooling after
Mt. Pinatubo in the 1990s). Attention to observable impacts
such as temperature change, and neglect of more invisible
non-warming impacts such as CO_2 fertilization of plants, may
also be a result of a salience heuristic. Second, the failure of
political decisionmakers to consider effects on populations
outside their electoral jurisdictions—voices omitted from their
political calculus—may explain the emission of gases by some
countries that damage the environment of others. And it may
explain why policies in response to such damage seem to at-
tend primarily to the emitters' share of expected damages, perhaps worrying more about ultraviolet radiation and agricultural losses in the North than about food spoilage and
agricultural gains in the South. Third, the fragmented international policy apparatus may foster bounded decisionmaking. The United Nations Environment Program (UNEP)
addresses environmental problems, the World Health Organization (WHO) addresses human health, the U.N. Food and Agriculture Organization (FAO) addresses forests and farming,
but there is no truly integrated risk management entity dealing
with interconnected problems. Nor is there any international
system for agenda selection, comparing risks, prioritizing
problems, or choosing appropriate degrees of response to
problems of different severity. The UNEP, WHO, FAO, the U.N.
General Assembly, the U.N. Commission on Sustainable Development, and others compete to put issues on the international risk agenda, often through sporadically organized "intergovernmental negotiating committees" (INCs) such as the

ones that negotiated the Framework Convention on Climate Change and the Vienna and Montreal agreements on protection of the stratospheric ozone layer. Risk management at the international level is thus ad hoc and undisciplined (Esty 1994), and as or more vulnerable to risk tradeoffs and the "risk of the month" syndrome as domestic policy is.

One positive force has been the role of scientists in international assessment panels, such as the IPCC, which can give a complex topic the breadth of vision it deserves. The IPCC helpfully framed the issue comprehensively in terms of "Climate Change," not solely "global warming" or "CO_2 control," and calculated the GWP index for multiple greenhouse gases; these steps helped to ensure that the INC created to formulate policy would also address the topic broadly. Still, the INC would likely have adopted the narrow CO_2-only policy proposals had not key governments advocated a comprehensive approach, and the INC never did address the non-climate impacts of the greenhouse gases such as carbon fertilization of plant photosynthesis.

When adopting environmental policies, we are advised to "aim before we shoot," to choose our targets on the basis of their relative risk priority; by the same reasoning, we ought to "use a big scope" to see the numerous targets and tradeoffs in our firing range. Global policymakers should consider the tools of RTA to illuminate these tradeoffs and point the way to risk-superior opportunities.

11

Resolving Risk Tradeoffs

JONATHAN BAERT WIENER
JOHN D. GRAHAM

What can be done to redress the ubiquitous risk tradeoffs besetting the national campaign to reduce risk? As the case studies in this volume illustrate, risk tradeoffs are a pervasive and fundamental problem of decisionmaking. In contexts from the care of a single patient to the care of the entire earth, striving to solve one problem often invokes other problems. Each intervention to protect against a target risk can simultaneously generate countervailing risks; these risk tradeoffs at least reduce the gross benefits of the intervention and in some cases mean that the intervention will do more harm than good. And the case studies presented here reflect only a sampling of the full spectrum of risk tradeoffs.

We believe that risk tradeoffs are prevalent not because of an inescapable law of risk homeostasis, but because of systematic shortcomings in the ways in which decisions are considered and structured. Thus, our response is not to counsel inaction or deregulation in the face of risk, but to suggest ways to make risk-reduction decisions more intelligent and effective. In Chapter 1 we sketched a method for recognizing risk tradeoffs and a set of factors to be weighed in facing tradeoffs among risks. We then applied this method of risk tradeoff analysis in nine case studies (summarized in Table 1.3). In this chapter we collect the lessons of our case studies to furnish suggestions for ensuring that risk tradeoffs are better handled by decisionmakers. We also offer some promising indications that risk tradeoff analysis can be and is being used in real-world decisions.

We begin by exploring possible answers to the vexing question of *why* undesirable risk tradeoffs occur. In search of a diagnosis we examine several potential sources of risk tradeoffs: omitted voice, heuristics, bounded roles, old-technology bias, and compensating behavior.

In the following section we identify reforms, both ongoing and proposed, that can help the nation's campaign to reduce risk become a more responsible, reflective, and pragmatically effective enterprise. The challenge of risk tradeoffs should be met neither by denial, nor by simple appeal to "less" or "more" action or regulation. Like Hirschman (1991, pp. 42, 153), we find the problem of perverse effects, when considered in a serious and pragmatic (rather than ideological) fashion, to be both important and soluble through intelligent decision-making. We believe that there are constructive ways, through the use of risk tradeoff analysis, to make better policies that provide more protection of human health and the environment, and we outline how RTA should be incorporated into decisionmaking about medical treatment and government regulation (including legislative, administrative, and judicial functions). In these decisionmaking contexts we propose RTA as a means toward a more holistic paradigm with which decisionmakers would "treat the whole patient" instead of confining their thinking to bounded fragments of larger systems. To help make this "whole patient" paradigm a reality in government decisionmaking, we propose specific structural changes in governmental institutions to help policymakers avoid perverse risk tradeoffs.

It is worth repeating the point made in Chapter 1 that not all countervailing risks are equally serious. Efforts to protect our health and the environment could be paralyzed if every hint of a countervailing risk sufficed to halt the decision-making process; yet serious damage to our health and the environment can be done if countervailing risks are ignored. The key challenge is to identify the important countervailing risks in terms of their seriousness relative to the target risk. Identifying a countervailing risk that rivals the reduction in the target risk (or reduces the gross benefits so much that the policy's costs seem excessive) may counsel modifying rather than scrapping the policy. Even that process of identification, of course, requires a decision about how much information to collect—how many "ripples" in the pond to examine—which entails comparing the value of obtaining additional information to its costs in resources and delay. But we are optimistic that RTA can help dedicated decisionmakers substantially improve the outcomes of their efforts to reduce risk.

In the final section of this chapter we foresee, over the longer term, the emergence of a more holistic decisionmaking paradigm that respects countervailing risks alongside target risks as multiple facets of complex, interconnected problems. In many ways this paradigm is not new but is already embodied in several key areas of thought: medicine, Gestalt psychology, ecology, systems analysis, democratic pluralism, and international relations. In some ways this new outlook is just an elaboration of the original premise of the national campaign to reduce risk, which began by arguing that countervailing risks of industrial activity, such as environmental damages, were being left out of society's calculus. We do not presume to "propose" a cultural change, which we recognize cannot be instituted by fiat; rather we are optimistic that a paradigmatic change in the way people think about risk is already under way, and that by unmasking and analyzing the phenomenon of risk tradeoffs, we can help build a growing critical mass that will embrace a more holistic risk-management outlook, just as revelations about target risks have engendered cathartic societal reevaluations and policy reforms in the past.

Sources of Risk Tradeoffs

Risk tradeoffs are not merely the result of "wooden-headed folly" (Tuchman 1984). The case studies in this volume and other literature indicate that the phenomenon of risk tradeoffs is rooted in the ways decisions are informed and structured. As a very general matter, many risk tradeoffs may be said to result from "intervention failure," analogous to the phenomenon of "market failure." It is well recognized that private markets may permit excessive threats to health and the environment, when those threats are "external" to the decisionmaking about activities from which they arise. For example, if firms do not face the social costs of pollution they emit, they will overproduce polluting activities. But just as markets may fail to maximize social well-being because the full set of consequences is not faced by market decisionmakers, so too interventions intended to reduce risk may fail because the decisionmaker does not consider the full set of risk-related consequences. A policy may actually accomplish its target goal (such as reducing a market externality) but inadvertently or predictably cause another failure (of the same or different type from the market failure it was meant to attack). In his analysis of a range of such "government failures," Wolf (1988) termed this kind of government failure a "derived externality"—an adverse consequence that is itself derived from the government's effort to redress a market externality (see also Warren and Marchant 1993, pp. 387–391).

Likewise, we view many risk tradeoffs as "intervention failures" by decisionmakers. The upshot of the headache/aspirin example in Chapter 1 is that the problem of risk tradeoffs is a *fundamental problem of decisionmaking*. It is not limited to government decisions on public policy matters but is frequent in individual choices as well. Risk tradeoffs may be magnified by government decisions that affect larger populations, but they are no less analytically difficult or pivotal for the individual trying to decide how to deal with an illness or the family diet.

The question remains why intervention failures occur: why do decisionmakers act without accounting for the full consequences of their interventions? Decision theorists, political scientists, and others have explored a number of plausible explanations. We offer these as potential insights into the sources of risk tradeoffs, though there may be other causes as well.

Omitted Voice. One prominent source of narrow decision-making is what one might call "omitted voice": the absence of affected parties from the decision process and the concomitant disproportionate influence of organized interests. The benefits to a decisionmaker of acting against a target risk may be largely defined by the support or mollification of key constituencies clamoring for such action (Sapolsky 1990). The decisionmaker is unlikely to take account of countervailing losses imposed on constituencies who are not participating in the dialogue. Meanwhile, if any individual decisionmaker (or constituent) invested the additional effort to determine a more complete answer to a problem, others would share the benefits at no cost to themselves; realizing this, no individual decisionmaker (or constituent) has an adequate incentive to prepare a comprehensive accounting of risks and seek an overall solution. To put it another way, from the perspective of a public decisionmaker, some countervailing risks are externalities, and therefore the costs of research and analysis to shape a fully optimal policy may exceed the benefits to the decisionmaker of serving the vocal constituency which cares only about a target risk. For society at large, however, the benefits of the optimal policy would exceed these costs.

Government bodies (such as legislatures and administrative agencies) tend to hear a subset of interests in part because there are costs to private parties of making themselves heard: where the consequences of a decision are concentrated on a defined group, such as an industry or the raison d'être of an advocacy group, the incentives for that group to act will be large; but where the consequences are broadly distributed across the general public, the incentives for ordinary citizens to organize and speak will be small (Olson 1965; Eskridge 1988). These "forgotten groups" may be particularly vulnerable to small but widely spread risk transfers and risk substitutions because of their comparative inability to mobilize, even in situations where their general interest ought to be a paramount concern. Moreover, even if multiple groups do mobilize to make their voices heard, legislators tend to hear only part of the story because they are most responsive to the local interest groups from their territorial voting districts.

Omitted voice has also become a topic of controversy in the medical community. For example, critics argue that women have been omitted from clinical trials of new medications, even though some of the drugs were then prescribed for women and, interacting with the hormonal and metabolic processes of women's bodies, could produce unintended adverse side effects (GAO 1990; IOM 1994; Mastroianni et al. 1994); moreover, failing to test medications on women could result in errors in selecting the most effective medications. These critics charge that decisions on which diseases to treat, which surgery to recommend, and which illnesses to study have also tended to omit or downplay the maladies that affect women, particularly in poorer countries but in the United States as well (Holloway 1994). Others argue to the contrary that at least in this country, women are not omitted from medical research and decision-making, have received more and often better health care than have men, and in consequence have achieved during this century a life expectancy 10 percent longer than that for men (78 years versus 71 years) (Kadar 1994).

Several of our case studies found omitted voice to be an important source of risk tradeoffs. The analysis of drinking water policies in Chapter 7 illustrated how organized efforts to reduce the risk of cancer from disinfection chemicals could impose on a relatively unaware general public a substantially increased risk of microbial disease. In Chapter 9 we noted how the measures to reduce pesticide residues on foods may reduce risk to most food consumers, who are represented by active advocacy groups, but increase the risks faced by relatively unrepresented groups such as farm workers and poor consumers. Some policies to reduce the danger of global warming, as described in Chapter 10, may serve human ends but increase the risks faced by non-human (hence non-participatory) life forms in mature forests and coastal ecosystems.

In other case studies, problems of omitted voice might have threatened risk tradeoffs but were at least partially redressed. For example, the countervailing risks to senior citizens posed by restricting their driver's licences, examined in Chapter 4, may have been avoided because of the potent political voice of older people in this country. The risk to the general public of

highway accidents posed by CAFE policies intended to conserve energy, analyzed in Chapter 5, was initially omitted from
the public policy debate and only surfaced when the insurance
industry raised this issue on behalf of all insured motorists
and courts held NHTSA accountable. The problem of lead recycling (Chapter 8), meanwhile, revealed both the inclusion
and omission of unrepresented affected groups. When EPA
was initially intending to require increased recycling on
"common sense" grounds, it was the preparation of a more
thorough risk tradeoff analysis that made the agency realize
the substantial adverse impact such a policy would have on
people living near secondary smelters and therefore reconsider. Without this RTA, these affected populations might have
been exposed to a serious risk transfer because of their
omitted voice. At the same time, EPA noted in its RTA that
populations outside the United States would be exposed to
smelting operations under key scenarios, but assigned that
risk an arbitrary quantification of zero in its calculus. These
foreign citizens were intentionally omitted from the decision,
and would have little opportunity to be heard or to influence
EPA's decision.

The asymmetry in consideration of consequences that results from the omission of affected voices from the decisionmaking dialogue helps to explain why *coincident* risk reductions (unexpected bonus risk reductions that accompany
reductions in the target risk) are less likely to be prevalent
than are *countervailing* risks. Coincident risk reductions may
serendipitously complement an intervention to address a
target risk, but there are no systematic forces at work to encourage such unexpected pluses. For example, policies to reduce carbon monoxide (CO) and other emissions from motor
vehicles, aimed at the target risk of outdoor air pollution, had
the coincident benefit of reducing accidental and suicide fatalities from direct inhalation of CO exhaust (Shelef 1994);
but this result was unexpected, and its beneficiaries did not
advocate for CO controls in advance. If decisionmakers
foresaw opportunities to achieve coincident risk reductions,
they would be likely to seek support from the beneficiary con-

stituencies, or to try to pare their interventions to avoid providing uncompensated bonus reductions.

Omitted voice may be a particularly troubling source of risk tradeoffs because of its ethical implications. A powerful group in society may lobby to reduce a risk it deems to be a worthy target, through policies that transfer the risk to less influential members of society. This may be the case, for example, in the advocacy of increased lead recycling (Chapter 8) and reduced use of pesticides on fruits and vegetables (Chapter 9). "Not in my backyard" (NIMBY) efforts to block "locally undesirable land uses," such as hazardous waste sites or lead smelters, may shift these land uses to the neighborhoods of populations who are less powerful because of historical discrimination against them in areas such as politics, employment, education, and housing (Been 1994; Hamilton 1993). Or the population onto whom a countervailing risk is about to be transferred may find it not just costly to express its opposition, but impossible to anticipate: for example, an intervention might transfer a risk of latent illness or ecological imbalance to future populations who cannot be identified or speak today, or to non-human life forms which cannot participate in human decisionmaking institutions.

"Risk transfers" may thus be another way of describing dysfunctions in democratic processes, such as invidious discrimination, parochial rent-seeking, and political or economic concentration of power, in which affected constituencies or the general public are left out of the decisionmaking process and the interests of the powerful few come to dominate.

Heuristics. Even when a decisionmaker does face a fairly full set of interested parties and prospective consequences, he or she may still ignore risk tradeoffs. When confronted with enormous amounts of potentially relevant information and the need to make a prompt decision, people tend to use "heuristic" devices to order their thinking (Tversky and Kahneman 1974). These mental shortcuts help boil down information about risks, focusing attention on the problem of most immediate concern but leaving the larger picture for another day. For example, people address a problem by disaggregating it—dividing it up into conceptual "boxes"—and addressing one category as though it were unconnected to other categories. The consequence is a stream of unexpected side effects (some good but many bad) ensuing from each decision to reduce a target risk.

Thus, for example, as illustrated in Chapter 9, the Delaney Clause regulates the cancer risk of chemicals synthesized by humans and used in or on foods, but not the cancer risk of "natural" chemicals found in foods (many of which are far more potent and which furnish the great majority of the carcinogens ingested by the average American [Ames et al. 1990]), nor the cancer-preventing effects of some pesticides and food additives, nor the noncancer risks of such chemicals; and the current law regulates new pesticides more stringently than existing ones even if the former are less risky. Many state legislatures are now passing "toxics use reduction" legislation that targets listed substances without requiring chemical users to compare the risks of the substances they are restricting to the new substances that will be adopted in their stead (Laden and Gray 1993). In tort law, perverse increases in risk can conceivably result where the liability system is arranged to cover only the risks of certain products (such as stepladders or vaccinations) but not of substitute arrangements that may be more risky (such as chairs piled on top of tables, or going without protection against transmitting disease) (Williams 1993). In the global arena, as described in Chapter 10, policy fixed its gaze on CO_2 emissions from fossil fuels in part because CO_2 emissions represent the largest single piece of the greenhouse gas emissions pie, but then neglected the consequences of excluding smaller categories, such as methane emissions, that could increase in response. The lesson is that big "boxes" may attract the first concern, but policy interventions that address only those boxes can cause other, initially small boxes to grow.

Another common heuristic is to respond to the salience of a recent crisis (for example, an airline disaster) even if the baseline probability of that type of outcome has not changed. This dynamic encourages reactive "risk-of-the-month" remedies crafted in the wake of visible events, often focusing narrowly on the type of risk manifested in the crisis (Slovic 1986; Lave and Males 1989). Much of the risk legislation of the past few decades has been enacted in response to salient crises; examples include the enactment of Superfund in the wake of the uproar over Love Canal, the ban on ocean dumping after wastes washed up on beaches, and the Oil Pollution Act passed after the Exxon Valdez spill in Alaska (Krier and Ursin 1977; Kasperson 1992). Aggressive but ad hoc policymaking may give short shrift to the complexities of countervailing risks.

Risk tradeoffs sometimes result from fixation on a specific symptom. The national interest in eliminating cancer (popular at least since President Nixon's highly touted "War on Cancer") has often driven policy to the exclusion of attention to other risks. It lies behind such measures as the policy to advise against eating fish on the grounds of slight elevations in cancer risk from trace amounts of contaminants, despite the role of fish in preventing many times more cases of heart disease, as described in Chapter 6; the campaign to reduce chlorination of drinking water, despite the protection such disinfection confers against deadly microbial diseases (Chapter 7); and the restrictions on carcinogenic pesticides without regard to their health benefits for the food supply and for poor families in particular (Chapter 9). More generally, many laws governing toxic substances address cancer risks but ignore or regulate less stringently the noncancer risks of those substances, such as neurotoxicity, reproductive toxicity, and immune system dysfunction (Myers and Colborn 1991).

Likewise, singular focus on the warming impacts of CO_2, omitting the direct effects of CO_2 on plant growth, seems to emanate at least in part from the political salience of the warming risk during hotter-than-normal years (Chapter 10). And the adverse safety consequences of auto fuel efficiency regulations arise from congressional preoccupation with energy conservation to the exclusion of safety concerns (Chapter 5).

Bounded Oversight Roles. A related and powerful source of risk tradeoffs is rooted in the structure of organizations: the fragmentation of decisionmaking into specialized roles with bounded oversight responsibilities. Bounded oversight structures appear not only in government but also in medicine, business, and even within families. The specialization of decisionmaking into bounded oversight roles is consistent with (and reinforced by) both the influences of omitted voice and heuristic thinking, though it may also occur for more idiosyncratic reasons.

For example, the splintering of medical care into specializations and subspecializations has drawn considerable attention and criticism. Fewer than 30 percent of practicing physicians in the United States are now primary care generalists (including family practice, internal medicine, and pediatrics), as compared to over 50 percent in every other industrialized country (Schroeder and Sandy 1993); and the percentage of newly graduating medical students entering primary care in the United States has declined from 36 percent in 1982 to under 15 percent in 1992 (Rosenthal 1993). In part, young doctors finishing their residencies have been encouraged by the medical education system to choose specialties, such as surgery, orthopedics, or cardiology, which are portrayed as more lucrative and glamorous and which may offer more flexible work schedules (Rosenthal 1993). In addition, government financial policies, such as subsidized loans for medical students (Rosenthal 1993, quoting Enthoven), and Medicare fee schedules that pay specialists more than generalists for the same work (Hsiao et al. 1993), have tended to reward specialization. As the fraction of physicians going into specialties rises, there will be a growing oversupply of specialty skills as well as an undersupply of generalists (Weiner 1994), which in a competitive market will eventually reduce specialists' earnings and increase those of generalists, thus attracting medical students to reverse the trend away from primary care. Many health maintenance organizations (HMOs) are now intensively recruiting primary care physicians with higher salary offers, and some clinics are training nurse practitioners and physicians' assistants to fill broader roles (Rosenthal 1993). But this readjustment may be muted by noncompetitive billing structures and nonmonetary incentives in medical circles. To date medical students continue to enter specialties more than primary care, and the net incomes of specialists are still rising rapidly (Schroeder and Sandy 1993). In any case, this readjustment can take many decades to redress the current imbalance.

One beneficial result of specialization in medicine is increasing skill levels and greater research progress in understanding the ailments of specific organs and body parts. But another result may be a medical system less capable of interpreting and treating multiple symptoms of interrelated maladies or interrelated causes of an ailment—in a word, less capable of treating whole patients. The problem is not specialists per se, but specialists whose outlook on diagnosis and therapy is bounded—physicians who see only the patient's interface with their specialty area and do not analyze illness, treatments, or side effects in terms of the whole patient.

Bounded specialization in government decisionmaking about risk is similarly rampant. It is virtually pathological in the executive branch of the U.S. government (Litan and Nordhaus 1983). The jurisdictions of administrative agencies tend to be defined by categorical boundaries that countervailing risks do not respect. Authority has been divided and subdivided into innumerable agencies and subagencies, each dealing with a different part of the risk terrain: the workplace (OSHA), the environment (EPA), consumer products (CPSC), transportation (DOT), nuclear energy (NRC), biodiversity (FWS), fisheries (FWS, NMFS), forests (FWS, USFS, BLM), climate (EPA, NOAA, DOE, USDA), and so on. Transportation safety policy within DOT is divided into air traffic (FAA) and road traffic (NHTSA, which is further divided into sub-fiefdoms governing fuel efficiency and safety). EPA, already separated from the natural resource agencies and from oversight of the workplace, is itself internally subspecialized into medium-specific subagencies: Air (divided by stationary and mobile sources), Radiation, Water (divided by drinking water, freshwater, and ocean pollution), Pesticides, Toxic Substances, and Wastes (divided by solid and hazardous wastes). Policies aimed at protecting any one of these domains will inevitably affect others, but mission-oriented agencies tend to overpromote their target goals and neglect side effects (Warren and Marchant 1993, p. 391).

Decisionmaking in Congress is likewise divided into specialized committees and subcommittees, which have become vying fiefdoms shepherding the executive branch agencies they oversee. Committees do not necessarily consider the impacts of their proposals on other areas. Congress has tended to devise piecemeal policies governing one slice of the risk spectrum at a time, such as clean air, clean water, and safe waste disposal (Haigh and Irwin 1990; Landy, Roberts, and Thomas 1990). Despite years of criticism, cross-media shifts of pollution have only just begun to receive attention from environmental agency officials, as described in Chapter 8. Congress has given little serious consideration to proposals calling for integration of U.S. environmental laws and institutions. Meanwhile, the tendency of Congress to develop legislation piecemeal has been a major contributor to the jurisdictional splintering of the administrative agencies charged with implementing those laws—even when those agencies were originally intended to be holistic organizations, as President Nixon initially intended for EPA (Marcus 1991; Hornstein 1992, p. 580). Indeed, the executive branch agencies have often been structured in the fragmented images of their subcommittee creators (Wilson 1980).

Surely a substantial reason for this fragmentation of responsibilities, in both the agencies and Congress, is that specialization facilitates the digestion of information and the accumulation of skills (Krier and Brownstein 1992). But as we have attempted to show in this book, bounded specialization also tends to blind the decisionmaker to information about risks outside his or her jurisdiction, to hamper synoptic decisionmaking, and to encourage risk tradeoffs. If optimal policy is not the justification for the current extent of specialized fragmentation in government, we may look for causes in the incentives created by the structure of political institutions and how that structure influences regulatory outcomes (Rodriguez 1994).

It seems plausible that the subdivision of Congress partly reflects the rivalry among partisan and regional factions in the development of legislative initiatives, which has its healthy as well as its dysfunctional aspects. It may also be a manifestation of the incentives of the members of Congress, as full-time legislators, to provide themselves with as many roles and titles as possible—every member a subcommittee chair. In addition, the limited time frame of congressional terms encourages a focus on those issues that will be most salient over the next two years. The similar fragmentation of the executive branch agencies seems to occur in part because it serves Congress for the agencies to be beholden to congressional power centers (which wield the weapons of annual budget approval and oversight hearings, as well as the power to amend statutes) rather than being delegated a broader scope of authority to make policy and allocate resources. The White House, however, is likely to resist such fragmentation and seek coordinated, integrated solutions to problems, since the President represents not individual districts or interest groups but the vote of the entire populace, and since presidential tenure has a longer time horizon than that of a House member.

It may also be that the government is itself driven to subdivide by the special interest groups advocating for (and against) health and environmental protection, because these groups may prefer a disaggregated structure in which they can focus pressure on specific decisions and officeholders to achieve tangible influence over the bureaucracy, and may distrust a structure that accords broad discretion to government policymakers. These advocacy groups may in turn feel pressure from their constituents, in the competitive battle for fundraising dollars, to demonstrate quick and advertisable successes rather than to engage in a more textured inquiry into optimal policy. National environmental advocacy groups, which ostensibly have as their objective protection of the whole environment, at times have opposed looking at cross-media effects when championing policy options. Schneider (1993) reports that certain environmental groups seeking a ban on disposal of wastes at sea did so even though they knew that one likely consequence would be increased disposal and incineration of wastes on land, closer to potentially more vulnerable human and freshwater communities.

Beyond specialization within the federal government, efforts are often divided between federal and state governments and among states. Because environmental media do not respect state boundaries, environmental risks are frequently multistate problems. The existence of political boundaries within environmental boundaries (for example, states within airsheds and watersheds, or states sharing the use of a common resource such as the atmosphere or ocean) can make it more likely that policies undertaken by one state to reduce a target risk will shift the risk to another state. The celebrated problem of acid rain illustrates precisely this kind of risk transfer: states attempting to reduce local ambient levels of sulfur pollutants, as the states were required to do under the 1977 Clean Air Act, encouraged emitting facilities to erect tall smokestacks that would inject the sulfur into high wind currents and thereby transport it downwind to fall in other states (Vestigo 1985). This risk transfer prompted national outcry, and in 1990 Congress rewrote the Clean Air Act, replacing state responsibility for ambient sulfur control with a national system of emissions reductions.

Risk transfers can also occur when nations share an environmental system; acid rain from the United States and Canada afflicted each other, and in Europe acid rain has been a multinational problem. At the global level, with no supersovereign and with most power in the hands of the 150-plus national governments, the disaggregation of authority over regional and planetary risks is greater still (Hurrell and Kingsbury 1992; Haas, Keohane, and Levy 1993). Thus actions to reduce risk within one nation's boundaries can shift risk to others' domains. As noted in Chapter 10, efforts by developing countries to combat malnutrition and microbial infection by refrigerating food may trade off with efforts by industrialized countries to end the use of CFCs that deplete the stratospheric ozone layer. As with medical specialties, the problem is not local jurisdiction per se, but the bounded outlook of the decisionmaker and the failure to take into account consequences outside that bounded role.

New-Old Bias. Stringent controls are often imposed solely or especially on *new* technologies, often because well-organized and visible existing industry can influence the regulatory process more effectively than unorganized and inchoate potential new competitors (Huber 1983). Yet controls on new sources of risk do nothing about existing sources, and can even lengthen the life of existing technologies (by raising the price of newer alternatives) and thereby exacerbate their associated risks. Hence regulations that apply only to new cars (as described in Chapter 5), pesticides (Chapter 9), medicines, and industrial technology have had the perverse effect of keeping more hazardous older products in use longer (Crandall 1983; Huber 1983; Crandall et al. 1986; Gruenspecht 1992).

Behavioral Responses. Human behavioral responses play a powerful role in determining the levels and distributions of various risks. Behavioral responses can negate intended reductions in the target risk while creating countervailing risks that were not anticipated. Anti-smoking advocates have always downplayed the promise of a "safe" cigarette, in part because of a fear that the availability of safer tobacco products would sanction or encourage smoking. Car safety devices intended to protect motor vehicle occupants (such as automatic seatbelts) may induce drivers to drive more aggressively or recklessly on the highway (Lave 1968; Peltzman 1975). When improved interstate highways were constructed after World War II, with limited access and divided traffic streams to reduce collision risks, drivers traded some of the extra safety for greater speed, reduced travel times, and longer travel distances (Graham 1988). Parents knowing that their car has airbags may now be less reluctant to allow their teenagers to borrow the car on weekend nights. Well-marked crosswalks may invite some pedestrians to cross without looking both ways. And medicine bottles with "child-safe" caps may encourage parents to leave those bottles nearer to children's hands or to leave the entire medicine cabinet unlocked (Viscusi 1992).

The behavioral feedback also works in reverse—for example, people are more likely to fasten safety belts in small cars than large cars, in part because of the greater injury risk in small cars (Evans 1985). Risk compensation behaviors can offset some or all of the intended reductions in the target risk to occupants, while creating countervailing risks for other road users. Well-protected drivers may prove more dangerous to bi-

cyclists and pedestrians. Although the extent of offsetting behavior will not always be large (Chirinko and Harper 1993),
efforts to reduce target risks can be complicated by unexpected behavioral compensation.

Toward Solutions. The solutions to these sources of risk
tradeoffs will vary with the context and institutions involved.
But it is worth pointing out that we do *not* think the solution
is to require everyone to be trained in all skills, or to have all
generalists and no specialists, or to have central global planning of regulation. Central planning is likely to be more rather
than less clumsy in achieving overall results (to say nothing of
its negative implications for liberty and political responsiveness), and specialization does bring certain advantages in
skills and research. Critics of integration have often been worried about the centralization of technocratic authority over
public value judgments (Krier and Brownstein 1992). Since
risk tradeoffs arise when decisionmakers fail to take account
of the impacts of their actions on others, the direction for reform is to devise and inculcate a broader method of decisionmaking by actors at all levels. Performance- or outcome-
oriented incentives to "treat the whole patient," coupled with
the freedom for flexible, decentralized decisionmaking to enable creative entrepreneurial solutions based on both expertise and value choices, are the likely avenues for improvement.

Incorporating RTA into Decisionmaking

There is both exaggeration and truth in the quip of the eminent
nineteenth-century pathologist Rudolf Virchow that "politics
is nothing but medicine on a grand scale" (Moynihan 1993,
p. 355). From that perspective, risk tradeoffs can be seen as a
type of iatrogenesis—increased risk resulting from therapy itself—fostered in large part by the inability of our institutions
to see and treat the "whole patient." Whether the "patient" is
an individual human or an ecosystem, those charged with reducing risk have subspecialized their roles into such finely tar-
geted elements of the nation's risk portfolio that they have
great difficulty anticipating and resolving the countervailing
consequences of their efforts to reduce risk.

Resolving risk tradeoffs would be more viable if decision-making institutions adopted a "whole patient" outlook for selecting the policies within their authority, and if some innovations in organizational structures were adopted to better link subspecialists to one another. The analytic core of the former proposal is embodied in our suggestion that decisionmakers employ risk tradeoff analysis to analyze countervailing risks as well as target risks. But because so many risk tradeoffs in decisionmaking are driven by structures that induce narrow and bounded decisions, proposing a new method of analysis will have only limited impact unless it is complemented by institutional reforms that enable and impel decisionmakers to pursue a more comprehensive analysis of risk.

Progress in Medical Decisions

Medicine has generally aimed to "treat the whole patient," and it is from this setting that we draw our exhortation. The Hippocratic oath commands physicians to "do no harm," an axiom that draws attention to the potential injuries caused by medical interventions. Moreover, a market economy gives health care providers substantial incentives to treat the whole patient, because it will do little good (in terms of health, reputation, and revenues from future care) if the physician fixes one symptom but the patient dies of the side effects, or if surviving patients are so displeased by the side effects that they switch providers.

In practice, though, there are distortions in the provision of medical care. Reimbursement rates may favor one procedure over another, or a patient's insurance status, which influences compensation to the provider for services rendered, may drive treatment choices. Even when fiscal incentives to the provider are not a factor, countervailing risks that are either subjective in character or long-term in nature may be shortchanged by physicians who focus on responding only to a target condition. But the basic problem remains of multiple specialists trying to work in concert, and it is made graphic by the high frequency of treatment-induced injury and illness in hospitals, sometimes accompanied by negligent physician behavior but also often the result of organizational failures of hospital management (Brennan et al. 1991; Leape et al. 1991; Johnson et al. 1992).

After heading toward bounded specialization for the past two decades, today the health care system is showing renewed interest in treating the whole patient. The role of the primary care physician—a general practitioner, family doctor, internal medicine physician, or pediatrician—is reentering the limelight. Whereas the fee-for-service system has been tending toward increasing specialization, health maintenance organizations (HMOs) tend to be staffed by more primary care physicians and fewer specialists. The primary care physicians at HMOs typically talk to or see the patient regularly, keep track of all symptoms, and act as gatekeepers and dispatchers for the specialists (Grumbach and Fry 1993), though cost-containment pressures at HMOs under managed care may hinder patient access to and satisfaction with their primary physicians (Gelb-Safran et al. 1994). Congress instituted reforms of the Medicare payment schedules in 1989 but left many distortions in place that still inflate the returns to specialists (Hsiao et al. 1993); many have called on the federal government to adjust these reimbursement rates to increase the returns to primary care services (for example, see ASIM 1993). And beyond financial returns, the medical education establishment is starting to renew the message that primary care and a "whole patient" approach can be glamorous. As one example, George Sheldon, surgery chairman at the University of North Carolina–Chapel Hill, has received acclaim from physicians and the news media for his "complete approach" to treating injuries through prevention (including public policies to reduce automobile traumas and violence), treatment, and research (O'Neill 1994).

Women's health is also receiving more inclusive attention. The National Institutes of Health recently established an Office for Research on Women's Health, and researchers are paying increased attention to gender in selecting their subjects for clinical trials (Holloway 1994). The case study of menopause therapy described in Chapter 2 indicates ways in which the medical community, together with patients, is working to think through and quantify a variety of target and counter-vailing risks that may affect a woman's overall health, including osteoporosis, heart disease, uterine cancer, breast cancer, vaginal and urinary dysfunctions, and mental and emotional problems. This analysis of both target and counter-vailing risks has not generated a consensus on a single "best" treatment regimen, in large part because the ideal prescription depends on the individual patient's characteristics (for example, family history of propensities for different diseases) and personal preferences. What RTA has done is to make the doctor and the patient more fully aware of the ramifications of different choices, and enable them to tailor a therapeutic strategy to the patient's portfolio of risks and preferences.

Even in the case of clozapine therapy for severe schizo-phrenia, where patient decisionmaking is impaired, counter-vailing risks are being considered in conjunction with target risks. As indicated in Chapter 3, the Food and Drug Admin-istration and the principal manufacturer of clozapine (Sandoz) began with an elaborate blood monitoring scheme to protect patients from the potentially fatal adverse side effects on the bone marrow. Blood monitoring requirements are now being relaxed to some extent, as physicians and families appear to be increasingly well informed about the potentially serious side effects of this drug. Indeed, the clozapine experience sug-gests that the drug diffusion process may be overly sensitive to countervailing risks. The drug's availability may be more restricted than necessary, since it now appears that a larger fraction of the schizophrenic population might experience overall reductions in risk if placed on clozapine therapy rather than current alternatives.

Medical decision analysts are also addressing the difficulty of comparing dissimilar risk outcomes and subjective factors, two of the analytic hurdles confronting formal use of RTA. Multi-attribute utility theory has given rise to concepts such as "quality-adjusted life years" (Weinstein and Fineberg 1980) that assist experts in the comparison of patient outcomes. As such tools become more fully developed, they will facilitate quantitative comparison of different adverse health outcomes on a single numerical scale (Pliskin et al. 1980; Loomes and

McKenzie 1989). Meanwhile, physicians are exploring patients' personal evaluations of risk tradeoffs. For example, using the drugs heparin and streptokinase in combination is somewhat more effective at reducing the target risk of blood clots in the thigh than is heparin alone, but adding streptokinase introduces a small countervailing risk of bleeding in the central nervous system that might be fatal. In order to help decide which treatment was preferable, physicians at the University of North Carolina decided to survey prospective blood clot patients. The survey indicated that in this case patients overwhelmingly preferred taking heparin alone in order to avoid the countervailing risk while tolerating more target risk (O'Meara 1994).

Progress in Government Decisions

To pursue the "whole patient" analogy for government institutions, the federal risk management staff could be seen as a hospital full of specialists but lacking a doctor in the house who can evaluate the best course of treatment for a patient with multiple organs and symptoms. American medicine is sounding the alarm when only a third of its ranks are generalists; the unfortunate reality is that in the federal government, there simply is no primary care staff for risk analysis and management at all.

One tempting yet dangerous solution to subspecialization in government would be more centralization of power in the hands of some unitary national or international agency—a "physician king" entrusted, like Plato's philosopher kings, with the power to resolve risk tradeoffs by sagely choosing a single best strategy. Such proposals are of dubious value. No one person or agency can process all the information needed to make every decision (Krier and Brownstein 1992). If a superagency were created, information costs and political forces might divide it into subagencies, and it is quite possible that the problem of neglected countervailing risks would reemerge. Meanwhile, centralization of power to deal with risk tradeoffs would itself pose significant countervailing risks. The founders of the American republic saw advantages in a diversity of power centers, including a safeguard against tyranny, the scope to experiment with different approaches and ideas, and responsiveness and accountability to local citizens.

The solution seems to us to lie not in pell-mell centralization but in improved decisionmaking skills, structures, and incentives at every level. Division of labor and freedom to experiment are useful; the challenge is to have decisionmakers in each component take into account their impacts on the larger whole.

A modest form of centralization of oversight in the federal government might nevertheless be useful. Supreme Court Justice Stephen Breyer has argued that a small group of expert risk managers, deployed in the White House after accumulating experience in numerous programs and agencies, would promote more competence and consistency in regulating risk (Breyer 1993). Although it might take twenty years or more to cultivate such a group, Breyer's vision of a cadre of expert public servants on the model of the French *conseil d'état* is worthy of serious consideration. The simple step of training experts in the risk analysis problems faced in each part of governent (Congress, the agencies, and so on) and then requiring that such multidisciplinary risk analysis expertise be located in the White House could be a major step toward incorporation of the insights of RTA into national policy. If this expert cadre would oversee the agencies' technocracy and report to the President, who is elected by the public, its existence at a central point in government could serve to strengthen rather than undermine the democratic accountability of regulatory power.

Without changes in how Congress and the regulatory agencies do their business, however, expert advisers in the White House and intelligently prepared RTAs might be ignored or never consulted in the first place. The *structure* of decisionmaking needs to direct attention to the substantive problem of risk tradeoffs. Only then will regulators be impelled to adopt methods of practice that treat the whole patient—risk-management approaches that employ RTA as a tool for diagnosis and therapy of health and environmental risks. In the following sections we discuss some specific strategies for institutionalizing RTA in the various branches of government.

Legislatures. The U.S. Congress has in the past demonstrated an awareness of risk tradeoffs. Its move in the 1970s to block the FDA's ban on saccharin (as a carcinogen) was motivated by saccharin's popularity but also by concern that alternative sweeteners posed countervailing risks of weight gain (Lave 1981). In a number of environmental statutes, Congress has paid some attention to the countervailing risks of its own actions. After enacting separate laws governing air pollution in 1970 and water pollution in 1972, thus encouraging cross-media pollution shifts, Congress made an unusual "finding" in enacting the 1976 law governing land-based solid waste disposal (RCRA): it acknowledged that one of the causes of the rising tide of solid wastes was "sludge and other pollution treatment residues" created "as a result of the Clean Air Act, the [Clean Water Act], and other Federal and State laws respecting public health and the environment" (42 U.S.C. 6901(b)(3)). Unfortunately, this finding was not sufficient to move Congress to integrate its laws into a multi-media pollution reduction approach.

More than a decade later, in the 1990 Clean Air Act provisions requiring technology-based controls of toxic air pollution, Congress did require EPA to prepare a report on its progress, including (among many other things) "any negative health or environmental consequences to the community of efforts to reduce such risks" (42 U.S.C. 7412(f)(1)(C)). Requiring such a report does not compel EPA to take such countervailing risks into account in regulating air toxics, but it certainly generates information that can influence regulatory choices. In the Clean Water Act, Congress instructed EPA to take into account (among many other factors) "non-water quality environmental impacts" when setting technology-based effluent limitations (33 U.S.C. 1314(b)(1)(B), (b)(2)(B), (b)(4)(B)), but left some ambiguity concerning whether such "impacts" are impacts of the effluent or of the effluent limitation measure. (Similar provisions on "non-air quality health and environmental impacts" appear in the Clean Air Act, 42 U.S.C. 7411(a)(1), 7412(d)(2), 7479(3).)

The 104th Congress is currently awash in proposed legislation aimed at reforming the risk management efforts of the federal government. None of these bills would integrate the fragmented structure of the medium-specific environmental laws or of the EPA's internal organization. (Indeed, the bill introduced in the 103rd Congress to raise EPA to cabinet status, S.171, would actually *increase* the number of piecemeal subfiefdoms within EPA.) But some of the bills would require analysis of countervailing risks when taking regulatory action. For example, Title III of H.R.9, the legislative embodiment of the Republican "Contract with America," would require agencies to assess "substitution risks" posed by regulations. Similarly, in the 103rd Congress, Senator Moynihan's (D–New York) amendments to the Safe Drinking Water Act reauthorization, S.1547, would have directly addressed the risk tradeoff described in Chapter 7 of this book. In section 1412(b) of the Act, he would allow EPA to modify its maximum contaminant levels for carcinogens if the original standard "would result in an increase in the overall health risk from drinking water by (i) increasing the concentration of other contaminants in drinking water; or (ii) interfering with the efficacy of drinking water treatment techniques . . ." EPA would be required to set the maximum contaminant level to "minimize the overall risk of adverse health effects, including the risk from the contaminant and the risk from other contaminants the concentrations of which may be affected by the use of treatment techniques and processes that would be employed to attain the maximum contaminant level." Other amendments would chart a broader course and require EPA to issue "periodic reports" that "evaluate risk management decisions under Federal environmental laws, including [but not limited to] the Safe Drinking Water Act, that present inherent and unavoidable choices between competing risks, including risks of controlling microbial versus disinfection contaminants in drinking water." Each such report shall discuss "the most appropriate methods of weighing and analyzing such risks," including the factors of severity, certainty, timing, and distribution of risk across the population. In section 1442, Senator Moynihan would ask EPA to conduct research on, among other things, "how to weigh and analyze competing risks" (1442(c)(3)); and he would ask EPA to prioritize its large research effort based, among other things, on targeting each "regulation [that] has the potential of imposing adverse impacts on public health" (1442(d)(6)).

There appears to be significant room for improvement in the way legislatures like the U.S. Congress consider risk tradeoffs. As described earlier, a fundamental source of risk tradeoffs is the piecemeal policies enacted by legislatures. Members are prone to the "risk of the month" syndrome that causes them to latch on to a particular target risk and pursue its elimination despite the dangers of countervailing risks (Lave and Males 1989), and they have created a panoply of subcommittees, each with its own fragmentary jurisdiction over risk policy, and a proliferation of separate issue-specific laws.

Surprisingly, unlike federal agencies proposing regulations, the U.S. Congress has not been required to formally assess or weigh the costs and benefits of proposed legislation. Agencies are required to do so under Presidential Executive Order 12866 (formerly 12291). As a first step, Congress should pass a law requiring that an RTA be commissioned and a public report of risk tradeoffs made at a meaningful step in the legislative process, such as when a bill is reported out of committee or subcommittee or conference or is brought up for action on the floor. Technical assistance to Congress might be provided by a relevant committee's staff, or by experts at offices affiliated with Congress: the Office of Technology Assessment (OTA), the Congressional Research Service (CRS), the Congressional Budget Office (CBO), or the General Accounting Office (GAO). Such analysis would help avoid new laws that cause more problems than they solve. And because risk tradeoffs are often a consequence of the omission from the risk management dialogue of groups burdened by countervailing risks, performing RTA in Congress would help bolster democratic pluralism and civic responsibility at the same time that it improved policy outcomes.

The fragmentation of Congress could be addressed by creating a Joint House-Senate Committee on Risk (Sunstein 1992). This committee might oversee all the risk policy activities of the existing committees, striving for a holistic picture that would avoid risk tradeoffs across programs, laws, and committee jurisdictions. Alternatively, the current morass of risk-related committee jurisdictions in each house of Congress could be replaced by a House Committee on Risk Policy and a Senate Committee on Risk Policy. These committees would handle all risk policy, much as the Ways and Means Committee handles all tax policy.

Several existing environmental laws have been held to prevent or constrain agencies from basing their decisions on the costs and benefits of action. Given the important detriment to the nation's campaign to reduce risk presented by risk trade-offs—a campaign often waged via legislation—legislators should revise these statutes to require agencies to base their decisions on evaluations of costs and benefits, including the use of RTA to assess net benefits. Congress could also revise the Administrative Procedures Act (APA) to clarify that rational, nonarbitrary rulemaking requires that account be taken of the countervailing risks of an agency's action. (This may already be required under the current APA language, as discussed below.)

Furthermore, Congress should revise the narrative instructions it uses in statutes that empower and direct agencies to manage risks. Many statutes currently require agencies to set standards at levels that "protect the public health" or ensure "no material harm" or "an ample margin of safety," all of which have been perplexing phrases to interpret and have triggered years of wasteful litigation without major improvements in public health (Graham 1985; Dwyer 1990). Instead Congress should legislate, as it did in the Clean Air Act for CFC-substitutes (see Chapter 10) and as it is considering doing in the Safe Drinking Water Act, that agencies act to "reduce overall risk" (or, as in the Toxic Substances Control Act, "prevent unreasonable risk"). Statutes could further define this formulation by expressly requiring an analysis and careful weighing, based on the factors in RTA, of both target and countervailing risks.

Executive Branch. The earliest RTAs were performed by academics and private consulting firms in an effort to influence executive branch regulatory policy. For example, the relative risks of alternative energy sources—taking into account risks throughout the fuel cycle from mining and transportation to generation, emissions, and waste disposal—were analyzed by advocates of nuclear power who hoped to demonstrate its net risk superiority (Inhaber 1979; Wilson 1979). More recently, RTAs of alternative vehicle fuels and cloth versus disposable diapers have been commissioned by interest groups seeking to influence regulatory policy. But the number of RTAs actually performed by analysts within the executive branch of the federal government is not well documented and is probably quite small.

Fortunately, there are encouraging signs. Not long before this book was completed, EPA decided to conduct a risk analysis of drinking water chlorination that approximates the full RTA suggested in Chapter 7, examining the effects of chlorination and several alternatives on the risks of cancer, microbial disease, acute toxicity, and other factors. There has been discussion of reforming EPA's risk analyses of pesticides to resemble more the RTA described in Chapter 9, considering not only the cancer risk of the subject pesticide but also the risk of the pesticide it would replace, as well as the risks of pests and carcinogens in foods. And EPA has recently released a study of electric vehicles (EVs), showing that the use of EVs to reduce urban air pollution can actually increase pollution, or shift it to other populations, depending on the location of and fuel used by the facility generating the electricity to charge the EVs (Suris 1994); thus the optimal use of EVs depends heavily on recognizing and managing these risk tradeoffs. As for global warming, analysts at EPA, DOE, and other federal agencies have begun nascent analyses of risk tradeoffs (Stewart and Wiener 1992; Tirpak and Ahuja 1990). While it is too early to assess the significance or permanence of these developments in EPA practice, it appears that the need for RTA is being recognized to a growing extent.

EPA has also begun to focus more attention on the problem of cross-media pollution resulting from regulatory fragmentation (Haigh and Irwin 1990; Davies 1992). A promising development is the use of "clusters," committees made up of staff and managers of various regulatory programs within the agency, to set priorities to coordinate assessment of the impact of major regulatory initiatives (Clealand-Hamnet and Retzer 1993). Clusters have been convened to address particular industries affected by multiple regulatory programs (for example, the pulp and paper industry), broad policy issues like environmental equity, and individual chemicals like lead. EPA has also endeavored to bring a multimedia theme to its enforcement actions, by simultaneously charging a facility with violations of air, water, and waste laws and seeking a global settlement (Dudek, Stewart, and Wiener 1992). The agency's increasing emphasis on "pollution prevention" and recycling programs also reflects an attempt to get out of the "shell game," although, as the lead acid battery problem discussed in Chapter 8 revealed, these programs are not immune to cross-media pollutant shifts. EPA and Amoco's joint study of the company's plant in Yorktown, Virginia, released in 1993 with much fanfare, helped demonstrate the opportunities for more flexible, cost-effective multimedia pollution reductions. The new "Common Sense Initiative," announced by administrator Carol Browner in 1994, includes a promise to bring more comprehensive, multimedia thinking to EPA's regulations; it will focus on overall pollution reductions in broad industry groupings, such as auto manufacturing, computers and electronics, iron and steel, and printing. The progress of such initiatives, however, remains to be seen.

EPA's emerging policy on CFC-substitutes is perhaps the best indication to date of both the capability of an expert agency to make complex RTA-based decisions in a situation of multiple risk endpoints, and its enthusiasm about doing so once given legislative authorization. Pursuant to a congressional requirement in the Clean Air Act that EPA regulate CFC-substitutes so as to "reduce[ ] the overall risk to human health and the environment" (section 612(c)), in May 1993 the EPA issued notice of new regulations to govern the CFC-substitutes (such as HCFCs and HFCs) now coming onto the market as CFCs are phased out in order to protect the stratospheric ozone layer. EPA addressed the risk tradeoffs surrounding CFCs and their substitutes (described in Chapter 10 of this volume) by proposing to compare alternative CFC-substitutes in terms of several risks: ozone depletion potential, toxicity, global warming potential, workplace illness, and impacts on air and water quality. EPA said it could not employ a single numerical index of net risk to rank the chemicals, but would consider quantitative measures of each risk endpoint as well as the quality of the evidence, certainty, and other information (U.S. EPA 1993).

There are several promising reforms that might move agencies closer to a "whole patient" perspective. We believe these reforms are practical and can be implemented in the foreseeable future. Recall that it was only fifteen years ago that agencies did not even have to evaluate the economic costs and benefits of proposed actions in a rigorous fashion, until such analyses were required by the Carter administration under the Paperwork Reduction Act of 1978, President Reagan under Executive Order 12291 (February 1981), and President Clinton under Executive Order 12866 (September 1993, replacing EO 12291). The agencies and White House offices are staffed by highly trained expert risk analysts and managers, and have more time to devote to analytic tasks than does the Congress. These attributes suggest their capacity to improve their analytic methods with only a short lag behind the progress observed in the academic and think-tank communities.

One avenue for reform is the rules established by the President for oversight of regulatory decisions. A Presidential Executive Order should state with specificity a requirement to perform RTA, obliging agency analysts to incorporate explicitly into estimates of the net benefits of proposed actions the effects of increases in countervailing risks (and, where relevant, reductions in coincident risks). President Reagan's Executive Order 12291, although it required analysis of the costs ("including any adverse effects," section 3(d)(2)) and benefits of agency proposals, and empowered OMB's Office of Information and Regulatory Affairs (OIRA) to supervise agency analyses, did not explicitly direct agencies or OMB to evaluate potential risk tradeoffs. President Clinton's Executive Order 12866, while reinforcing OIRA's role and the requirement to analyze costs and benefits, now does require a form of RTA: among the "costs anticipated from the regulatory action" which agencies are required to analyze are "any adverse effects on the efficient functioning of the economy, private markets . . ., *health, safety, and the natural environment*" (section 6(a)(3)(C)(ii); emphasis added). If this requirement is forcefully implemented by OMB/OIRA, it could be an important tool in identifying and reducing countervailing risks caused by regulatory actions. It would have been preferable to have covered countervailing risks in the section referring to assessment of the net benefits of a regulation rather than its costs (for both analytic and legal reasons, the latter discussed below), but for the moment this provision in EO 12866 is a bold stroke for progress against risk tradeoffs.

In most cases an agency's technical staff should be able to conduct a fairly complete RTA in its initial evaluation of a policy proposal, just as it today assesses economic costs and benefits. Agency conduct of RTA and White House oversight would in some cases require an iterative process of analysis by the agency, review by OMB/OIRA, and reanalysis by the proponent agency, because OIRA might identify pathways for risk tradeoffs that the agency had not considered or addressed. For example, OIRA might perceive a countervailing risk that the agency had neglected to address, perhaps because the agency made a heuristic omission of risks not within its jurisdiction, perhaps because OIRA's economic analysis uncovered behavioral responses to the proposal, or perhaps because the agency recognized the issue but felt it did not have the in-house expertise to do the analysis. If this responsibility is to be discharged competently, OIRA's technical staff will need to be expanded to include additional disciplines as well as economists. Or OIRA could undertake its RTA review function in consultation with other bodies with appropriate expertise, such as the White House Office of Science and Technology Policy (OSTP) or the agency whose constituency would be injured by the countervailing risk.

Agencies and subagencies should at least identify, consider, and publicize the effects of their policies on other (countervailing) risks. This policy could be imposed by the agencies themselves, in the form of internal RTA guidelines, or by the White House or Congress. Agencies would then perform RTA and inform the public of the potential risk tradeoffs (offsets, substitutions, transfers, transformations) that might accompany their proposed actions. This variant of a "right-to-know" policy would notify the potential victims of countervailing risks about their impending danger. Without such notification, constituencies affected by countervailing risks are unlikely to be mobilized quickly enough to influence policy choices.

For example, suppose an EPA program office dealing with air pollution performed RTA for a planned restriction on an air pollutant and found that the restriction would be likely to increase emissions of certain hazardous substances inside the factory workplace—a risk transfer to workers. The EPA office should notify OSHA and publish this finding, perhaps with its notice of proposed rulemaking. This kind of linkage would invite OSHA, workers, and affected communities to enter the policy dialogue, and would encourage a joint risk-reduction approach that intelligently balances and achieves protection of both the outdoor and indoor environment. The notice requirement might induce the EPA office to work with OSHA to resolve the tradeoff prior to publication. The same pattern would be played out with appropriate institutional bodies for risk transfers (for instance, from air to waterways), risk substitutions (reductions in one air pollutant but increases in another), and so forth.

In addition, the array of risk-protection institutions in the executive branch of the federal government could be better integrated. In the early 1990s the governments of the United Kingdom and Mexico consolidated their pollution and resource management agencies into more integrated environmental policy departments. Short of creating a single "super risk-protection agency," which might have countervailing drawbacks of centralization, a better integration of existing agencies could be achieved. For example, when the same chemical (such as formaldehyde) is regulated to protect workers, consumers, and the public, it may make sense to attempt a single, comprehensive rule that represents the collaborative efforts of OSHA, CPSC, and EPA rather than having three rules drafted independently. OMB/OIRA could insist on such collaboration in the regulatory review process as a method to ensure that potential risk transfers and risk transformations are considered by the interested agencies.

More radical reform could include reorganizing the executive branch to integrate the array of health and environmental protection agencies (such as EPA, DOI, USDA/USFS, DOC/NOAA, DOT/NHTSA, FDA, OSHA, and DOE/NRC) toward comprehensive management of overall risk. Some of the current fragmentation arose from political quirks, such as the placement of NOAA in the Commerce Department during the Nixon administration, and the movement of USFS from DOI to USDA early in this century. A restructuring could create two much more holistic entities: a risk management agency combining EPA, FDA, OSHA, DOT/NHTSA, and DOE/NRC under one roof, and an ecological resource agency combining DOI, USDA, and DOC/NOAA. Such a reorganization would no doubt confront those with vested interests in the current allocation and division of power, and would be difficult to undertake once cabinet secretaries had been named who would fight for their turf; an ideal time might thus be the beginning of a President's second term.

An alternative to radical restructuring would be the establishment of a "primary care provider" in the regulatory apparatus dedicated to treating the "whole patient." This "primary risk manager" would handle intake of new problems, analyze risks using RTA, dispatch cases to specialists as needed, and track progress and symptoms. Agencies with specific bounded responsibilities would then act as specialists providing secondary and tertiary care. The line agencies would retain their functions and much of their autonomy, but they would be coordinated with one another, and the primary risk manager would keep track of the whole patient and the countervailing risks that might arise from various specific policies. This tiered structure would enable more comprehensive risk policy, without the administrative drawbacks of centralizing all decisions and information (Krier and Brownstein 1992). The primary risk manager would be situated in the White House, would have a multidisciplinary staff, and would work in consultation with an interagency committee. Such an official would, among other things, encourage the White House itself to take a holistic view of risk reduction policies, and would confer on White House oversight of regulatory agencies a supportive as well as restraining disposition. (The staff of this new primary risk manager could well be the cadre of experts proposed by Justice Breyer.) The primary risk manager could be located in any number of White House offices, including OMB/OIRA, OSTP, the Council on Environmental Quality (CEQ), the National Economic Council, the office of the Chief of Staff, or in a new office reorganizing or replacing some existing functions. Perhaps the optimal niche for this manager would be as an Assistant to the President, chairing a professional Council of Risk Analysts and a Risk Management Committee made up of the heads of these other White House Offices, and with the authority (pursuant to an Executive Order, and a close working relationship with the President) to review proposed risk management actions (including regulations and proposals for legislation) and make the hard decisions occasioned by weighing risk versus risk.

We are aware that the creation of new power centers in the White House may generate concerns of excessive politicization of an analytic function. It is therefore important that new power centers publish their analyses for public criticism as well as work internally with government officials. Moreover, we believe that the problems of risk tradeoffs are sufficiently important to warrant high-level attention. Furthermore, there is politics in risk management today—but politics distorted by special interest pressures on agencies—and the process of weighing and selecting among risks in RTA inherently involves value judgments (in addition to expert input) that we believe should be made by officials accountable to a democratically elected President.

A primary risk manager could also be established for a single complex agency, as an "Undersecretary for Risk Management" created to oversee several program offices. At EPA, for example, this office would oversee the Air, Radiation, Water, Wastes, Pesticides, Pollution Prevention, and Toxic

Substances offices, with a mandate to ensure that their policies take account of risk tradeoffs and thereby "reduce overall risk." The Undersecretary for Risk at EPA could be established in the very legislation lifting EPA to cabinet status.

Apart from the fragmented regulatory risk management activities of the agencies, their splintered scientific risk assessment activities might also be better coordinated if an expert unit of the executive branch were in charge of overseeing complex risk assessments of interest to multiple agencies or of major interest to society (Rosenthal et al. 1992). Today agencies are using inconsistent risk assessment methods to address common subjects. And agencies are sometimes using questionable assumptions and methods in their risk assessments without disclosing them to the regulators who must use these data; for example, some agency risk assessments present single-point estimates that obscure uncertainties (Finkel 1990; Bogen 1990), assume exposure to a hypothetical maximum exposed individual rather than projecting realistic exposure, and extrapolate biological effects from high doses to low doses (and animals to humans) without attention to biological understanding of how agents exert their effects. Although line agencies have substantial expertise in making regulatory (risk management) decisions, they do not always cultivate the norms of analytic objectivity and the requisite scientific expertise to perform sound risk assessments. Peer review of risk assessments would likely improve their rigor and legitimacy (Graham 1991). The result of coordinating and overseeing risk assessments is likely to be more consistent and unbiased risk assessments for decisionmaking and methods that are responsive to advances in scientific knowledge, resulting in less criticism of regulatory agencies for "cooking the numbers" to support their regulatory choices.

A coordinating and oversight unit for risk assessments could be housed, for example, at the White House Office of Science and Technology Policy (OSTP), or at the U.S. Public Health Service (PHS), or at a new Council of Risk Analysts in the White House. In any event it should be separate from the office that oversees regulatory risk management decisions, namely OIRA, in order to respect the important distinction between risk assessment and risk management (NAS 1983) and to keep the scientific work distinct from the much more political work of regulatory decisionmaking. OSTP, while a small White House office, is the logical place for oversight of scientific analyses made by the agencies, and it has recently beefed up its expertise in this area with the creation of a full Associate Director position for the Environment. Still, OSTP might require additional staff, or it could rely on PHS or on a staff supplied by detailees from line agencies (or both). Moreover, OSTP has perhaps the best contacts in the nongovernmental scientific community who can help keep it informed about new developments and can recruit experts in consulting or advisory capacities on especially complex issues.

Courts. Judges play a crucial role in reviewing the regulatory decisions made by administrative agencies in light of the statutes enacted by Congress (Melnick 1983). The courts have not, however, been a reliable source of leadership for more intelligent management of society's risk portfolio (Stewart 1986). Administrative agencies should retain the lead responsibility for societal risk management, because large expert agencies are far better equipped for this task than are generalist judges with small staffs and little ability to collect data or monitor results (Stewart 1986). But courts can play a much more constructive role in shaping the guidelines for agency decisionmaking. Judges can help bring rationality to the nation's risk reduction policies by recognizing the importance of risk tradeoffs and incorporating them into standard doctrines of judicial review.

Some courts are already moving in this direction. Recently the U.S. Court of Appeals for the Fifth Circuit held that EPA, acting under the Toxic Substances Control Act (TSCA), could not regulate the target risk of asbestos-related diseases without also considering countervailing risks (*Corrosion Proof Fittings v. EPA* 1991). The court noted that EPA was banning asbestos as a carcinogen, but had considered neither the carcinogenicity of substitutes for asbestos nor whether banning the use of asbestos in brake linings might increase traffic accidents due to longer braking distances. In TSCA, Congress required EPA to have a "reasonable basis to conclude that the [substance] will present an unreasonable risk of injury to health or the environment," 15 U.S.C. 2605(a), and specifically that EPA must consider "the benefits of such substance . . . and the availability of substitutes," 15 U.S.C. 2605(c)(1)(C). The court held that EPA's failure to consider the risk of substitutes "deprives its order of a reasonable basis" because "EPA cannot say with any assurance that its regulation will increase workplace safety when it refuses to evaluate the harm that will result from the increased use of substitute products." The court pointed out that *"eager to douse the dangers of asbestos, the agency inadvertently actually may increase the risk of injury Americans face"* (emphasis added). Hence the court remanded the regulation to EPA for reconsideration.

The Fifth Circuit's decision was based on the language in the Toxic Substances Control Act requiring EPA to have a "reasoned basis" for its action, but courts are applying the concept in broader settings as well. In a recent decision about automobile fuel efficiency rules, addressing the risk tradeoff covered in Chapter 5 of this book, the U.S. Court of Appeals for the District of Columbia Circuit held that the National Highway Traffic Safety Administration's rulemaking process was not "reasoned" when it focused on the environmental risks of excessive fuel use but failed to confront the countervailing risk of occupant injury in automobile crashes resulting from the use of smaller vehicles (*CEI v. NHTSA* 1992). Applying the general doctrine that an agency must provide a "reasoned analysis" for its decision, the court stated that NHTSA could have "seriously examined" both risks, "faced the [risk] tradeoff," and explained "its judgment [that] the trade-off was worth it" (pp. 323–324). But the court found that NHTSA had not done so; the defect was "not . . . NHTSA's judgment call, but . . . NHTSA's attempt to paper over the need to make a call" (p. 323). The upshot of the court's ruling is that under bedrock principles of administrative law, agencies must confront risk tradeoffs and weigh risk versus risk.

Since these are recent cases in a large body of administrative law, their long-term significance is unclear. Some court decisions have upheld agency decisions not to regulate in the face of large countervailing risks, but few have required agencies to weigh countervailing risks where the agency had not done so (see Warren and Marchant 1993, p. 428). Courts could strengthen their approach to risk tradeoffs in several ways. Confirming the holding in *CEI v. NHTSA*, courts could hold that an agency rulemaking is "arbitrary and capricious" under the Administrative Procedures Act (APA) (5 U.S.C. 706), as a failure to undertake "reasoned analysis," if it ignores important countervailing risks. The Supreme Court's decision in the 1984 airbags case, *Motor Vehicle Manufacturers Association v. State Farm Insurance* (1983), made clear that agencies must conduct a "reasoned analysis" and furnish a "reasoned basis" for their decisions. Our suggestion would offer a specific analytic yardstick for judging whether the agency's approach has been reasoned: the agency would satisfy the "reasoned analysis and basis" test if it applied RTA by considering the risk tradeoff, weighing risk versus risk, and making a reasoned judgment about the preferred course in that context (including the possibility of "risk-superior" moves). The court would not be required to judge the substantive reasonableness of the agency's conclusion, only to ensure that the agency confronted the risk tradeoff.

In cases where increases in countervailing risks are so great that they actually outweigh the reduction in the target risk, in total or at the margin, courts might question the substantive reasonableness of the agency's conclusion and find such a decision to be "arbitrary and capricious" (in violation of the APA). The Fifth Circuit adopted this approach nominally under the "substantial evidence" test, but its reasoning seems equally applicable to the more typical and less stringent "arbitrary and capricious" standard of review. In such cases the agency would be proposing to do "more harm than good," which seems at least intuitively "arbitrary and capricious" (Warren and Marchant 1993).

Our point is not that courts should take on the task of estimating countervailing risks and selecting what they believe to be optimal risk strategies. As we have noted throughout this book, those tasks require both substantial expertise and attention to public valuations of different risks, and are therefore better performed by technically competent agencies accountable to elected officials. Furthermore, oversight of agencies' risk tradeoff analyses and decisions would best be handled by the executive branch, employing one or more of the oversight measures we described earlier, such as a White House risk oversight body to review RTAs and to provide primary risk management direction, or primary risk managers in each agency.

There may nevertheless be times when the executive branch apparatus fails to address important risk tradeoffs, and it is in circumstances like these that judicial review is the last bulwark of sound administrative government. If courts do not stand ready to insist on consideration of countervailing risks, agencies may neglect important side effects of their decisions, as in *CEI v. NHTSA*, or decide to impose ostensibly risk-reducing rules that actually generate more risk than they prevent. The prospect and occasional reality of judicial review can help instill in agencies diligent attention to risk tradeoffs. It would still be the responsibility of interested parties to present such information to the agency during its rulemaking, and of the agency to face and weigh the tradeoffs in its competent discretion. Generalist courts would simply review the agency's administrative record, as they normally do, and assess whether the agency conducted a "reasoned analysis" and avoided "arbitrary and capricious" decisions in view of the guideposts of risk tradeoff analysis.

In addition to principles of administrative law and the APA, courts also ensure adherence to the terms of the regulatory statute under which the agency is acting. Courts should find RTA obligatory under many existing statutes. There may be isolated cases (for example, the draconian Delaney Clause described in Chapter 9) in which the statute proscribes RTA or insists on decreases in a target risk regardless of countervailing risks. But if the statute provides for prevention of "unreasonable risk" or for balancing of costs and benefits, then there are ample grounds for requiring the agency to undertake RTA. For example, the Toxic Substances Control Act (TSCA) calls for protection against "unreasonable risk" (15 U.S.C.

2605(a)), the Occupational Safety and Health Act requires standards set that are "reasonably necessary or appropriate to provide safe or healthful employment" (29 U.S.C. 652(8)), and the Clean Water Act says effluent limitations shall "result in reasonable further progress" toward clean water goals (33 U.S.C. 1311(b)(2)(A)). Other examples of such language can be found in the Federal Insecticide, Fungicide, and Rodenticide Act (FIFRA) and the Consumer Product Safety Act. Courts have often interpreted the words "reasonable" or "unreasonable risk" to require that the burdens of agency action be justified by gains, that is, to mean that an increment of risk is "unreasonable" only where it would be worthwhile (benefits justify costs) to prevent it (for example, *ATMI v. Donovan* 1981, pp. 510–511; *UAW v. OSHA* 1991, pp. 1319–1320; *AquaSlide 'N Dive Corp. v. CPSC* 1978, p. 839). That has long been the standard of "reasonableness" in tort law as well (*U.S. v. Carroll Towing Co.* 1947, p. 173). Under these circumstances, it is a modest step for courts to say that "reasonable" policy requires at least consideration of countervailing risks that the policy might itself cause, and it is just a clarification of current law to say that a policy is substantively "unreasonable" where its net benefits, accounting for countervailing as well as target risks, do not justify its costs. When courts apply these principles in judging agency action under "reasonable risk" statutes, they should recognize that RTA requires both technical expertise and sensitive value judgments, making considerable deference to agency decisions appropriate.

RTA should not be precluded, however, under statutes that prohibit cost-benefit analysis or consideration of cost. Such statutes prohibit consideration of financial cost and require the agency to look solely at health-based factors or maximum feasible environmental improvement (for example, *NRDC v. EPA* 1989; *ATMI v. Donovan* 1981). Courts should nonetheless require RTA under these laws, because risk tradeoffs are part of the health-based or environment-based calculus—a feature of the effectiveness of the rule in attaining its risk-reduction goals—rather than a financial cost of the rule. While full policy analysis addresses cost-benefit tradeoffs, RTA addresses the set of risks reduced and increased at a given level of social opportunity cost—the net benefits. Recall that in the head-ache/aspirin example in Chapter 1, we did not ask how much a dose of aspirin (or acetaminophen, or ibuprofen) costs to purchase, though surely that would matter for any complete decision; we asked about the full portfolio of risks affected by an equivalent dose of each of the analgesics—a question that is often missed in more complex choices. Consequently courts could and should require the evaluation of countervailing risks as part of the risk-reduction analysis that supports such a rule. It is also for this reason that President Clinton's EO 12866 would have avoided confusion if it had classified coun-tervailing risks to health, safety, and the environment as part of the benefits assessment rather than part of the costs as-sessment.

To remedy the problem of risk transfers caused by omitted voice, one approach would be to confer on victims of counter-vailing risks arising from agency actions the standing to chal-lenge such actions. Victims of risk tradeoffs might be excluded from such lawsuits because by definition they are not victims of the target risk, and the Supreme Court has held that for a litigant to have standing to sue to challenge agency actions in federal court, he or she must, unless Congress provides dif-ferently in a particular statute, be "within the zone of interests" meant to be protected by the statute (*Association of Data Pro-cessing Service Organizations v. Camp* 1970). Although this test has sometimes been downplayed, the Court occasionally applies it to bar litigants from challenging policies meant to protect other interests (Menell and Stewart 1994, pp. 833–834; see *Clarke v. Securities Industry Ass'n* 1987, pp. 397–400). The Court derived the "zone of interests" test from the APA, which entitles to judicial review any person who is "ad-versely affected . . . by agency action within the meaning of a relevant statute" (5 U.S.C. 702). But the very difficulty of coun-tervailing risks is that they are often outside the ambit of the statute's stated scope or objective or even inconsistent with the statute's intention. Giving victims of countervailing risks such standing (presumably by clarification of the APA, or through a clarifying Supreme Court decision) might help force agencies to consider the victims of risk transfers. On the other hand, more lawsuits can be dysfunctional: litigation directed at administrative agencies can add more to paralysis and to rulemaking costs (and thereby discourage public rulemaking as a policy vehicle) than it improves the prospect for intelligent decisions (Graham, Green, and Roberts 1988).

Another way to enable litigants to challenge the countervailing risks of risk-management decisions would be judicial reform of the "functional equivalence" doctrine for environmental impact statements (EISs). Under the National Environmental Policy Act (NEPA), all federal agencies undertaking major actions must prepare EISs. Congress has exempted certain environmental regulatory actions from the requirement to perform an EIS (for example, actions under the Clean Air Act, 15 U.S.C. 793(c)(1), and the Clean Water Act, 33 U.S.C. 1371(c)), and by regulation EPA has exempted itself from EIS requirements under RCRA (40 C.F.R. 124.9(b)(6)). The courts have gone further, holding that a regulatory action undertaken by EPA, because it necessarily relies on consideration of environmental protection, is the "functional equivalent" of an EIS (for example, *EDF v. EPA* 1973). Courts have asserted that EPA's internal structure would assure attention to risk tradeoffs (*Weyerhauser v. Costle* 1978, p. 1053). The difficulty, of course, is that regulatory actions aimed at a target environmental risk may increase countervailing risks (to the environment or to other endpoints), and EPA's internal fragmentation often foments rather than prevents such tradeoffs. Given the purpose of EISs under NEPA to ensure recognition of all important environmental impacts of government action, courts could and should relax the "functional equivalence" exemption in cases where a prima facie case can be made that the environmental regulatory action would pose the risk of significant adverse effects on the environment (in the same or other media as the regulation would address).

International Institutions. The fragmentation and bounded specialization of government decisionmaking that drives many risk tradeoffs in the United States is also apparent at the global level, as detailed in Chapter 10. For example, the primary mission of the World Health Organization (WHO) in combating disease may have contributed to its neglect of the environmental side effects of using DDT to eliminate malaria (see Chapter 9), and the primary mission of the United Nations Environment Programme (UNEP) in protecting the global environment may have contributed to the arguable tradeoff between preventing ozone depletion and allowing food spoilage in the treaty that UNEP spearheaded to phase out CFCs (see Chapter 10).

Integrating the risk management functions of these international institutions might help solve global risk tradeoffs. Proposals such as those by Esty (1994) for a "global environmental organization," integrating the current agencies designed to protect the environment (UNEP) and human health (WHO) and to manage forests and agricultural land use (FAO), would go a long way in this regard. But to take comprehensive account of risk tradeoffs, such an entity ought to include as well attention to other risks, such as risks in the occupational, product use, and medical areas, even if there is no international regulatory regime to direct policy for such local risks. Integrating UNEP, WHO, and FAO into a large global organization could exacerbate risk tradeoffs in the categories not governed by the new entity's mission.

But the major risk tradeoffs identified in Chapter 10 resulted largely from causes other than institutional fragmentation. For example, the focus on global warming (and on carbon dioxide from energy sources in particular) of the Intergovernmental Panel on Climate Change (IPCC) and the subsequent treaty negotiating committee is difficult to explain as bounded specialization given these institutions' broad aegis, and might be better explained on the basis of heuristic decisionmaking frameworks. The key to moderating these kinds of risk tradeoffs at the global level is not necessarily integration of current mission-oriented institutions, though that might be helpful, but a method of analysis practiced at each decisionmaking point which internalizes the side effects of pursuing the target mission. A new global agency would not necessarily address the problems of heuristics, and might still fall prey to myopic focus on an ad hoc risk agenda. And it might find, as the U.S. EPA did, that initially synoptic intentions cannot hold back the political and administrative pressures for internal bureaucratic fragmentation. Furthermore, the benefits of integrated decisionmaking need to be considered in light of the disadvantages of centralizing power, especially at the international level where decisionmakers may be especially unaccountable to the public interest.

For these reasons the substantive application of risk tradeoff analysis to global decisionmaking appears to be a prior and more fundamental reform than a structural merger of existing institutions. The kinds of structural changes discussed here and earlier in the domestic context—such as integration of fragmented agencies, establishment of primary risk managers, and review of agency risk management decisions by executive and judicial authorities—could, if deployed appropriately, be quite helpful tools to ensure that international institutions employ risk tradeoff analysis and internalize a vision of "overall risk reduction."

Toward a New Paradigm for Risk Reduction

These analytic and structural reforms, important as they are, will ultimately not succeed without some cultural maturation. Under a new "whole patient paradigm," the first inclination would no longer be to strike impetuously at a target risk, but rather to understand better the complex interrelations of systems and gain more mastery over the broad terrain of countervailing risks.

This cultural change is not so remote or abstract as it might at first seem. The very basis for the creation of the risk-regulation institutions in the United States today—EPA, FDA, OSHA, CPSC, and others—was a recognition of the imperfections of market decisionmaking and a pivotal cultural change that turned to public policy to ensure that market decisionmakers took into account impacts (such as pollution) that they had heretofore viewed as external. That cultural change built slowly throughout this century, culminating in a major paradigm shift in risk policy around 1970. Similarly, the stated aim of the 1969 National Environmental Policy Act (NEPA) was to inculcate a culture of environmental risk awareness into all federal decisionmaking. It is no accident that NEPA, the modern Clean Water and Clean Air Acts, and their related institutions were all created around 1970, riding a cultural shift in the nation's attitudes toward human health and the environment.

But it is ironic that these very regulatory institutions, those responsible for promoting health and environmental values in society, can themselves create countervailing risks. Fortunately, we think, the cultural shift of the 1970s has reached a point of sufficient maturity and accomplishment that the system can now embrace the complex phenomenon of risk tradeoffs. New analytic methods and reformed institutions will be manifestations of the transition to this more holistic outlook.

The new culture we are envisaging is actually not so new. It has its intellectual roots in several crucial twentieth-century developments in thought and practice. It is these much broader forces that have laid the basis for the use of a new tool, risk tradeoff analysis, as we have described it.

First, as discussed earlier, RTA is quite apparent in the medical community's renewed enthusiasm for the primary care provider, who looks at all outcomes affecting the "whole patient." Formal analysis of clinical decisions and the full panoply of patient outcomes, aided by methods such as decision theory, is currently a major growth industry in schools of medicine and public health.

Second, RTA can be seen as a renewed expression of the ecological ethic that underlies American environmental policy. As the ecologist John Muir wrote in 1869, "When we try to pick out anything by itself, we find it hitched to everything else in the universe" (Muir 1988, p. 110). That basic insight motivates the entire discussion of risk tradeoffs. And that insight has always been foremost in the minds of leading ecologists and public health experts who recognize the danger in preoccupation with a single symptom or problem in isolation. Our environmental politics is now beginning to recognize the wisdom in Muir's statement as a caution against simple preoccupation with each target risk that happens to capture the attention of the mass media. Moreover, the modern science of chaos mathematics is in a way formalizing Muir's idea that everything is interconnected, and that even seemingly small actions in one part of a system will affect other parts. In addition, environmental policy is coming to incorporate Charles Darwin's related insight that biological communities survive in perpetual evolutionary dynamism and interaction, and that humans are part of this community—one of many species evolved from common ancestors, sharing the globe. Darwin's thesis implies that human activity has complex interfaces with other ecological activity, that it does not occur in isolation, that there is no simple categorical difference between "nature" and human beings (much as later ecological ethicists, like Aldo Leopold and William Devall, have argued from a very different perspective), and therefore that outcomes for each species (including our own) depend on the consequences of many individual actions and environmental interactions over time (Botkin 1990). The RTA framework offers a chance to account for this complexity and dynamism as we adopt a more encompassing view of the campaign to reduce risk and of our world as a whole.

Third, the new culture we describe derives from fundamental principles of social science developed in this century. The call for seeing and treating the "whole patient" draws not only on physical medicine but also on Gestalt psychology: the idea that perceptions of the whole are qualitatively different from perceptions of each piece taken at a time. The ideas that leverage on a target risk can increase other risks, and that there are tradeoffs and potentially perverse feedbacks, are essential features of integrated systems analysis. The attention drawn to omitted voices as a source of dysfunctional risk tradeoffs, and the point that weighing risk tradeoffs depends not just on quantitative factors estimated by technocrats but on values and ethics that vary from community to community and person to person, are essential foundations of democratic pluralism. The realization that actions in one locale may transfer risk to others, and that such consequences are of concern to us all, is part of an evolution of human political identity from towns to nation-states to global interdependence.

The challenge of risk tradeoffs is thus a challenge to remake the paradigm for risk policy. The new paradigm recognizes that systems are complex and chaotic, without teleological directions, in discord as often as in harmony. It rejects simple laws of inexorable progress or perverse intransigence. It rejects complete reliance on science or complete reliance on popular will, on objective expertise or on subjective values. It rejects inaction—in the face of either target risks or countervailing risks—and counsels enlightened intervention. Faced with complex, multidimensional realities, the new paradigm resists the temptation to despair or to be satisfied with piecemeal responses, and urges confidence in the capacity of human reason to confront and resolve risk tradeoffs. As our society's paradigm is changing from yesterday's fragmented, bounded approach to a more integrated, whole-patient culture, our effort should be to fashion useful tools, like RTA, that can translate the new mind-set into practical decisions. This experiment in pragmatism may hold the key to saving the national campaign to reduce risk from itself.

References

1. Confronting Risk Tradeoffs

Adler, Jonathan H. 1992. "Clean Fuels, Dirty Air." In *Environmental Politics: Public Costs, Private Awards,* ed. Michael S. Greve and Fred L. Smith, pp. 19–45. New York: Praeger.

Ames, Bruce N., Renae Magaw, and Lois Swirsky Gold. 1987. "Ranking Possible Carcinogenic Hazards." *Science,* vol. 236, April 17, pp. 271–280.

Ames, Bruce N., Margie Profet, and Lois Swirsky Gold. 1990a. "Nature's Chemicals and Synthetic Chemicals: Comparative Toxicology." *Proceedings of the National Academy of Sciences USA,* vol. 87, pp. 7782–7786.

———— 1990b. "Dietary Pesticides (99.9% All Natural)." *Proceedings of the National Academy of Sciences,* vol. 87, pp. 7777–7781.

Ames, Bruce N., and Lois Swirsky Gold. 1993. "Another Perspective . . . Nature's Way," *Consumer's Research,* vol. 76, no. 8, August, p. 20.

Anderson, Christopher. 1991. "Cholera Epidemic Tied to Risk Miscalculation." *Nature,* vol. 354, November 28, p. 255.

Anderton, D. L., et al. 1994. "Hazardous Waste Facilities: Environmental Equity Issues in Metropolitan Areas." *Evaluation Review,* vol. 18, pp. 123–140.

Angier, Natalie. 1992. "Debate on Buildings: to Scrub or Not." *New York Times,* Jan. 14, p. C1.

Associated Press (AP). 1994. "U.S. Warns About Drug for Cancer." *New York Times,* April 9, p. 9.

Bartel, Ann T., and Lacy G. Thomas. 1985. "Direct and Indirect Effects of Regulation: A New Look at OSHA's Impact." *Journal of Law and Economics,* vol. 28, pp. 1–25.

Been, Vicki. 1994. "Locally Undesirable Land Uses in Minority Neighborhoods: Disproportionate Siting or Market Dynamics?" *Yale Law Journal,* vol. 103, pp. 1383–1415.

Bowman, Karlyn H., and Everett C. Ladd, eds. 1993. "Public Opinion and Demographic Report." *The American Enterprise,* May/June, pp. 100–101.

Breyer, Stephen G. 1982. *Regulation and Its Reform.* Cambridge, Mass.: Harvard University Press.

Brody, Jane E. 1994. "Strong Views on Origins of Cancer." *New York Times,* July 5, pp. B5–B9.

Brown, David L., ed. 1992. *Risk and Outcome in Anesthesia.* Philadelphia: Lippincott.

Bullard, Robert D. 1990. *Dumping in Dixie: Race, Class, and Environmental Quality.* Oxford: Westford Press.

Bunker, J. P., B. Barnes, and F. Mosteller, eds. 1977. *Costs, Risks, and Benefits of Surgery.* New York: Oxford University Press.

Bureau of the Census, U.S. Department of Commerce. 1992. *Statistical Abstract of the United States 1992.*

Burger, Edward J. 1990. "Health as a Surrogate for the Environment." *Daedalus,* vol. 119, no. 4, Fall, pp. 133–154.

Centers for Disease Control (CDC), U.S. Department of Health and Human Services, Public Health Service. 1993. *Monthly Vital Statistics Report,* vol. 41 (7), Supplement, Jan. 4.

Centers for Disease Control (CDC), Public Health Service, U.S. Department of Health and Human Services. 1991. *Fact Book.* Atlanta.

Chirinko, Robert S., and Edward P. Harper. 1993. "Buckle Up or Slow Down? New Estimates of Offsetting Behavior and Their Implications for Automobile Safety Regulation." *Journal of Policy Analysis and Management,* vol. 12, pp. 270–298.

Corrosion Proof Fittings v. U.S. Environmental Protection Agency (EPA), 947 F.2d 1201 (5th Cir. 1991).

Council of Economic Advisers (CEA), Executive Office of the President. 1994. *Economic Report of the President 1994,* Washington, D.C.

Crandall, Robert C. 1983. *Controlling Industrial Pollution: The Economics and Politics of Clean Air.* Washington, D.C., Brookings.

Crandall, Robert C., Howard K. Gruenspecht, Theodore Keeler, and Lester Lave. 1986. *Regulating the Automobile.* Washington, D.C.: Brookings.

Crouch, Edmund, and Richard Wilson. 1982. *Risk-Benefit Analysis.* Cambridge, Mass.: Ballinger.

Davies, J. Clarence (Terry). 1988. "The Environmental Protection Act." Second Draft, September. Washington, D.C.: The Conservation Foundation.

Dudek, Daniel J., Alice LeBlanc, and Peter Miller. 1990. "Sulphur Dioxide and Carbon Dioxide: Consistent Policymaking in the Greenhouse." Working Paper, Environmental Defense Fund, New York.

Dudek, Daniel J., Richard B. Stewart, and Jonathan B. Wiener. 1992. "Environmental Policy for Eastern Europe: Technology-Based Versus Market-Based Approaches." *Columbia Journal of Environmental Law,* vol. 17, pp. 1–52.

Duke, Steven B. 1993. *America's Longest War: Rethinking Our Tragic Crusade Against Drugs.* New York: Putnam's Sons.

Dunlap, Riley E. 1991. "Public Opinion in the 1980s: Clear Consensus, Ambiguous Commitment." *Environment,* October, pp. 10–37.

Economist magazine. 1994. "Display Technology: City Lights." September 3, pp. 80–81.

Edelson, Ed. 1991. "What a Relief." *American Health,* vol. 10, no. 9, November, p. 9.

Evans, Leonard. 1985. "Driver Behavior Revealed in Relations Involving Car Mass." In *Human Behavior and Traffic Safety,* ed. Leonard Evans and Richard Schwing. New York: Plenum Press, pp. 337–352.

Fisher, Jeffrey A. 1994. *The Plague Makers: How We Are Creating Catastrophic New Epidemics—And What We Must Do to Avert Them.* New York: Simon and Schuster.

Frey, Christopher H. 1992. "Quantitative Analysis of Uncertainty and Variability in Environmental Policy Making." Draft report, U.S. Environmental Protection Agency, Washington, D.C., September.

Fuchs, Victor. 1986. *The Health Economy.* Cambridge, Mass.: Harvard University Press.

Geiser, Kenneth. 1991. "The Greening of Industry: Making the Transition to a Sustainable Economy." *Technology Review,* August/September, pp. 64–72.

Graham, John D., ed. 1988. *Preventing Automobile Injury: New Findings from Evaluation Research.* Dover, Mass.: Auburn House.

Graham, John D. 1990. *Auto Safety: Assessing America's Performance.* Dover, Mass.: Auburn House.

———— 1991. "Improving Chemical Risk Assessment." *Regulation,* Fall, pp. 14–17.

Graham, John D., Bei-Hung Chang, and John D. Evans. 1992. "Poorer Is Riskier." *Risk Analysis,* vol. 12, no. 3, pp. 333–337.

Graham, John D., and George M. Gray. 1993. "Optimal Use of 'Toxic Chemicals.' " In *Risk in Perspective,* Harvard Center for Risk Analysis, vol. 1, no. 2, May.

Grossman, Gene M., and Alan B. Krueger. 1991. "Environmental Impacts of a North American Free Trade Agreement." Princeton University Department of Economics, October 8.

Gruenspecht, Howard K. 1992. "Differentiated Regulation: The Case of Auto Emissions Standards." *American Economic Review,* vol. 72 (Papers and Proceedings), May, pp. 328–331.

Guruswamy, Lakshman. 1991. "The Case for Integrated Pollution Control." *Law and Contemporary Problems,* vol. 54, no. 4, pp. 41–56, Autumn.

Hahn, Robert, and Eric Males. 1990. "Can Regulatory Institutions Cope with Cross Media Pollution?" *Journal of the Air and Waste Management Association,* vol. 40 (1), pp. 24–31.

Haigh, Nigel, and Frances Irwin, eds. 1990. *Integrated Pollution Control in Europe and North America.* Washington, D.C.: The Conservation Foundation.

Hamilton, James T. 1993. "Politics and Social Costs: Estimating the Impact of Collective Action on Hazardous Waste Facilities." *RAND Journal of Economics,* vol. 24, pp. 101–125.

Hammitt, James, and Jonathan A. K. Cave. 1991. *Research Planning for Food Safety: A Value-of-Information Approach.* Santa Monica, Calif.: RAND Corporation.

Harrington, Winston. 1989. *Acid Rain: Science and Policy.* Washington, D.C.: Resources for the Future, p. 16.

Health Effects Institute (HEI), Asbestos Research. 1991. *Asbestos in Public and Commercial Buildings: A Literature Review and Synthesis of Current Knowledge.* Cambridge, Mass.

Hileman, Bette. 1994. "Environmental Estrogens Linked to Reproductive Abnormalities, Cancer." *Chemical and Engineering News,* January 31, pp. 19–23.

Hird, John. 1993. "Environmental Policy and Equity: The Case of Superfund." *Journal of Policy Analysis and Management,* vol. 12, no. 2, pp. 323–343.

Hirschman, Albert O. 1991. *The Rhetoric of Reaction: Perversity, Futility, Jeopardy.* Cambridge, Mass.: Harvard University Press.

Hopkins, Thomas D., ed. 1992. *Regulatory Policy in Canada and the*

United States. Conference Proceedings, Rochester Institute of Technology, Rochester, N.Y.

Hornstein, Donald T. 1992. "Reclaiming Environmental Law: A Normative Critique of Comparative Risk Analysis." *Columbia Law Review,* vol. 92, pp. 562–633.

Hoskin, Alan F., J. Paul Leigh, and Thomas W. Planek. 1994. "Estimated Risk of Occupational Fatalities Associated with Hazardous Waste Site Remediation." *Risk Analysis,* vol. 14, no. 6 (December), pp. 1011–1017.

Huber, Peter. 1983. "The Old-New Division in Risk Regulation." *Virginia Law Review,* vol. 69, no. 6, September, pp. 1025–1107.

Kaminer, Wendy. 1994a. "Crime and Community." *The Atlantic Monthly,* May, pp. 111–120.

——— 1994b. "Federal Offense." *The Atlantic Monthly,* June, pp. 102–114.

Keeney, Ralph L. 1990. "Mortality Risks Induced by Economic Expenditures." *Risk Analysis,* vol. 10, no. 1, pp. 147–159.

——— 1994. "Sounding Board: Decisions about Life-Threatening Risks." *New England Journal of Medicine,* vol. 331, no.3, July 21, pp. 193–196.

Keeney, Ralph L., and Howard Raiffa. 1976. *Decisions with Multiple Objectives: Preferences and Value Tradeoffs.* New York: John Wiley and Sons.

Keeney, Ralph L., and Detlof von Winterfeldt. 1986. "Why Indirect Health Risks of Regulations Should Be Examined." *Interfaces,* vol. 16, pp. 13–27.

Kellerman, A. L., and D. T. Reay. 1986. "Protection or Peril: An Analysis of Firearm-Related Deaths in the Home." *New England Journal of Medicine,* vol. 314, pp. 1557–1560.

Kellerman, A. L., et al. 1993. "Gun Ownership as a Risk Factor for Homicide in the Home." *New England Journal of Medicine,* vol. 329, pp. 1084–1091.

Kleiman, Mark A. R. 1992. *Against Excess: Drug Policy for Results.* New York: Basic Books.

Krimsky, Sheldon, and Dominic Golding, eds. 1992. *Social Theories of Risk.* Westport, Conn.: Praeger.

Kuhn, Thomas S. 1970. *The Structure of Scientific Revolutions,* 2d ed. Chicago: University of Chicago Press.

Lancaster, John. 1991. "Weighing the Gain in Oil-Spill Cures: Harm from Aggressive Hot-Water Cleanup May Eclipse the Environmental Benefits." *Washington Post,* April 22, p. A3.

Landy, Marc, Marc J. Roberts, and Stephen Thomas. 1990. *The En-*

vironmental Protection Agency: Asking the Wrong Questions. New York: Oxford University Press.

Lave, Lester B. 1981. *The Strategy of Social Regulation: Decision Frameworks for Policy.* Washington, D.C.: Brookings.

Lave, Lester B., and Eric H. Males. 1989. "At Risk: The Framework for Regulating Toxic Substances." *Environmental Science and Technology,* vol. 23, no. 4, pp. 386–391.

Loy, Wesley. 1993. "Dredging for Lessons from the Tragedy in Prince William Sound." *Washington Post,* Feb. 15, p. A3.

Morgan, M. Granger, and Max Henrion. 1990. *Uncertainty: A Guide to Dealing with Uncertainty in Quantitative Risk and Policy Analysis.* New York: Cambridge University Press.

Moynihan, Daniel Patrick. 1993. "Iatrogenic Government: Social Policy and Drug Research." *American Scholar,* Summer, pp. 351–362.

National Academy of Sciences. 1981. *Risk and Decision Making: Perspectives and Research.* Washington, D.C.

Neff, Joseph. 1994. "More Lockups Fail to Reduce Violent Crime, Study Says." *Raleigh News and Observer,* June 6, p. 3A.

Nemecek, Sasha. 1994. "Backfire: Could Prozac and Elavil Promote Tumor Growth?" *Scientific American,* vol. 271, no. 3, September, pp. 22–23.

New York Times. 1994. "New Whooping Cough Vaccine Is Said to Eliminate Side Effects." Nov. 25, p. A20.

Office of Management and Budget (OMB), Executive Office of the President. 1990–1991. *Regulatory Program of the U.S. Government.* Washington, D.C.

Ottoboni, M. Alice. 1991. *The Dose Makes the Poison,* 2d ed. New York: Van Nostrand Reinhold.

Peltzman, Sam. 1975. "The Effects of Automobile Safety Regulation." *Journal of Political Economy,* vol. 83, no. 4, pp. 677–725.

——— 1985. *The Regulation of Automobile Safety.* Washington, D.C.: American Enterprise Institute for Public Policy Research.

Pirkle, James L., et al. 1994. "The Decline in Blood Lead Levels in the United States: the National Health and Nutrition Examination Surveys (NHANES)." *Journal of the American Medical Association,* vol. 272, no. 4, July 27, pp. 284–291.

Poore, Patricia. 1992. "Disposable Diapers are O.K.: The Real World." *Garbage,* Oct./Nov., pp. 27–31.

Portney, Paul R. 1988. "Reforming Environmental Regulation: Three Modest Proposals." *Issues in Science and Technology,* vol. 4, no. 2, Winter, pp. 74–81.

Rice, Faye. 1992. "Next Steps for the Environment." *Fortune,* October 19, pp. 98–100.

Roe, David. 1989. "An Incentive-Conscious Approach to Toxic Chemical Controls." *Economic Development Quarterly,* vol. 3, no. 3, August, pp. 179–187.

Roy, Manik, and Hillel Gray. 1992. "Toxics Use Reduction: The Critical Issues." *Pollution Prevention Review,* Spring, pp. 181–188.

Russell, Milton, E. William Colglazier, and Mary R. English. 1991. "Hazardous Waste Remediation: The Task Ahead." University of Tennessee, Knoxville, December, p. 16.

Samet, Jonathan, and John Spengler, eds. 1991. *Indoor Air Pollution: A Health Perspective.* Baltimore: Johns Hopkins University Press.

Schneider, Keith. 1991. "Harm to Nature from Valdez Spill is Now Seen as Far Worse by U.S." *New York Times,* April 10, p. A1.

——— 1993. "Sea-Dumping Ban: Good Politics, but Not Necessarily Good Policy." *New York Times,* March 22, p. A1.

Schumpeter, Joseph A. 1942. *Capitalism, Socialism and Democracy.* New York: Harper.

Sedjo, Roger A. 1993. "Global Consequences of U.S. Environmental Policies." *Journal of Forestry,* vol. 91, no. 4, April, pp. 19–21.

Sen, Amartya. 1993. "The Economics of Life and Death." *Scientific American,* May, pp. 40–47.

Slovic, Paul. 1986. "Informing and Educating the Public about Risk." *Risk Analysis,* vol. 6, pp. 403–415.

Starr, Chauncey, and Christopher Whipple. 1980. "Risks of Risk Decisions." *Science,* vol. 208, p. 1114.

Taylor, Humphrey. 1992. "Prospects for Prevention." *Health Management Quarterly,* vol. 14, pp. 21–24.

Tolley, George, Donald Kenkel, and Robert Fabian, eds. 1994. *Valuing Health for Policy: An Economic Approach.* Chicago and London: University of Chicago Press.

Tuchman, Barbara W. 1984. *The March of Folly: From Troy to Vietnam.* New York: Ballantine Books.

Tversky, A., and D. Kahneman. 1974. "Judgement under Uncertainty: Heuristics and Biases." *Science,* vol. 185, p. 1124.

U.S. Department of Agriculture (USDA). 1992. "Americans Are Eating More Fruits and Vegetables." *Farmline,* July, pp. 8–9, 12.

U.S. Department of Health and Human Services (HHS). 1992. *Health USA and Prevention Profile.* Hyattsville, Md.: U.S. Public Health Service.

U.S. Environmental Protection Agency (EPA). 1990. *Environmental Investments: The Cost of a Clean Environment.* Washington, D.C.

Viscusi, W. Kip. 1992. *Fatal Tradeoffs: Public and Private Responsibilities for Risk.* New York: Oxford University Press.

———— 1993. *Product-Risk Labeling: A Federal Responsibility.* Washington, D.C.: American Enterprise Institute.

Viscusi, W. Kip, et al. 1994. Symposium on "Mortality Costs of Regulatory Expenditures." *Journal of Risk and Uncertainty,* vol. 8, no. 1.

Viscusi, W. Kip, Wes Magat, and Joel Huber. 1991. "Pricing Environmental Health Risks: Survey Assessments of Risk-Risk and Risk-Dollar Tradeoffs for Chronic Bronchitis." *Journal of Environmental Economics and Management,* vol. 21, pp. 32–51.

Whipple, Christopher. 1985. "Redistributing Risk." *Regulation,* May/June, pp. 37–44.

Wiener, Norbert. 1993. *Invention: The Care and Feeding of Ideas.* Cambridge, Mass.: MIT Press.

Wildavsky, Aaron. 1979. "No Risk Is the Highest Risk of All." *American Scientist,* vol. 67, p. 32.

———— 1980. "Richer Is Safer." *The Public Interest,* no. 60, Summer, pp. 23–39.

———— 1988. *Searching for Safety.* New Brunswick: Transaction Publishers.

Wilde, Gerald S. 1985. "Risk Homeostasis in an Experimental Context." In *Human Behavior and Traffic Safety,* ed. Leonard Evans and Richard Schwing, pp. 119–143. New York: Plenum Press.

Wilson, Edward O. 1992. *The Diversity of Life.* Cambridge, Mass.: Harvard University Press.

Wilson, James Q. 1975. *Thinking About Crime.* New York: Basic Books.

Wolf, Charles. 1988. *Markets or Governments: Choosing Between Imperfect Alternatives.* Cambridge, Mass.: MIT Press.

Wolfson, Adam. 1985. "Profits with Honor." *Policy Review,* Spring, pp. 50–52.

Yoon, Carol Kaesuk. 1994. "Thinning Ozone Layer Implicated in Decline of Frogs and Toads." *New York Times,* March 1, p. B12.

Zeckhauser, Richard J., and W. Kip Viscusi. 1990. "Risk Within Reason." *Science,* vol. 248, May 4, pp. 559–564.

Zimmerman, Rae. 1993. "Social Equity and Environmental Risk." *Risk Analysis,* vol. 13, pp. 649–666.

———— 1994. "Issues of Classification in Environmental Equity: How

We Manage Is How We Measure." *Fordham Urban Law Journal*, vol. 21, pp. 633–669.

2. *Estrogen Therapy for Menopause*

American College of Physicians. 1992. "Guidelines for Counseling Postmenopausal Women about Preventive Hormone Therapy." *Annals of Internal Medicine*, vol. 117, pp. 1038–1041.

Baber, R. J., and J. W. Studd. 1989. "Hormone Replacement Therapy and Cancer." *British Journal of Hospital Medicine*, vol. 41, pp. 142–149.

Birkenfeld, A., and N. G. Kase. 1991. "Menopause Medicine: Current Treatment Options and Trends." *Comprehensive Therapy*, vol. 17, pp. 36–45.

Brody, J. E. 1992. "Can Drugs 'Treat' Menopause? Amid Doubt, Women Must Decide." *New York Times*, May 19, pp. C1, C8.

Ditkoff, E. C., W. G. Crary, M. Cristo, and R. A. Lobo. 1991. "Estrogen Improves Psychological Function in Asymptomatic Postmenopausal Women." *Obstetrics and Gynecology*, vol. 78, pp. 991–995.

Gambrell, R. D. 1992. "Update on Hormone Replacement Therapy." *American Family Physician*, vol. 46, pp. 87S–96S.

Grady, D., and V. Ernster. 1991. "Does Postmenopausal Hormone Therapy Cause Breast Cancer?" *American Journal of Epidemiology*, vol. 134, pp. 1396–1400.

Grady, D., S. M. Rubin, D. B. Petitti, C. S. Fox, D. Black, B. Ettinger, V. L. Ernster, and S. R. Cummings. 1992. "Hormone Therapy to Prevent Disease and Prolong Life in Postmenopausal Women." *Annals of Internal Medicine*, vol. 117, pp. 1016–1037.

Harlap, S. 1992. "The Benefits and Risks of Hormone Replacement Therapy: An Epidemiologic Overview." *American Journal of Obstetrics and Gynecology*, vol. 166, pp. 1986–1992.

Hillard, T. C., S. Whitcroft, M. C. Ellerington, and M. I. Whitefield. 1991. "The Longterm Risks and Benefits of Hormone Replacement Therapy." *Journal of Clinical Pharmacy and Therapeutics*, vol. 16, pp. 231–245.

Hillner, B. E. 1992. "Estrogen Therapy for Geriatric Osteoporosis: Just One Ball in a Complex Juggling Act." *Southern Medical Journal*, vol. 85, pp. 2S10–2S16.

Nabulsi, A. A., A. R. Folsom, A. White, W. Patsch, G. Heiss, K. K. Wu, and M. Szklo. 1993. "Association of Hormone-Replacement Therapy with Various Cardiovascular Risk Factors in Postmenopausal Women." *New England Journal of Medicine,* vol. 328, pp. 1069–1075.

Studd, J. 1992. "Complications of Hormone Replacement Therapy in Post-Menopausal Women." *Journal of the Royal Society of Medicine,* vol. 85, pp. 376–377.

Torrance, G. W. 1986. "Measurement of Health State and Utilities for Economic Appraisal: A Review." *Journal of Health Economics,* vol. 5, pp. 1–30.

Ubell, E. 1993. "Should You Take Estrogen?" *Parade,* May 9, pp. 10–11.

Wile, A. G., R. W. Opfell, and D. A. Margileth. 1993. "Hormone Replacement Therapy in Previously Treated Breast Cancer Patients." *American Journal of Surgery,* vol. 165, pp. 372–375.

3. Clozapine Therapy for Schizophrenia

Allebeck, P., and B. Wistedt. 1986. "Mortality in Schizophrenia: A Ten-Year Follow-up Based on the Stockholm County Inpatient Register." *Archives of General Psychiatry,* vol. 43, pp. 650–653.

Alstrom, C. H. 1942. "Mortality in Mental Hospitals with Especial Regard to Tuberculosis." *Acta Psychiatrica et Neurologica,* vol. 24, Supplementum, pp. 1–422.

Babigian, H. M., and C. L. Odoroff. 1969. "The Mortality Experience of a Population with Psychiatric Illness." *American Journal of Psychiatry,* vol. 126, pp. 470–480.

Beck, M. N.. 1968. "Twenty-five and Thirty-five Year Follow Up of First Admissions to Mental Hospital." *Canadian Psychiatry Association Journal,* vol. 13, pp. 219–229.

Black, D. W., G. Warrack, and G. Winokur. 1985a. "The Iowa Record-Linkage Study: I. Suicides and Accidental Deaths among Psychiatric Patients." *Archives of General Psychiatry,* vol. 42, pp. 71–75.

———— 1985b. "The Iowa Record-Linkage Study: II. Excess Mortality among Patients with Organic Mental Disorders." *Archives of General Psychiatry,* vol. 42, pp. 78–81.

———— 1985c. "The Iowa Record-Linkage Study: III. Excess Mortality among Patients with 'Functional' Disorders." *Archives of General Psychiatry,* vol. 42, pp. 82–88.

Bleuler, M. 1978. *The Schizophrenic Disorders: Longterm Patient and Family Studies,* trans. S. Clemens. New Haven: Yale University Press.

Bromet, E., M. Davies, and S. C. Schulz. 1988. "Basic Principles of Epidemiologic Research in Schizophrenia." Chapter 8 in M. T. Tsuang and J. C. Simpson, eds., *Nosology, Epidemiology and Ge-*

netics of Schizophrenia, vol. 3 of *Handbook of Schizophrenia,* ed. H. A. Nasrallah. New York: Elsevier.

Claghorn, J., G. Honigfeld, F. S. Abuzzahab, R. Wang, R. Steinbook, V. Tuason, and G. Klerman. 1987. "The Risks and Benefits of Clozapine versus Chlorpromazine." *Journal of Clinical Psychopharmacology,* vol. 7, pp. 377–384.

Davis, J. M., C. B. Schaffer, G. A. Killian, C. Kinard, and C. Chan. 1980. "Important Issues in the Drug Treatment of Schizophrenia." *Schizophrenia Bulletin,* vol. 6, pp. 70–87.

Davison, G. C., and J. M. Neale. 1982. *Abnormal Psychology,* 3rd ed. New York: John Wiley & Sons.

Drake, R. E., C. Gates, A. Whitaker, and P. G. Cotton. 1985. "Suicide among Schizophrenics: A Review." *Comprehensive Psychiatry,* vol. 26, pp. 90–100.

Eichelman, B., and A. Hartwig. 1990. "Ethical Issues in Selecting Patients for Treatment with Clozapine: A Commentary." *Hospital and Community Psychiatry,* vol. 41, pp. 880–882.

Fischer-Cornelssen, K. A., and U. J. Ferner. 1976. "An Example of European Multicenter Trials: Multispectral Analysis of Clozapine." *Psychopharmacology Bulletin,* vol. 12, pp. 34–39.

Green, A. I., and C. Salzman. 1990. "Clozapine: Benefits and Risks." *Hospital and Community Psychiatry,* vol. 41, no. 4, pp. 379–380.

Hastings, D. W. 1958. "Follow-up Results in Psychiatric Illness." *American Journal of Psychiatry,* vol. 114, pp. 1057–1066.

Heinrichs, D. W., E. T. Hanlon, and W. T. Carpenter, Jr. 1984. "The Quality of Life Scale: An Instrument for Rating the Schizophrenic Deficit Syndrome." *Schizophrenia Bulletin,* vol. 10, pp. 388–398.

Herrman, H. E., J. A. Baldwin, and D. Christie. 1983. "A Record-Linkage Study of Mortality and General Hospital Discharge in Patients Diagnosed as Schizophrenic." *Psychological Medicine,* vol. 13, pp. 581–593.

Honigfeld, G., J. Patin, and J. Singer. 1984. "Clozapine: Antipsychotic Activity in Treatment-Resistant Schizophrenics." *Advances in Therapy,* vol. 1, pp. 77–97.

Kane, J., G. Honigfeld, J. Singer, and H. Meltzer. 1988a. "Clozapine for the Treatment-Resistant Schizophrenic: A Double-Blind Comparison with Chlorpromazine." *Archives of General Psychiatry,* vol. 45, pp. 789–796.

——— 1988b. "Clozapine in Treatment-Resistant Schizophrenics." *Psychopharmacology Bulletin,* vol. 24, no. 1, pp. 62–67.

Langfeldt, G. 1969. "Schizophrenia: Diagnosis and Prognosis." *Behavioral Science,* vol. 14, pp. 173–182.

Lehman, A. F. 1983. "The Well-Being of Chronic Mental Patients:

Assessing Their Quality of Life." *Archives of General Psychiatry,* vol. 40, pp. 369–373.

Lindelius, R., and D. W. K. Kay. 1973. "Some Changes in the Pattern of Mortality in Schizophrenia, in Sweden." *Acta Psychiatry Scandinavica,* vol. 49, pp. 315–323.

Marder, S. R., and T. Van Putten. 1988. "Who Should Receive Clozapine?" *Archives of General Psychiatry,* vol. 45, pp. 865–867.

Martin, R. L., C. R. Cloninger, S. B. Guze, and P. J. Clayton. 1985a. "Mortality in a Follow-up of 500 Psychiatric Outpatients: I. Total Mortality." *Archives of General Psychiatry,* vol. 42, pp. 47–54.

—— 1985b. "Mortality in a Follow-up of 500 Psychiatric Outpatients: II. Cause-Specific Mortality." *Archives of General Psychiatry,* vol. 42, pp. 58–66.

Medicine & Health. 1991. "Medicaid Programs to Cover Clozaril." Vol. 45, no. 22, June 3, p. 2.

Meltzer, H. Y. 1990. "Commentary: Defining Treatment Refractoriness in Schizophrenia." *Schizophrenia Bulletin,* vol. 14, no. 4, pp. 563–565.

Meltzer, H. Y., S. Burnett, B. Bastani, and L. F. Ramirez. 1990. "Effects of Six Months of Clozapine Treatment on the Quality of Life of Chronic Schizophrenic Patients." *Hospital and Community Psychiatry,* vol. 41, no. 8, pp. 892–897.

Neale, J. M., T. F. Oltmanns, and G. C. Davison. 1982. *Case Studies in Abnormal Psychology.* New York: John Wiley & Sons.

Niswander, G. D., G. M. Haslerud, and G. D. Mitchell. 1963. "Changes in Cause of Death of Schizophrenic Patients." *Archives of General Psychiatry,* vol. 9, pp. 229–234.

Pelonero, A. L. and R. L. Elliott. 1990. "Ethical and Clinical Considerations in Selecting Patients Who Will Receive Clozapine." *Hospital and Community Psychiatry,* vol. 41, no. 8, pp. 878–880.

Robb, C. 1991. "Change in Rule Reduces Price of Schizophrenia Drug." *The Boston Globe,* June 10, p. 4.

Safferman, A. Z. 1991. "Clozaril Test Change May Endanger Patients" (letter). *The Wall Street Journal,* April 10, p. A23.

Shopsin, B., H. Klein, M. Aaronsom, and M. Collora. 1979. "Clozapine, Chlorpromazine, and Placebo in Newly Hospitalized, Acutely Schizophrenic Patients: A Controlled, Double-Blind Comparison." *Archives of General Psychiatry,* vol. 36, pp. 657–664.

Terkelsen, K. G., and R. C. Grosser. 1990. "Estimating Clozapine's Cost to the Nation." *Hospital and Community Psychiatry,* vol. 41, no. 8, pp. 863–869.

Tsuang, M. T. 1978. "Suicide in Schizophrenics, Manics, Depressives, and Surgical Controls: A Comparison with General Population Suicide Mortality." *Archives of General Psychiatry*, vol. 35, pp. 153–155.

Tsuang, M. T., S. V. Faraone, and M. Day. 1988. "Schizophrenic Disorders." Chapter 13 in A. M. Nicholi, ed., *The New Harvard Guide to Psychiatry*. Cambridge, Mass.: Harvard University Press.

Tsuang, M. T., and R. F. Woolson. 1977. "Mortality in Patients with Schizophrenia, Mania, Depression and Surgical Conditions." *The British Journal of Psychiatry*, vol. 130, pp. 162–166.

Tsuang, M. T., R. F. Woolson, and J. A. Fleming. 1980. "Premature Deaths in Schizophrenia and Affective Disorders." *Archives of General Psychiatry*, vol. 37, pp. 979–983.

U.S. Food and Drug Administration (FDA), Department of Health and Human Services. 1990. "Summary Basis of Approval, Clozaril, Sandoz Pharmaceutical."

Wallis, C., and J. Willwerth. 1992. "Schizophrenia: A New Drug Brings Patients Back to Life." *Time*, July 6, pp. 53–57.

Westermeyer, J. F., and M. Harrow. 1988. "Course and Outcome in Schizophrenia." Chapter 10 in M. T. Tsuang and J. C. Simpson, eds., *Nosology, Epidemiology and Genetics of Schizophrenia*, vol. 3 of *Handbook of Schizophrenia*, ed. H. A. Nasrallah. New York: Elsevier.

4. Licensing the Elderly Driver

Aronson, M. K., W. L. Ooi, D. L. Geva, et al. 1991. "Dementia: Age-Dependent Incidence, Prevalence and Mortality in the Old." *Archives of Internal Medicine*, vol. 151, pp. 989–992.

Avorn, J. 1988. "Medications and the Elderly." In *Geriatric Medicine*, ed. J. W. Rowe and R. W. Besdine. Boston: Little, Brown.

Barr, R. A., and J. Eberhard. 1994. "Older Drivers: A Different Problem, A Different Solution?" *Alcohol, Drugs and Driving*, vol. 10, pp. 93–100.

California Department of Health Services (DHS). 1990. *Reporting Alzheimer's Disease and Related Disorders: Guidelines for Physicians.*

Carp, Frances M. 1988. "Significance of Mobility for the Well-Being of the Elderly." In National Research Council (NRC), Transportation Research Board, *Transportation in an Aging Society: Improving Mobility and Safety for Older Persons*, Special Report 218, vol. 2, pp. 1–20. Washington, D.C.

Carr, D., T. Jackson, and P. Alquire. 1990. "Characteristics of an

Elderly Driving Population Referred to a Geriatric Assessment Center." *Journal of the American Geriatric Society,* vol. 38, pp. 1145–1150.

Centers for Disease Control and Prevention (CDC), U.S. Department of Health and Human Services. 1991. *Injury Mortality Atlas of the United States, 1979–1987.* Atlanta, Ga.

Doege, T., and A. Engelberg. 1986. *Medical Conditions Affecting Drivers.* Chicago: American Medical Association.

Drachman, D. 1988. "Who May Drive? Who May Not? Who Shall Decide?" *Annals of Neurology,* vol. 24, pp. 787–788.

Evans, D. A., H. H. Funkenstein, M. S. Albert, et al. 1989. "Prevalence of Alzheimer's Disease in a Community Population of Older Persons." *Journal of the American Medical Association,* vol. 262, pp. 271–286.

Evans, Leonard. 1988a. "Older Driver Involvement in Fatal and Severe Traffic Crashes." *Journal of Gerontology,* vol. 43, pp. 5186–5193.

——— 1988b. "Risk of Fatality from Physical Trauma versus Sex and Age." *Journal of Trauma,* vol. 28, pp. 368–378.

——— 1991. *Traffic Safety and the Driver.* New York: Van Nostrand Reinholdt.

——— 1993. "How Safe Were Today's Older Drivers When They Were Younger?" *American Journal of Epidemiology,* vol. 137, pp. 769–775.

Findley, L. J., W. Weiss, and E. R. Jabour. 1991. "Drivers with Untreated Sleep Apnea: A Cause of Death and Serious Injury." *Archives of Internal Medicine,* vol. 151, pp. 1451–1452.

Friedland, R., E. Koss, A. Kumar, et al. 1988. "Motor Vehicle Crashes in Dementia of the Alzheimer Type." *Annals of Neurology,* vol. 23, p. 782–786.

Frisbee, T. 1991. "Keeping Over-The-Hill Drivers in the Game." *Traffic Safety,* vol. 1, pp. 10–13.

Gilley, D. W., R. S. Wilson, D. A. Bennett, et al. 1991. "Cessation of Driving and Unsafe Motor Vehicle Operation by Dementia Patients." *Archives of Internal Medicine,* vol. 151, pp. 941–946.

Gillins, L. 1990. "Yielding to Age: When the Elderly Can No Longer Drive." *Journal of Geriatric Nursing,* vol. 16, pp. 12–15.

Graca, J. 1987. "Driving Regulations and the Elderly." *Journal of the American Geriatric Society,* vol. 35, p. 90.

Gregory, D. R. 1982. "The Physician's Role in Highway Safety-Reporting Requirements." In Cyril H. Wecht, ed., *Legal Medicine,* pp. 257–256. Philadelphia: W. B. Saunders.

Hakamies-Blomqvist, L. E. 1993. "Fatal Accidents of Older Drivers." *Accident Analysis and Prevention*, vol. 25, pp. 19–27.

Hansotia, P., and S. K. Broste. 1991. "The Effect of Epilepsy or Diabetes Mellitus on the Risk of Automobile Accidents." *New England Journal of Medicine*, vol. 324, p. 22.

Holton, Lisa. 1990. "Older Drivers Face Tough Road: Balancing Independence, Impairment." *American College of Physicians Observer*, vol. 10, no. 6, p. 18.

Hundenski, R. J. 1992. "Public Transport Passenger Accidents: An Analysis of the Structural and Functional Characteristics of Passenger and Vehicle." *Accident Analysis and Prevention*, vol. 24, pp. 133–142.

Janke, M. J. 1991. "Accidents, Mileage, and the Exaggeration of Risk." *Accident Analysis and Prevention*, vol. 23, pp. 183–188.

Keeler, Theodore E. 1994. "Highway Safety, Economic Behavior, and Driving Environment." *American Economic Review*, vol. 84, no. 3, June, pp. 684–693.

Krumholz, A., R. S. Fisher, R. P. Lesser, and A. Hauser. 1991. "Driving and Epilepsy: A Review and Reappraisal." *Journal of the American Medical Association*, vol. 265, pp. 622–626.

Leigh-Smith, J., D. T. Wade, and R. L. Hewer. 1986. "Driving after Stroke." *Journal of the Royal Society of Medicine*, vol. 79, pp. 200–203.

Lucas-Blaustein, M., L. Fillip, C. Dungan, and L. Tune. 1988. "Driving in Patients with Dementia." *Journal of the American Geriatrics Society*, vol. 36, pp. 1087–1091.

Meier, B. 1992. "Safety and the Older Driver: When Difficult Issues Collide." *New York Times*, May 4, p. 1.

National Highway Traffic Safety Administration (NHTSA), U.S. Department of Transportation. 1989. *Older Drivers, the Age Factor in Traffic Safety.* Report no. DOT HS 807 402.

——— 1991. *Fatal Accident Reporting System, 1990.* Washington, D.C., December.

National Research Council (NRC), Transportation Research Board. 1988. *Transportation in an Aging Society: Improving Mobility and Safety for Older Persons.* Special Report 218, Washington, D.C.

National Safety Council. 1993. *Accident Facts.* Chicago, Ill.

Persson, D. 1993. "The Elderly Driver: Deciding When to Stop." *The Gerontologist*, vol. 33, pp. 88–91.

Popkin, C. L., and C. Little. 1990. *Developing Local Resources for the Safe Transportation of the Elderly Driver.* University of North Carolina Highway Traffic Research Center, Report no. HSRC-PR178.

Reuben, D. B., R. A. Silliman, and M. Traines. 1988. "The Aging Driver: Medicine, Policy, and Ethics." *Journal of the American Geriatrics Society,* vol. 36, pp. 1135–1142.

Schlag, B. 1993. "Elderly Drivers in Germany—Fitness and Driving Behavior." *Accident Analysis and Prevention,* vol. 25, pp. 47–55.

Stephens, T., and C. A. Schoenborn. 1988. *Adult Health Practices in the United States and Canada.* Comparative and International Vital and Health Statistics Reports, Series 5, No. 3, National Center for Health Statistics (DHHS Publication 88–1479), Hyattsville, Md.

Strickberger, A. S., C. A. Cantillon, and P. F. Friedman. 1991. "When Should Patients with Lethal Ventricular Arrhythmias Resume Driving?" *Annals of Internal Medicine,* vol. 115, pp. 560–563.

Tinetti, M. E., and M. Speechley. 1989. "Prevention of Falls among the Elderly." *New England Journal of Medicine,* vol. 320, pp. 1055–1059.

Underwood, M. 1992. "The Older Driver: Clinical Assessment and Injury Prevention." *Archives of Internal Medicine,* vol. 152, pp. 735–740.

Waller, P. F. 1985. "Preventing Injury to the Elderly." In *Aging and Public Health,* ed. H. T. Phillips and S. A. Gaylord, pp. 103–146. New York: Springer.

——— 1988. "Renewal Licensing of Older Drivers." In National Research Council (NRC), Transportation Research Board, *Transportation in an Aging Society: Improving Mobility and Safety for Older Persons.* Special Report 218, vol. 2, pp. 72–100. Washington, D.C.

Williams, A. F., and O. Carter. 1989. "Driver Age and Crash Involvement." *American Journal of Public Health,* vol. 79, pp. 326–327.

5. Saving Gasoline and Lives

Competitive Enterprise Institute (CEI) v. NHTSA, 956 Fed. 2d 321 (D.C. Cir. 1992).

Council of Economic Advisers (CEA), Executive Office of the President. 1994. *Economic Report of the President 1994.* Washington, D.C.

Crandall, Robert C., and John D. Graham. 1984. "Automobile Safety Regulation and Offsetting Driver Behavior: Some New Empirical Estimates." *American Economic Review,* vol. 74, p. 328.

———— 1989. "The Effect of Fuel Economy Standards on Automobile Safety." *Journal of Law and Economics*, vol. 32, pp. 97–118.

———— 1991. "New Fuel Economy Standards?" *The American Enterprise*, Mar./Apr., p. 68.

Crandall, Robert C., Howard K. Gruenspecht, Theodore E. Keeler, and Lester Lave. 1986. *Regulating The Automobile*. Washington, D.C.: Brookings Institution.

Environmental Protection Agency (EPA). 1990. *Environmental Investments: The Cost of a Clean Environment*. Washington, D.C.

Evans, Leonard. 1985a. "Driver Behavior Revealed in Relations Involving Car Mass." In *Human Behavior and Traffic Safety*, ed. L. Evans and R. Schwing, pp. 337–352. New York: Plenum Press.

———— 1985b. "Involvement Rate in Two-Car Crashes versus Driver Age and Car Mass of Each Involved Car." *Accident Analysis and Prevention*, vol. 17, p. 155.

———— 1991. *Traffic Safety and the Driver*. New York: Plenum Press.

Evans, Leonard, and Michael Frick. 1991. "Driver Fatality Risk in Two-Car Crashes—Dependence on Masses of Driven and Striking Car." 13th International Technical Conference on Experimental Safety Vehicles, Paris.

Graham, John D. 1983. "Automobile Safety: An Investigation of Occupant Protection Policies." Ph.D. dissertation, Carnegie Mellon University.

———— 1984. "Technology, Behavior, and Safety: An Empirical Study of Automobile Safety Regulation." *Policy Sciences*, vol. 17, pp. 141–151.

———— 1992. "The Safety Risks of Proposed Fuel Economy Legislation." *Risk: Issues in Health and Safety*, vol. 3, Spring, pp. 95–126.

Greene, D. 1978–79. "CAFE or Price? An Analysis of the Effects of Federal Fuel Economy Regulations and Gasoline Price on New Car MPG." *Journal of Energy*, vol. 11, p. 37.

Gruenspecht, Howard K. 1992. "Differentiated Regulation: The Case of Auto Emissions Standards." *American Economic Review*, vol. 72 (Papers & Proceedings), May, pp. 328–331.

Insurance Institute for Highway Safety (IIHS). 1991. "Comparison Shows Downsizing Plays a Dramatic Role in Occupant Death Rates." *Status Report: Highway Loss Reduction*, March 16, p. 4.

Jorgensen, Dale W., and Peter J. Wilcoxen. 1992. "Reducing CO_2 Emission: The Cost of Different Goals." In John R. Moroney, ed., *Advances in the Economics of Energy and Resources*, vol. 7, pp. 125–158. Greenwich: JAI Press.

Kahane, C. 1990. "Effect of Car Size on the Frequency and Severity of Rollover Crashes." In *The Effect of Car Size on Fatality and Injury Risk in Single-Vehicle Crashes,* vol. 28. National Highway and Traffic Safety Administration (NHTSA), Washington, D.C.

Leigh, J. Paul, and A. L. Frank. 1987. "Tax Gasoline to Save Lives." *New England Journal of Medicine,* vol. 316, p. 316.

Leigh, J. Paul, and James T. Wilkinson. 1991. "The Effect of Gasoline Taxes on Highway Fatalities." *Journal of Policy Analysis and Management,* vol. 10, pp. 474–481.

National Academy of Sciences (NAS). 1992. *Automotive Fuel Economy: How Far Should We Go?* Washington, D.C.: National Academy Press.

National Highway Traffic Safety Administration (NHTSA), U.S. Department of Transportation. 1990. *The Effect of Car Size on Fatality and Injury Risk in Single-Vehicle Crashes.* Washington, D.C.

——— 1991. *Fatal Accident Reporting System.* Washington, D.C., December.

——— 1992. *Fatal Accident Reporting System,* Annual Report. Washington, D.C.

National Research Council (NRC). 1992. *Rethinking the Ozone Problem in Urban and Regional Air Pollution.* Washington, D.C.: National Academy Press.

Office of Technology Assessment (OTA). 1991. *Improving Automobile Fuel Economy: New Standards, New Approaches.* Washington, D.C., U.S. Congress.

Robertson, Leon. 1991. "How to Save Fuel and Reduce Injuries in Automobiles." *Journal of Trauma,* vol. 31, p. 107.

Society of Auto Engineers. 1977. *Passenger Car Occupant Death Rates.* Tech. Paper Series 770808.

6. *Eating Fish*

Bang, H. O., et al. 1980. "The Composition of the Eskimo Food in Northwestern Greenland." *American Journal of Clinical Nutrition,* vol. 33, pp. 2657–2661.

Bang, H. O., and J. Dyerberg. 1972. "Plasma Lipids and Lipoprotein in Greenlandic West Coast Eskimos." *Acta Medica Scandinavica,* vol. 192, pp. 85–94.

Bureau of the Census, U.S. Department of Commerce. 1990. *Statistical Abstract of the United States: 1988.*

Cad, J. A. 1985. "Fish, Fatty Acids, and Human Health." *New Eng-*

land *Journal of Medicine,* vol. 312, no. 19, pp. 1253–1254.

Consumers Union (CU). 1992. "Is Our Fish Fit to Eat?" *Consumer Reports,* February, pp. 103–120.

Curb, J. D., and D. M. Red. 1985. "Fish Consumption and Mortality from Coronary Heart Disease." *New England Journal of Medicine,* vol. 313, p. 821.

Environmental Protection Agency (EPA). 1989. *Assessing Human Health Risks from Chemically Contaminated Fish and Shellfish: A Guidance Manual.* EPA-503/8-89-002, Appendix F.

Fora, J. A., and B. S. Glenn. 1991–92. "Reducing the Health Risks of Sport Fish." *Issues in Science and Technology,* Winter, pp. 73–77.

Hirai, A., et al. 1980. "Eiscosapentaenoic Acid and Platelet Function in Japanese." *Lancet,* vol. 2, pp. 1132–1133.

Institute of Medicine (IOM). 1991. *Sea Food Safety.* Washington, D.C.: National Academy Press.

Johnson, Kevin. 1992. "At Reservation, Fish Risk Hits Home." *USA Today,* December 3, p. 11A.

Kagawa, Y., et al. 1982. "Eicosapolyenoic Acid of Serum of Lipids of Japanese Islanders with Low Incidence of Cardiovascular Disease." *Journal of Nutritional Science and Vitaminology,* vol. 28, pp. 441–453.

Keys, A. 1980. *Seven Countries: A Multivariate Analysis of Death and Coronary Heart Disease.* Cambridge, Mass.: Harvard University Press.

Kromhout, D., et al. 1985. "The Inverse Relation between Fish Consumption and 20-Year Mortality from Coronary Heart Disease." *New England Journal of Medicine,* vol. 312, no. 19, pp. 1205–1209.

Lee, T. H., et al. 1985. "Effect of Dietary Enrichment with Eicosapentaenoic and Docosahexaenoic Acids on In Vitro Neutrophil and Monocyte Leukotriene Generation and Neutrophil Function." *New England Journal of Medicine,* vol. 312, no. 19, pp. 1217–1224.

National Research Council (NRC). 1989. *Diet and Health: Implications for Reducing Chronic Disease Risk.* Washington, D.C.: National Academy Press.

Phillipson, B. E., et al. 1985. "Reduction of Plasma Lipids, Lipoprotein, and Apoproteins by Dietary Fish Oils in Patients with Hypertriglyceridemia." *New England Journal of Medicine,* vol. 312, no. 19, pp. 1210–1216.

Reinert, R. E., et al. 1991. "Risk Assessment, Risk Management, and

Fish Consumption Advisories in the United States." *Fisheries,* vol. 16, no. 6, pp. 5–12.

Shahar, Eyal, et al. 1994. "Dietary n-3 Polyunsaturated Fatty Acids and Smoking-Related Chronic Obstructive Pulmonary Disease." *New England Journal of Medicine,* vol. 331, no. 4, July 28, pp. 228–233.

Simopoulos, A. P. 1991. "Omega-3 Fatty Acids in Health and Disease and in Growth and Development." *American Journal of Clinical Nutrition,* vol. 54, pp. 438–463.

Tolley, George, Donald Kenkel, and Robert Fabian, eds. 1994. *Valuing Health for Policy: An Economic Approach.* Chicago and London: University of Chicago Press.

Tyson, Rae. 1992. "EPA 'Glosses Over' Risk of Fish." *USA Today,* December 3, p. 1A.

U.S. Senate, Select Committee on Nutrition and Human Needs. 1977. *Dietary Goals for the United States.* Washington, D.C.: U.S. Government Printing Office.

Vollset, S. E., et al. 1985. "Fish Consumption and Mortality from Coronary Heart Disease." *New England Journal of Medicine,* vol. 313, pp. 820–821.

Wheeler, Timothy B. 1992. "Many Fish Pose Risk at Table." *Baltimore Sun,* December 3, p. 1C.

7. Seeking Safe Drinking Water

Abdel-Rahman, M., D. Couri, and R. Bull. 1984. "Toxicity of Chlorine Dioxide in Drinking Water." *Journal of the American College of Toxicology,* vol. 3, pp. 277–284.

Abdel-Rahman, M., D. Suh, and R. Bull. 1984. "Toxicity of Monochloramine in the Rat: An Alternative Drinking Water Disinfectant." *Journal of Toxicology and Environmental Health,* vol. 13, pp. 825–834.

Akin, Elmer W., John C. Hoff, and Edwin C. Lippy. 1982. "Waterborne Outbreak Control: Which Disinfectant?" *Environmental Health Perspectives,* vol. 46, pp. 7–12.

Amato, Ivan. 1993. "The Crusade Against Chlorine." *Science,* vol. 261, July 9, pp. 152–154.

American Water Works Association. 1984. *Introduction to Water Treatment: Principles and Practices of Water Supply Operations,* vol. 2. Denver, Colo.

Anderson, Christopher. 1991. "Cholera Epidemic Traced to Risk Miscalculation." *Nature,* vol. 354, November 28, p. 255.

Assaad, F., and I. Borecka. 1977. "Nine-Year Study of WHO Virus

Reports on Fatal Virus Infections." *Bulletin of the World Health Organization,* vol. 55, pp. 445–453.

Bellar, T. A., J. J. Lichtenberg, and R. C. Kroner. 1974. "The Occurrence of Organohalides in Chlorinated Drinking Water." *Journal of the American Water Works Association,* vol. 66, pp. 703–706.

Brooke, James. 1991. "Cholera Kills 1,100 in Peru and Marches On, Reaching the Brazilian Border." *New York Times,* April 19, p. A3.

Bull, Richard J. 1982. "Health Effects of Drinking Water Disinfectants and Disinfectant By-Products." *Environmental Science and Technology,* vol. 16, pp. 554–559.

Bull, Richard J., Janice M. Brown, Earle A. Meierhenry, Ted A. Jorgenson, Merrel Robinson, and Judith A. Stober. 1986. "Enhancement of the Hepatotoxicity of Chloroform in B6C3F1 Mice by Corn Oil: Implications for Chloroform Carcinogenesis." *Environmental Health Perspectives,* vol. 69, pp. 49–58.

Calabrese, Edward J., and Charles E. Gilbert. 1989. "Drinking Water Quality and Water Treatment Practices: Charting the Future." In Edward J. Calabrese, Charles E. Gilbert, and Harris Pastides, eds., *Safe Drinking Water Act,* pp. 113–142. Chelsea, Mich.: Lewis.

Cantor, Kenneth P., Robert Hoover, Patricia Hartge, Thomas J. Mason, Debra T. Silverman, Ronald Altman, Donald F. Austin, Margaret A. Child, Charles R. Key, Loraine D. Marrett, Max H. Myers, Ambati S. Narayana, Lynn I. Levin, J. W. Sullivan, G. Marie Swanson, David B. Thomas, and Dee W. West. 1987. "Bladder Cancer, Drinking Water Source, and Tap Water Consumption: A Case-Control Study." *Journal of the National Cancer Institute,* vol. 79, pp. 1269–1279.

Carpenter, Betsy. 1991. "Is Your Water Safe? Turning on the Faucet May Be Fraught with Health Risks." *U.S. News & World Report,* vol. 111, July 29, pp. 48–55.

Centers for Disease Control (CDC). 1991. *Fact Book,* p. 7. Atlanta: Department of Health and Human Services, Public Health Service.

Clark, Robert M., James A. Goodrich, and John C. Ireland. 1984–1985. "Costs and Benefits of Drinking Water Treatment." *Journal of Environmental Systems,* vol. 14, pp. 1–30.

Cotruvo, Joseph A., and Marlene Regelski. 1989. "Issues in Developing National Primary Drinking Water Regulations for Disinfection and Disinfection By-Products." In Edward J. Calabrese, Charles E. Gilbert, and Harris Pastides, eds., *Safe Drinking Water Act,* pp. 57–69. Chelsea, Mich.: Lewis.

Craun, Gunther F. 1986. *Waterborne Diseases in the United States.* Boca Raton, Fla.: CRC Press.

—— , ed. 1993. *Safety of Water Disinfection: Balancing Chemical and Microbial Risks.* Washington, D.C.: International Life Sciences Institute Press.

Crump, Kenny S., and Harry A. Guess. 1982. "Drinking Water and Cancer: Review of Recent Epidemiological Findings and Assessment of Risks." *Annual Review of Public Health,* vol. 3, pp. 339–357.

Dowd, Ann Reilly. 1994. "Environmentalists Are on the Run." *Fortune,* September 19, pp. 91–100.

Environmental Protection Agency (EPA). 1977. "National Interim Primary Drinking Water Regulations." *U.S. Code of Federal Regulations,* Title 40, part 141.

—— 1981. Drinking Water Research Division. "Chlorine, Is There a Better Alternative?" *The Science of the Total Environment,* vol. 18, pp. 235–243.

—— 1985. *Health Assessment Document for Chloroform.* Washington, D.C.

—— 1986. "Protecting Our Water Supply." *EPA Journal,* September, pp. 1–28.

—— 1994a. "National Primary Drinking Water Regulations: Disinfectants and Disinfection By-products, Proposed Rule." *Federal Register,* vol. 59, no. 145, pp. 38668–38829, July 29.

—— 1994b. "National Primary Drinking Water Regulations: Enhanced Surface Water Treatment Requirements" (proposed rule). *Federal Register,* vol. 59, no. 145, pp. 38832–38858, July 29.

Food Chemical News. 1993. "Seventh Cholera Pandemic Continues Unabated in Much of World." Vol. 35, no. 19, July 5.

Fowle, John R., III, and Frederick C. Kopfler. 1986. "Water Disinfection: Microbes versus Molecules—An Introduction of Issues." *Environmental Health Perspectives,* vol. 69, pp. 3–6.

Galbraith, P. 1989. "National Survey of Environmental Health Priorities of State Public Health Commissioners." Connecticut Department of Health Services, Hartford, Conn., 1987, as cited in Edward J. Calabrese, Charles E. Gilbert, and Harris Pastides, eds., *Safe Drinking Water Act,* p. 114. Chelsea, Mich.: Lewis.

Gerba, Charles P., and Charles N. Haas. 1988. "Assessment of Risks Associated with Enteric Viruses in Contaminated Drinking Water." In *Chemical and Biological Characterization of Sludges, Sediments, Dredge Spoils, and Drilling Muds,* ed. J. J. Lichtenberg, J. A. Winter, C. I. Weber, and L. Fradkin. ASTM STP 976, pp. 489–494. Philaadelphia: American Society for Testing and Materials.

Glass, R. I., M. Libel, and A. D. Brandling-Bennett. 1992. "Epidemic Cholera in the Americas." *Science,* vol. 256, June 12, pp. 1524–1525.

Herren-Freund, S. L., M. A. Pereira, and G. Olson. 1987. "The Carcinogenicity of Trichloroethylene and Its Metabolites, Trichloroacetic Acid and Dichloroacetic Acid, in Mouse Liver." *Toxicology and Applied Pharmacology,* vol. 90, pp. 183–189.

Heywood, R., R. J. Sortwell, P. R. B. Noel, A. E. Street, D. E. Prentice, F. J. C. Roe, P. F. Wadsworth, A. M. Worden, and N. J. Van Abbe. 1979. "Safety Evaluation of Toothpaste Containing Chloroform: III. Long-term Study in Beagle Dogs." *Journal of Environmental Pathology and Toxicology,* vol. 2, pp. 835–851.

Hoff, John C., and Elmer W. Akin. 1986. "Microbial Resistance to Disinfectants: Mechanisms and Significance." *Environmental Health Perspectives,* vol. 69, pp. 7–13.

International Life Sciences Institute (ILSI). 1991. *News,* vol. 9, July/August.

Jorgenson, T. A., E. F. Meierhenry, C. J. Rushbrook, R. J. Bull, and M. Robinson. 1985. "Carcinogenicity of Chloroform in Drinking Water to Male Osborne-Mendel Rats and Female B6C3F1 Mice." *Fundamentals of Applied Toxicology,* vol. 5, pp. 760–769.

Kjellstrand, C., J. Eaton, Y. Yawata, H. Swoffard, C. Kolpin, T. Buselmeier, B. von Hartitzsch, and H. Jacob. 1974. "Hemolysis in Dialysized Patients Caused by Chloramines." *Nephron,* vol. 13, pp. 427–433.

Lee, Gary. 1993. "Public Seen as Uninformed about Tap Water Problems; Study: Contamination May Kill 900 Each Year." *Washington Post,* September 27, p. A11.

Levine, William C., and Gunther F. Craun. 1990. "Waterborne Disease Outbreaks, 1986–1988." *Morbidity and Mortality Weekly Report,* vol. 39, no. SS-1, March, pp. 1–13.

Manwaring, J. F. 1985. "Public Drinking Water and Chemicals." In *Safe Drinking Water: The Impact of Chemicals on a Limited Resource,* ed. R. G. Rice, pp. 21–31. Chelsea, Mich.: Lewis.

Maxwell, Nancy Irwin, David E. Burmaster, and David Ozonoff. 1991. "Trihalomethanes and Maximum Contaminant Levels: The Significance of Inhalation and Dermal Exposures to Chloroform in Household Water." *Regulatory Toxicology and Pharmacology,* vol. 14, pp. 297–312.

McKone, Thomas E. 1987. "Human Exposure to Volatile Organic

Compounds in Household Tap Water: The Indoor Inhalation Pathway." *Environmental Science and Technology,* vol. 21, pp. 1194–1201.

Moore, Gary S., and Edward J. Calabrese. 1980. "The Health Effects of Chloramines in Potable Water Supplies: A Literature Review." *Journal of Environmental Pathology and Toxicology,* vol. 4, pp. 257–263.

National Academy of Sciences (NAS). 1987. *Drinking Water and Health: Disinfectants and Disinfectant By-Products.* Washington, D.C.

National Cancer Institute (NCI). 1976. "Report on Carcinogenesis Bioassay of Chloroform, PB-164018." Springfield, Va.: National Technical Information Service.

National Research Council (NRC). 1977. *Drinking Water and Health.* Washington, D.C.: National Academy Press.

Nature. 1991. "Cholera Marches On." Vol. 350, April, p. 640.

Palmer, A. K., A. E. Street, F. J. C. Roe, A. N. Worden, and N. J. Van Abbe. 1979. "Safety Evaluation of Toothpaste Containing Chloroform: II. Long-term Studies in Rats." *Journal of Environmental Pathology and Toxicology,* vol. 2, pp. 821–833.

Roe, F. J. C., A. K. Palmer, A. N. Worden, and N. J. Van Abbe. 1979. "Safety Evaluation of Toothpaste Containing Chloroform: I. Longterm Studies in Mice." *Journal of Environmental Pathology and Toxicology,* vol. 1, pp. 799–819.

Rook, J. J. 1974. "Formation of Haloforms during Chlorination of Natural Waters." *Journal of the Society of Water Treatment and Examination,* vol. 23, pp. 234–243.

Rose, Joan B., and Charles P. Gerba. 1991. "Use of Risk Assessment for Development of Microbial Standards." *Water Science Technology,* vol. 24, pp. 29–34.

Rose, Joan B., Charles N. Haas, and Stig Regli. 1991. "Risk Assessment and Control of Waterborne Giardiasis." *American Journal of Public Health,* vol. 81, pp. 709–713.

Shih, K. L., and J. Lederberg. 1976. "Chloramine Mutagenesis in *Bacillus subtilis.*" *Science,* vol. 192, pp. 1141–1143.

Simmon, Vincent F., and Robert G. Tardiff. 1978. "The Mutagenic Activity of Halogenated Compounds Found in Chlorinated Drinking Water." In *Water Chlorination: Environmental Impact and Health Effects,* ed. Robert J. Jolley, Hend Gorchev, and D. Heyward Hamilton, Jr., pp. 417–431. Ann Arbor, Mich.: Ann Arbor Scientific Publications.

Slovic, Paul. 1987. "Perception of Risk." *Science,* vol. 236, pp. 280–285, April 17.

Stout, Janet E., Victor L. Yu, Paul Muraca, Jean Joly, Nancy Troup, and Lucy S. Tompkins. 1992. "Potable Water as a Cause of Sporadic Cases of Community-Acquired Legionnaires' Disease." *New England Journal of Medicine,* vol. 326, pp. 151–155.

Terry, Sara. 1993. "Drinking Water Comes to a Boil." *New York Times Magazine,* September 26, pp. 42–65.

Walker, Bailus. 1989. "Achieving Safe Drinking Water: Summary and Recommendations." In *Safe Drinking Water Act,* ed. Edward J. Calabrese, Charles E. Gilbert, and Harris Pastides, pp. 1–2. Chelsea, Mich.: Lewis.

White, George Clifford. 1978. "Current Chlorination and Dechlorination Practices in the Treatment of Potable Water, Wastewater and Cooling Water." In *Water Chlorination: Environmental Impact and Health Effects,* ed. Robert L. Jolley, vol. 1, pp. 1–15. Ann Arbor, Mich.: Ann Arbor Science Publishers.

Williamson, S.J. 1981. "Epidemiological Studies on Cancer and Organic Compounds in U.S. Drinking Waters." *The Science of the Total Environment,* vol. 18, pp. 187–203.

Wilson, Richard. 1980. "Measuring and Comparing Risks to Establish a De Minimis Risk Level." *Regulatory Toxicology and Pharmacology,* vol. 8, pp. 267–282.

Wones, R. G., L. Mieczkowski, and L. A. Frohman. 1989. "Drinking Water and Human Lipid and Thyroid Metabolism." In Robert L. Jolley, ed., *Water Chlorination: Chemistry, Environmental Impact and Health Effects,* vol. 6. Chelsea, Mich.: Lewis.

World Bank. 1992. *World Development Report: Environment and Development.* Washington, D.C.

Zeighami, E. A., A. P. Watson, and G. F. Craun. 1990. "Chlorination, Water Hardness and Serum Cholesterol in Forty-six Wisconsin Communities." *International Journal of Epidemiology,* vol. 19, no. 1, pp. 49–58.

8. Recycling Lead

Barnett, Phillip. 1991. House Subcommittee on Health and the Environment. Personal communication to Katherine Walker, Harvard Center for Risk Analysis, December 16.

Battery Council International. 1992. "National Recycling Rate Study." Chicago, April.

Centers for Disease Control and Prevention (CDC). 1991. *Preventing*

Lead Poisoning in Young Children. Atlanta: U.S. Department of Health and Human Services/Public Health Service.

Davis, J. M. 1992. "Current Issues in Assessing the Health Risks of Lead." *The Toxicologist,* vol. 12, no. 1, p. 246.

Dudek, Daniel J., Richard B. Stewart, and Jonathan B. Wiener. 1992. "Environmental Policy for Eastern Europe: Technology-Based Versus Market Based Approaches." *Columbia Journal of Environmental Law,* vol. 17, no. 1, pp. 17–52.

Environmental Protection Agency (EPA). n.d. "Fact Sheet: Negotiated Rulemaking/Regulatory Negotiation."

——— 1989a. "Risk Analysis to Support Municipal Waste Combustor New Source Performance Standard and Emission Guideline Development." Office of Air Quality Planning and Standards, Environmental Standards Division, Research Triangle Park, North Carolina. As cited in EPA, 1991c.

——— 1989b. "Standards of Performance for New Stationary Municipal Waste Combustors; Proposed Rule and Notice of Public Hearing." *Federal Register,* vol. 54, no. 243, December 20, pp. 52209–52304.

——— 1990a. "Intent to Form an Advisory Committee to Negotiate Recycling of Lead Acid Batteries and Announcement of Organizational Meeting." *Federal Register,* vol. 55, no. 247, December 24, p. 52884.

——— 1990b. *Reducing Risk: Setting Priorities and Strategies for Environmental Protection.* Science Advisory Board, SAB-EC-90-021, September.

——— 1990c. "The Nation's Hazardous Waste Management Program at a Crossroads: The RCRA Implementation Study." 20S-0001, Office of Solid Waste and Emergency Response, July.

——— 1991a. "Cost Analysis of Options to Enhance Lead-Acid Battery Recycling." Draft Report, Regulatory Impacts Branch, Economics and Technology Division, Office of Toxic Substances, August.

——— 1991b. "Establishment and Open Meeting of the Negotiated Rulemaking Advisory Committee for the Lead Acid Battery Recycling Rule." *Federal Register,* vol. 56, January 25, pp. 2885–2886.

——— 1991c. "Lead Acid Battery Recycling Risk Assessment." Draft, September.

——— 1991d. "Standard of Performance for New Stationary Sources: Municipal Waste Combustors; Final Rule." *Federal Register,* vol. 56, February 11, pp. 5488–5527.

———— 1991e. "U.S. Environmental Protection Agency Strategy for Reducing Lead Exposure." February 21.

———— 1994. "National Emissions Standards for Hazardous Air Pollutants (NESHAP) (Secondary Lead Smelters); Notice of Proposed Rule; Notice of Public Hearing." *Federal Register,* vol. 59, June 9, pp. 29750–29778.

Fortuna, Richard C. 1991. "Comments on Strategies for Managing Present and Future Wastes." From Workshop on Hazardous Wastes, *Risk Analysis,* vol. 11, no. 1, pp. 83–88.

Franklin Associates. 1988. "Characterization of Products Containing Lead and Cadmium in Municipal Solid Waste in the United States, 1970–2000." October 17. As cited in EPA, 1991c.

Hahn, Robert W., and Eric H. Males. 1990. "Can Regulatory Institutions Cope with Cross Media Pollution?" *Journal of the Air and Waste Management Association,* vol. 40, no. 1, pp. 24–31.

Haigh, Nigel, and Frances Irwin, eds. 1990. *Integrated Pollution Control in Europe and North America.* Washington, D.C.: The Conservation Foundation.

Kunreuther, H. 1991. "Managing Hazardous Wastes." *Risk Analysis,* vol. 11, no. 1, pp. 19–26.

Males, Eric H. 1989. "Cross-Media Pollution Problems and the Role of Regulatory Analysis." Qualifier part A, Department of Engineering and Public Policy, Carnegie Mellon University, Pittsburgh, January 10. Unpublished.

National Commission on the Environment. 1993. *Choosing a Sustainable Future: The Report of the National Commission on the Environment.* Washington, D.C.: World Wildlife Fund.

Ottoboni, M. Alice. 1991. *The Dose Makes the Poison: A Plain-Language Guide to Toxicology,* 2nd ed. New York: Van Nostrand Reinhold.

President's Council on Competitiveness. 1990. "Fact Sheet on Recycling Requirement in the Municipal Waste Combustors Rule." Washington, D.C.: Office of the Vice President, December 19.

9. Regulating Pesticides

Ames, Bruce N. 1992. "Pollution, Pesticides and Cancer." *Journal of AOAC International,* vol. 75, pp. 1–5.

Ames, Bruce N., and Lois S. Gold. 1990. "Too Many Rodent Carcinogens: Mitogenesis Increases Mutagenesis." *Science,* vol. 249, August 31, pp. 970–971.

Brown, David. 1994. "When Disease Resists." *Washington Post,* February 14, p. A3.

Calabrese, E. J. (ed.). 1994. *Biological Effects of Low Level Exposures: Dose-Response Relationships.* Ann Arbor: Lewis.

Carpenter, W. D. 1991. "Insignificant Risks Must Be Balanced against Great Benefits." In Chemical and Engineering News Forum on Risk Assessment of Pesticides, *Chemical and Engineering News,* vol. 69, January 7, pp. 37–39.

Carr, C. J., and A. C. Kolbye, Jr. 1991. "A Critique of the Use of the Maximum Tolerated Dose in Bioassays to Assess Cancer Risk from Chemicals." *Regulatory Toxicology and Pharmacology,* vol. 14, pp. 78–87.

Carson, Rachel. 1962. *Silent Spring.* Boston: Houghton Mifflin.

Chambers, P. L., D. Henschler, and F. Oesch. 1987. "Mouse Liver Tumors: Relevance to Human Cancer Risk." *Archives of Toxicology,* Supplement 10.

Drogin, Bob. 1992. "Deadly Malaria Returns with a Vengeance." *Washington Post,* November 10, p. Z11.

Environmental Protection Agency (EPA). 1985. "Captan Special Review Position Document 2/3." Office of Pesticides and Toxic Substances, June.

—— 1986. "Guidelines for Carcinogen Risk Assessment." *Federal Register,* vol. 51, Sept. 26, pp. 33992–34003.

—— 1987. "Notice of Intent to Initiate Special Review of the Ethylene Bisdithiocarbamate (EBDC) Pesticides." *Federal Register,* vol. 52, July 17, pp. 27172–27177.

—— 1989a. "Captan: Intent to Cancel Registrations; Conclusion of Special Review; Notice of Final Determination." *Federal Register,* vol. 54, Feb. 24, pp. 8116–8149.

—— 1989b. "EBDC Special Review Technical Support Document, Position Document 2/3." Office of Pesticides and Toxic Substances, December.

—— 1992. "Ethylene Bisdithiocarbamates (EBDCs): Notice of Intent to Cancel and Conclusion of Special Review." *Federal Register,* vol. 57, March 2, pp. 7484–7580.

Evans, John S., John D. Graham, George M. Gray, Adrienne Hollis, B. Ryan, Andrew Smith, Mark Smith, and A. Taylor. 1992. "Summary of a Workshop to Review an OMB Report on Regulatory Risk Assessment and Management." *Risk: Issues in Health and Safety,* vol. 3, pp. 71–83.

General Accounting Office (GAO), U.S. Congress. 1991. "Pesticides: EPA's Use of Benefit Assessments in Regulating Pesticides." March.

——— 1992. "Hired Farmworkers: Health and Well-being at Risk." HARD-92–46, February.

Graham, John D. 1993. Testimony on pesticide reform legislation before Joint Hearing of the House Subcommittee on Health and Environment and the Senate Committee on Labor and Human Resources. Washington, D.C., September 21.

Holland, Charles D., and Robert L. Sielken, Jr. 1991. "Cancer Modeling and Risk Assessment." Special Report, The Texas Institute for the Advancement of Chemical Technology Inc.

Huber, Peter. 1983. "The Old-New Division in Risk Regulation." *Virginia Law Review,* vol. 69, no. 6, September, pp. 1025–1107.

Keeney, Ralph L. 1990. "Mortality Risks Induced by Economic Expenditures." *Risk Analysis,* vol. 10, pp. 147–159.

Kilman, S. 1989. "Spreading Poison: Fungus in Corn Crop, A Potential Carcinogen Invades Food Supplies, Regulators Fail to Stop Sales of Last Fall's Harvest Laden with Aflatoxin." *Wall Street Journal,* February 23, pp. A1, A8–A9.

Kurtz, E. A. 1990. Personal communication; letter to EPA special review branch from Edward A. Kurtz, EAK AG Inc., Agricultural Consultants, May.

Les v. Reilly, 968 F.2d 985 (9th Cir. 1992).

National Research Council (NRC), Environmental Studies Board. 1980. *Regulating Pesticides.* Washington, D.C.: National Academy Press.

——— , Board on Agriculture. 1987. *Regulating Pesticides in Food: The Delaney Paradox.* Washington, D.C.: National Academy Press.

——— 1989. *Field Testing Genetically Modified Organisms: Framework for Decisions.* Washington, D.C.: National Academy Press.

——— , Committee on Risk Assessment Methodology, Board on Environmental Studies and Toxicology, Commission on Life Sciences. 1993. *Issues in Risk Assessment.* Washington, D.C.: National Academy Press.

Office of Management and Budget (OMB), Executive Office of the President. 1991. "Current Regulatory Issues in Risk Assessment and Risk Management." In *Regulatory Program of the United States Government, April 1, 1990–March 1, 1991,* Washington, D.C.

Office of Science and Technology Policy (OSTP), Executive Office of the President. 1992. "Exercise of Federal Oversight Within Scope of Statutory Authority: Planned Introductions of Biotechnology

Products into the Environment." *Federal Register,* vol. 57, February 27, pp. 6753–6762.

Ottoboni, M. A. 1991. *The Dose Makes the Poison: A Plain-Language Guide to Toxicology,* 2nd ed. New York: Van Nostrand Reinhold.

Quest, John A., Karen L. Hamernik, Reto Engler, William L. Burnam, and Penelope A. Fenner-Crisp. 1991. "Evaluation of the Carcinogenic Potential of Pesticides: 3. Aliette." *Regulatory Toxicology and Pharmacology,* vol. 14, pp. 3–11.

Reinert, J. C., S. G. Slotnick, and D. J. Viviani. 1990. "A Discussion of the Methodologies Used in Pesticide Risk-Benefit Analysis." *The Environmental Professional,* vol. 12, pp. 94–100.

Rosenthal, Alon, George M. Gray, and John D. Graham. 1992. "Legislating Acceptable Cancer Risk from Exposure to Toxic Chemicals." *Ecology Law Quarterly,* vol. 19, pp. 269–362.

Steinmetz, K. A., and J. D. Potter. 1991. "Vegetables, Fruit, and Cancer: I. Epidemiology." *Cancer Causes and Control,* vol. 2, pp. 325–357.

United Nations Environment Programme (UNEP). 1992. *Methyl Bromide: Its Atmospheric Science, Technology, and Economics.* June.

Upton, Arthur C. 1988. "Are There Thresholds for Carcinogens? The Thorny Problem of Low-Level Exposure." *Annals of the New York Academy of Sciences,* vol. 534, pp. 863–884.

U.S. Department of Agriculture (USDA), National Agricultural Pesticide Impact Assessmemnt Program. 1992. "A Preliminary Draft of a Biological and Economic Assessment of Methyl Bromide." May.

Whipple, Chris. 1985. "Redistributing Risk." *Regulation,* May/June, pp. 37–44.

Yeh, F. S., M. C. Yu, C. C. Mo, S. Luo, M. J. Tong, and B. E. Henderson. 1989. "Hepatitis B Virus, Aflatoxins, and Hepatocellular Carcinoma in Southern Guangxi, China." *Cancer Research,* vol. 49, pp. 2506–2509.

Zilberman, David, Andrew Schmitz, Gary Sasterline, Erik Lichtenberg, and Jerome B. Siebert. 1991. "The Economics of Pesticide Use and Regulation." *Science,* vol. 253, pp. 518–522.

10. *Protecting the Global Environment*

Adams, Richard M., J. David Glyer and Bruce A. McCarl. 1989. "The Economic Effects of Climate Change on U.S. Agriculture: A Preliminary Assessment." In *The Potential Effects of Global Climate Change on the United States,* ed. Joel B. Smith and Dennis A.

Tirpak. U.S. Environmental Protection Agency, EPA-230-05-89-053, Appendix C: Agriculture, vol. 1, June, pp. 4-1 through 4-56.

Adams, Richard M., Cynthia Rosenzweig, et al. 1990. "Global Climate Change and U.S. Agriculture." *Nature*, vol. 345, May 17, pp. 219–223.

Arbatov, A. 1990. USSR Academy of Sciences, communication to U.S. EPA, Office of Global Change.

Balling, Robert C. 1992. *The Heated Debate: Greenhouse Predictions versus Climate Reality.* San Francisco: Pacific Research Institute for Public Policy.

Bazzaz, Fakhri A., and Eric D. Fajer. 1992. "Plant Growth in a CO_2-Rich World." *Scientific American*, January, pp. 68–74.

Bernard, Harold. 1980. *The Greenhouse Effect.* Cambridge, Mass.: Ballinger.

Bradley, Richard A., Edward C. Watts, and Edward R. Williams. 1991. *Limiting Net Greenhouse Gas Emissions in the United States.* U.S. Department of Energy, September.

Brookes, Warren. 1990. "Global Warming Benefits?" *Washington Times*, March 12, p. F1.

Bruhl, C., and Paul J. Crutzen. 1989. "On the Disproportionate Role of Tropospheric Ozone as a Filter Against Solar UV-B Radiation." *Geophysical Research Letters*, vol. 16, pp. 703–706.

Budyko, M. I. 1982. *Earth's Climate: Past and Future.* New York: Academic Press.

Bureau of National Affairs (BNA). 1991. "Commission Asked to Make Formal Proposal on Energy Tax to Address Climate Change." *BNA International Environment Reporter: Current Report*, December 18, p. 670.

Burniaux, Jean-Marc, John P. Martin, et al. 1992. "The Costs of Reducing CO_2 Emissions: Evidence from GREEN." Economics Department Working Paper No. 115, Organization for Economic Co-operation and Development (OECD), Paris.

Chandler, David. 1992. "Fear Expressed of Runaway Greenhouse Effect." *Boston Globe*, February 10, p. 3.

Cline, William R. 1992. *The Economics of Global Warming.* Washington, D.C.: Institute for International Economics.

Congressional Budget Office (CBO). 1990. "Carbon Charges as a Response to Global Warming: The Effects of Taxing Fossil Fuels." August.

Crutzen, Paul J. 1991. "Methane's Sinks and Sources." *Nature*, vol. 350, April 4, pp. 380–381.

———— 1992. "Ultraviolet on the Increase." *Nature,* vol. 356, March 12, pp. 104–105.

Department of Energy (DOE). 1990. "The Economics of Long-Term Global Climate Change: A Preliminary Assessment." Report of a U.S. Interagency Task Force (chaired by CEA), DOE/PE-0096P, September.

Department of Justice (DOJ). 1991. "A Comprehensive Approach to Addressing Potential Climate Change." Report of a U.S. Interagency Task Force, February.

Dockery, D. W., et al. 1993. "An Association between Air Pollution and Mortality in Six U.S. Cities." *New England Journal of Medicine,* vol. 329, December 9, pp. 1753–1759.

Dower, Roger, and Mary Beth Zimmerman. 1992. *The Right Climate for Carbon Taxes.* Washington, D.C.: World Resources Institute, August.

Drake, Bert G., and P. W. Leadley. 1991. "Canopy Photosynthesis of Crops and Native Plant Communities Exposed to Long-term Elevated CO_2." *Plant, Cell, and Environment,* vol. 14, pp. 853–860.

Dudek, Daniel J. 1987. "Assessing the Implications of Changes in Carbon Dioxide Concentrations and Climate for Agriculture in the United States." New York: Environmental Defense Fund.

Dudek, Daniel J., and Alice LeBlanc. 1990. "Offsetting New CO_2 Emissions: A Rational First Greenhouse Policy Step." *Contemporary Policy Issues,* vol. 8, July, pp. 29–42.

Edmonds, Jae, Marshall Wise, and Chris MacCracken. 1994. "Advanced Energy Technologies and Climate Change: An Analysis Using the Global Change Assessment Model (GCAM)," draft version 2.0, April 27. Washington, D.C.: Pacific Northwest Laboratories, Global Environmental Change Program.

Environmental Protection Agency (EPA). 1993. "Protection of Stratospheric Ozone." *Federal Register,* vol. 58, no. 90, May 12, pp. 28094–28192.

Esty, Daniel C. 1994. "The Case for a Global Environmental Organization." In Peter B. Kenen, ed., *Managing the World Economy.* Washington, D.C.: Institute for International Economics.

European Communities (EC). 1991a. *Commission of the EC: JOULE Program.* May.

———— 1991b. COHERENCE, Report for the Commission of the European Communities, Directorate General XII, "Cost-Effectiveness Analysis of CO_2 Reduction Options: Synthesis Report." May.

Falk, Jim, and Andrew Brownlow. 1989. *The Greenhouse Challenge: What's to Be Done?* Ringwood, Victoria, Australia: Penguin Books.

Farman, J. C., B. G. Gardiner, and J. D. Shanklin. 1985. "Large Losses of Total Ozone in Antarctica Reveal Seasonal ClO_x/NO_x Interaction." *Nature*, vol. 315, pp. 207–210.

German Bundestag Study Commission. 1989. *Protecting the Earth's Atmosphere: An International Challenge.* Bonn, Germany.

——— 1990. *Protecting the Earth's Atmosphere.* Bonn, Germany, November 7.

Glantz, Michael. 1991. "Winners and Losers." Boulder, Colo.: National Center for Atmospheric Research.

Gray, C. Boyden. 1992. "Put the Forests First." *Washington Post,* June 2, p. A19.

Gribbin, John. 1982. *Future Weather and the Greenhouse Effect.* New York: Delacourt Press.

Grodzinski, Bernard 1992. "Plant Nutrition and Growth Regulation by CO_2 Enrichment." *BioScience*, vol. 42, no. 7, July/August, pp. 517–525.

Hallett, Frederick H. 1993. "Is the Sky Falling Down?" Letter, *Washington Post,* May 8, p. A20.

Harmon, M., W. Ferrell, and J. Franklin. 1990. "Effects on Carbon Storage of Conversion of Old-Growth Forests to Young Forests." *Science,* vol. 247, February 9, p. 699.

Hirsh, Nancy. 1988. "Nuking Global Warming." *Environmental Action,* vol. 20, no. 2, September–October, pp. 7–8.

Hoffman, John. 1991. Director, Office of Global Change, U.S. EPA. Personal communication.

Hogan, Kathleen, John Hoffman, and Ann Thompson. 1991. "Methane on the Greenhouse Agenda." *Nature*, vol. 354, November 21, pp. 181–182.

Hoyle, Fred. 1981. *Ice: The Ultimate Human Catastrophe.* New York: Continuum.

Idso, Sherwood, and Bruce Kimball. 1991. "Doubling CO_2 Triples Growth Rate of Sour Orange Trees." DOE Research Summary no. 13, CDIAC/ORNL, December.

Intergovernmental Panel on Climate Change (IPCC). 1990a. *Climate Change: The IPCC Scientific Assessment,* ed. J. T. Houghton, G. J. Jenkins, and J. J. Ephraums. Cambridge: Cambridge University Press.

——— 1990b. *Climate Change: The IPCC Impacts Assessment,* ed. W. J. Tegart, G. W. Sheldon, and D. C. Griffiths. Canberra: Australian Government Printing Service.

——— 1990c. *Climate Change: The IPCC Response Strategies.* Washington, D.C.: Island Press.

——— 1992. *Climate Change 1992: The Supplementary Report to the*

IPCC Scientific Assessment. Cambridge: Cambridge University Press.

Jones, P. D., and T. M. L. Wigley. 1990. "Global Warming Trends." *Scientific American,* vol. 263, pp. 84–91.

Kane, Sally M., John M. Reilly, and James Tobey. 1992a. "A Sensitivity Analysis of the Implications of Climate Change for World Agriculture." In *Economic Issues in Global Climate Change: Agriculture, Forestry, and Natural Resources,* ed. John M. Reilly and Margot Anderson, pp. 117–131. Boulder, Colo.: Westview Press.

—— 1992b. "An Empirical Study of the Economic Effects of Climate Change on World Agriculture." *Climatic Change,* vol. 21, May, pp. 1–16.

Karl, Thomas, et al. 1991. "Global Warming: Evidence for Asymmetric Diurnal Temperature Change." *Geophysical Research Letters,* vol. 18, December, pp. 2253–2256.

Kerr, James, C. T. McElroy, et al. 1993. "Evidence for Large Upward Trends of Ultraviolet-B Radiation Linked to Ozone Depletion." *Science,* vol. 262, November 12, pp. 1032–1034.

Kerr, Richard. 1992. "Huge Impact Tied to Mass Extinction." *Science,* vol. 257, August 14, pp. 878–880.

Kiehl, Jeffrey T. 1992. "Cold Comfort in the Greenhouse." *Nature,* vol. 355, February 27, p. 773.

Krupnick, Alan J., and Paul R. Portney. 1991. "Controlling Urban Air Pollution: A Benefit-Cost Assessment." *Science,* vol. 252, April 26, pp. 522–528.

Lascelles, David. 1992. "A Mission to Make Polluters Pay." *Financial Times* (London), January 28, p. 16, col. 3.

Leggett, Jane. 1992. U.S. EPA, personal communication, May. Based on William Pepper, Jane Leggett, Jae Edmonds, Rob Swart et al., background paper for Emissions Scenarios, reported in IPCC 1992.

Levenson, Thomas. 1989. *Ice Time: Climate, Science, and Life on Earth.* New York: Harper & Row.

MacNeill, J., P. Winsemius, and T. Yakushiji. 1991. *Beyond Interdependence: The Meshing of the World's Economy and the Earth's Ecology.* New York: Oxford University Press.

Mitchell, Catherine, Jim Sweet, and Tim Jackson. 1990. "A Study of Leakage from the UK Natural Gas Distribution System." *Energy Policy,* vol. 18, November, pp. 809–818.

Molina, Mario J., and F. Sherwood Rowland. 1974. "Stratospheric Sinks for Chlorofluorocarbons: Chlorine Atomic-atalysed Destruction of Ozone." *Nature,* vol. 249, pp. 810–812.

Monastersky, R. 1992. "UV Hazard: Ozone Lost versus Ozone Gained." *Science News,* September 19, pp. 180–181.

Mooney, H. A., et al.. 1991. "Predicting Ecosystem Responses to Elevated CO_2 Concentrations." *BioScience,* vol. 41, no. 2, February, pp. 96–104.

Naj, Amal Kumar. 1991. "CFC Substitute Might be Toxic, Rat Study Finds." *Wall Street Journal,* July 2, p. B1, col.6.

National Academy of Sciences (NAS). 1991a. *Policy Implications of Greenhouse Warming.* Washington, D.C.

—— 1991b. *Policy Implications of Greenhouse Warming: Report of the Adaptation Panel.*

—— 1991c. *Policy Implications of Greenhouse Warming: Report of the Mitigation Panel.*

National Acid Precipitation Assessment Program (NAPAP). 1991. *1990 Integrated Assessment Report.* Washington, D.C., November.

National Research Council (NRC). 1991. *Rethinking the Ozone Problem in Urban and Regional Air Pollution.* Washington, D.C.

Netherlands. 1990. "Climate Change Policy in the Netherlands and Supporting Measures." Netherlands Ministry of Housing, Physical Planning and the Environment, Directorate General for Environment, November.

Noll, Roger G., and James E. Krier. 1990. "Some Implications of Cognitive Psychology for Risk Regulation." *Journal of Legal Studies,* vol. 19, pp. 747–779.

Nordhaus, William D. 1991. "To Slow or Not to Slow: The Economics of the Greenhouse Effect." *The Economic Journal,* vol. 101, no. 6, pp. 920–937.

Oren, Ram. 1994. School of the Environment, Duke University. Personal communication, May 4.

Pearce, Fred. 1992. "Grain Yields Tumble in Greenhouse World." *New Scientist,* April 18, p. 4 (reporting study by Martin Parry).

Peters, Robert L., and Thomas E. Lovejoy (eds.). 1992. *Global Warming and Biological Diversity.* New Haven: Yale University Press.

Ponte, Lowell. 1976. *The Cooling.* Englewood Cliffs, N.J.: Prentice-Hall.

Quay, P. D., B. Tilbrook, and C. S. Wong. 1992. "Oceanic Uptake of Fossil Fuel CO_2: Carbon-13 Evidence." *Science,* vol. 256, April 3, p. 74.

Rabchuk, Victor I., and Nicolay I. Ilkevich. 1991. "A Study of Methane Leakage in the Soviet Natural Gas Supply System." Paper prepared for Siberian Energy Institute, USSR Academy of Sciences, and Batelle Pacific Northwest Laboratory, Washington, D.C., May.

Ramanathan, Veerabhadran. 1975. "Greenhouse Effect Due to Chlorofluorocarbons: Climatic Implications." *Science,* vol. 190, October 3, pp. 50–52.

Ramanathan, V., R. J. Cicerone, H. B. Singh, and J. T. Kiehl. 1985. "Trace Gas Trends and Their Potential Role in Climate Change." *Journal of Geophysical Research,* vol. 90, pp. 5547–5566.

Ramaswamy, V., M. D. Schwarzkopf, and K. P. Shine. 1992. "Radiative Forcing of Climate from Halocarbon-Induced Global Stratospheric Ozone Loss." *Nature,* vol. 355, February 27, pp. 810–812.

Reilly, John M. 1992. "Climate Change Damage and the Trace Gas Index Issue." In *Economic Issues in Global Climate Change: Agriculture, Forestry, and Natural Resources,* ed. John M. Reilly and Margot Anderson, pp. 72–88. Boulder, Colo.: Westview Press.

Reinsch, Anthony, and Jennifer Considine. 1992. "Challenging OPEC: World Oil Market Projections, 1992–2007." Canadian Energy Research Institute, Calgary, July.

Rensberger, Boyce. 1993. " 'Greenhouse Effect' Seems Benign So Far: Warming Most Evident At Night, in Winter." *Washington Post,* June 1, p. A1 (reporting studies by Patrick Michaels, James Hansen, P. D. Jones, and K. R. Briffa).

Rodhe, Henning. 1990. "A Comparison of the Contribution of Various Gases to the Greenhouse Effect." *Science,* vol. 248, June 8, pp. 1217–1219.

Rosenberg, Norman. 1991. "Comments." In *Global Warming: Economic Policy Responses,* ed. Rudiger Dornbusch and James M. Poterba, pp. 330–334. Cambridge, Mass.: MIT Press.

Rosenberg, Norman, et al. 1990. "From Climate and CO_2 Enrichment to Evapotranspiration." In *Climate Change and U.S. Water Resources,* ed. Paul Waggoner, pp. 151–175. New York: John Wiley & Sons.

Rosenberg, Norman, et al. 1991. "Processes for Identifying Regional Influences of and Responses to Increasing Atmospheric CO_2 and Climate Change: the MINK Project." U.S. Department of Energy, August.

Rowland, F. Sherwood. 1989. "Chlorofluorocarbons and the Depletion of Stratospheric Ozone." *American Scientist,* vol. 77, January-February, pp. 36–45.

Rutherford, Thomas. 1992. "The Welfare Effects of Fossil Carbon Restrictions: Results from a Recursively Dynamic Trade Model." OECD Economics Department Working Papers No. 112, Paris.

Schelling, T. C. 1991. "Economic Responses to Global Warming: Prospects for Cooperative Approaches." In *Global Warming: Economic Policy Responses*, ed. Rudiger Dornbusch and James M. Poterba. Cambridge, Mass.: MIT Press.

Schneider, Stephen H. 1988. "Doing Something about the Weather." *World Monitor*, vol. 1, no. 3, December, pp. 28–37.

———— 1989a. "The Changing Climate." *Scientific American*, September, pp. 70–79.

———— 1989b. *Global Warming: Are We Entering the Greenhouse Century?* San Francisco: Sierra Club Books.

Seckmeyer, Gunther, and P. L. McKenzie. 1992. "Increased Ultraviolet Radiation in New Zealand." *Nature*, vol. 359, September 10, pp. 135–137.

Smith, Joel B., and Dennis A. Tirpak (eds.). 1989. *The Potential Effects of Global Climate Change on the United States.* U.S. Environmental Protection Agency (EPA), EPA-230-05-89-053, Washington, D.C.

Smith, R. C., et al. 1992. "Ozone Depletion: Ultraviolet Radiation and Phytoplankton Biology in Antarctic Waters." *Science*, vol. 255, February 21, pp. 952–958.

Solomon, Susan, and Daniel L. Albritton. 1992. "Time-dependent Ozone Depletion Potentials for Short- and Long-Term Forecasts." *Nature*, vol. 357, May 7, pp. 33–37.

Stevens, William K. 1992. "Plant Study Questions Nature of Ozone Risk." *New York Times*, August 25, p. C2.

Stewart, Richard B., and Jonathan B. Wiener. 1990. "A Comprehensive Approach to Climate Change." *American Enterprise*, vol. 1, no. 6, November-December, pp. 75–80.

———— 1992. "The Comprehensive Approach to Global Climate Policy: Issues of Design and Practicality." *Arizona Journal of International and Comparative Law*, vol. 17, pp. 84–113.

Stone, Peter H. 1992. "Forecast Cloudy: The Limits of Global Warming Models." MIT Center for Global Change Science, Report No. 12, March.

Tans, Pieter, et al. 1990. "Observational Constraints on the Global Atmospheric CO_2 Budget." *Science*, vol. 247, pp. 1431–1438.

Tobey, James, John M. Reilly, and Sally M. Kane. 1992. "Economic

Implications of Global Climate Change for World Agriculture." *Journal of Agricultural and Resource Economics*, vol. 17, no. 1, July, pp. 195–204.

Wallis, Max. 1991. "Leaking Gas in the Greenhouse." *Nature*, vol. 354, December 12, p. 428.

Weiner, Jonathan. 1990. *The Next One Hundred Years: Shaping the Fate of Our Living Earth.* New York: Bantam Books.

Weisskopf, Michael. 1992. "Study Finds CFC Alternatives More Damaging than Believed." *Washington Post*, February 23, p. A3.

Wigley, T. M. L. 1991. "Could Reducing Fossil-Fuel Emissions Cause Global Warming?" *Nature*, vol. 349, February 7, pp. 503–505.

Will, George F. 1992. "Chicken Littles: The Persistence of Eco-Pessimism." *Washington Post*, May 31, p. C7.

World Bank. 1992. *World Development Report: Environment and Development.* Washington, D.C.

World Meteorological Organization (WMO). 1991. *Scientific Assessment of Ozone Depletion.* Pre-print, December 17.

World Wildlife Fund. 1992. "Can Nature Survive Global Warming?" Washington, D.C., February.

Yoon, Carol Kaesuk. 1994. "Thinning Ozone Layer Implicated in Decline of Frogs and Toads." *New York Times*, March 1, p. B12 (citing study by Andrew Blaustein, John Hays, et al. in *NAS Proceedings*).

Zimmerman, Mary Beth. 1992. "Comparing the Costs and Benefits of Climate Policies." Working paper, Alliance to Save Energy, Washington, D.C.

11. Resolving Risk Tradeoffs

Ackerman, Bruce, and William Hassler. 1981. *Clean Coal/Dirty Air.* New Haven: Yale University Press.

American Society for Internal Medicine (ASIM). 1993. *Rebuilding Primary Care: A Blueprint for the Future.* Washington, D.C., March.

American Textile Manufacturers Institute, Inc. (ATMI) v. Donovan, 452 U.S. 490 (1981).

Aqua Slide 'N Dive Corp. v. Consumer Product Safety Commission (CPSC), 569 F.2d 831 (5th Cir. 1978).

Association of Data Processing Service Organizations v. Camp, 397 U.S. 150 (1970).

Bartel, Ann T., and Lacy G. Thomas. 1985. "Direct and Indirect Effects of Regulation: A New Look at OSHA's Impact." *Journal of Law and Economics*, vol. 28, pp. 1–25.

Been, Vicki. 1994. "Locally Undesirable Land Uses in Minority Neighborhoods: Disproportionate Siting or Market Dynamics?" *Yale Law Journal,* vol. 103, pp. 1383–1415.

Bogen, Kenneth. 1990. *Uncertainty in Environmental Health Risk Assessment.* New York: Garland.

Botkin, Daniel B. 1990. *Discordant Harmonies.* New York: Oxford.

Brennan, T. A., L. E. Hebert, N. M. Laird, A. Lawthers, K. E. Thorpe, L. L. Leape, A. R. Localio, S. R. Lipsitz, J. P. Newhouse, and P. C. Weiler. 1991. "Hospital Charactersitics Associated with Adverse Events and Substandard Care." *Journal of the American Medical Association,* vol. 265, no. 24, pp. 3265–3269.

Brennan, T. A., L. L. Leape, N. M. Laird, L. Hebert, A. R. Localio, A. G. Lawthers, J. P. Newhouse, P. C. Weiler, and H. H. Hiatt. 1991. "Incidence of Adverse Events and Negligence in Hospitalized Patients. Results of the Harvard Medical Practice Study 1." *New England Journal of Medicine,* vol. 324, no. 6, pp. 370–376.

Breyer, Stephen G. 1993. *Breaking the Vicious Circle: Toward Effective Risk Regulation.* Cambridge: Harvard University Press.

Clarke v. Securities Industries Association, 479 U.S. 388 (1987).

Clealand-Hamnett, Nancy, and Joseph Retzer. 1993. "Crossing Agency Boundaries." *Environmental Forum,* vol. 10, no. 2, pp. 17–21.

Competitive Enterprise Institute (CEI) v. National Highway Traffic Safety Administration (NHTSA), 956 F.2d 321 (D.C. Cir. 1992).

Corrosion Proof Fittings v. U.S. Environmental Protection Agency (EPA), 947 F.2d 1201 (5th Cir. 1991).

Crandall, Robert, and John D. Graham. 1991. "New Fuel Economy Standards?" *The American Enterprise,* vol. 2, April, pp. 68–69.

Cropper, Maureen, and Paul Portney. 1990. "Discounting and the Evaluation of Lifesaving Programs." *Journal of Risk and Uncertainty,* vol. 3, pp. 369–379.

Cropper, M. L., S. K. Aydede, and P. R. Portney. 1991. "Discounting Human Lives." *American Journal of Agricultural Economics,* vol. 73, pp. 1410–1415.

Davies, J. Clarence (Terry). 1988. "The Environmental Protection Act." Second Draft, September. Washington, D.C.: The Conservation Foundation.

——— 1992. "Some Thoughts on Implementing Integration." *Environmental Law,* vol. 22, pp. 139–148.

Dwyer, John. 1990. "The Pathology of Symbolic Legislation." *Ecology Law Quarterly,* vol. 17, pp. 233–316.

Environmental Defense Fund (EDF) v. EPA, 498 F.2d 1247, 1254–57 (D.C. Cir. 1973).

Eskridge, William. 1988. "Politics without Romance: Implications of Public Choice Theory for Statutory Interpretation." *Virginia Law Review*, vol. 74, pp. 275–338.

Esty, Daniel C. 1994. "The Case for a Global Environmental Organization." In Peter B. Kenen, ed., *Managing the World Economy*. Washington, D.C.: Institute for International Economics.

Finkel, Adam. 1990. *Confronting Uncertainty in Risk Management: A Guide for Decision Makers*. Resources for the Future, Washington, D.C., January.

Finkel, Adam, and John S. Evans. 1987. "Evaluating the Benefits of Uncertainty Reduction in Environmental Health Risk Management." *Journal of the Air Pollution Control Association*, vol. 37, pp. 1164–1171.

Fisher, Ann, Gary H. McClelland, and William D. Schulze. 1989. "Communicating Risk under Title III of SARA: Strategies for Explaining Very Small Risks in a Community Context." *Journal of Air and Waste Management Association*, vol. 39, no. 3, March, pp. 271–276.

Foran, Jeffrey, and Barbara F. Glenn. 1992. "Reducing the Health Risks of Sport Fish." *Issues in Science and Technology*, vol. 8, pp. 73–77.

Gelb-Safran, Dana, Alvin R. Tarlov, and William H. Rogers. 1994. "Primary Care Performance in Fee-for-Service and Prepaid Health Care Systems: Results from the Medical Outcomes Study." *Journal of the American Medical Association*, vol. 271, no. 20, May 25, pp. 1579–1586.

General Accounting Office (GAO), Congress of the United States. 1990. "National Institutes of Health: Problems in Implementing Policy on Women in Study Populations." Testimony of Mark V. Nadel, Associate Director, before House Committee on Energy and Commerce, Subcommittee on Health and Environment, June 18.

Goldstein, Bernard. 1989. "The Maximally Exposed Individual: An Inappropriate Basis for Public Health Decisionmaking." *Environmental Forum*, November/December, pp. 13–16.

Graham, John D. 1985. "The Failure of Agency-Forcing: The Regulation of Airborne Carcinogens under Section 112 of the Clean Air Act." *Duke Law Journal*, vol. 1985, February, pp. 100–150.

———— 1991. "Improving Chemical Risk Assessment." *Regulation*, Fall, pp. 14–17.

Graham, John D., Laura Green, and Marc J. Roberts. 1988. *In Search of Safety: Chemicals and Cancer Risk*. Cambridge, Mass.: Harvard University Press.

Gruenspecht, Howard G. 1992. "Differentiated Regulation: The Case of Auto Emissions Standards." *American Economic Review*, vol. 72 (Papers and Proceedings), May, pp. 328–331.

Grumbach, Kevin, and John Fry. 1993. "Managing Primary Care in the United States and in the United Kingdom." *New England Journal of Medicine*, vol. 328, no. 13, April 1, pp. 940–945.

Haigh, Nigel, and Frances Irwin, eds. 1990. *Integrated Pollution Control in Europe and North America*. Washington, D.C.: The Conservation Foundation.

Hammitt, James, and Jonathan A. K. Cave. 1991. *Research Planning for Food Safety: A Value-of-Information Approach*. Santa Monica: Rand Corporation.

Hass, Peter M., Robert O. Keohane, and Marc A. Levy (eds.). 1993. *Institutions for the Earth: Sources of Effective International Environmental Protection*. Cambridge, Mass.: MIT Press.

Hirschman, Albert O. 1991. *The Rhetoric of Reaction: Perversity, Futility, Jeopardy*. Cambridge, Mass.: Harvard University Press.

Holdren, John. 1990. "Energy in Transition." *Scientific American*, September, pp. 157–163.

Holloway, Marguerite. 1994. "Trends in Women's Health: A Global View." *Scientific American*, August, pp. 77–83.

Hornstein, Donald T. 1992. "Reclaiming Environmental Law: A Normative Critique of Comparative Risk Analysis." *Columbia Law Review*, vol. 92, pp. 562–633.

Hsiao, W. C., D. L. Dunn, and D. K. Verrilli. 1993. "Assessing the Implementation of Physician-Payment Reform." *New England Journal of Medicine*, vol. 328, no. 13, April 1, pp. 928–933.

Hurrell, Andrew, and Benedict Kingsbury (eds.). 1992. *The International Politics of the Environment*. Oxford: Oxford University Press.

Inhaber, H. 1979. "Risk with Energy from Conventional and Nonconventional Sources." *Science*, vol. 203, p. 718.

Institute of Medicine (IOM), National Academy of Sciences. 1994. *Women and Health Research*. Washington, D.C.: National Academy Press.

Johnson, W. G., T. A. Brennan, J. P. Newhouse, L. L. Leape, A. G. Lawthers, H. H. Hiatt, and P. C. Weiler. 1992. "The Economic Consequences of Medical Injuries: Implications for a No-Fault Insurance Plan." *Journal of the American Medical Association*, vol. 267, no. 18, pp. 2487–2492.

Kadar, Andrew G. 1994. "The Sex-Bias Myth in Medicine." *The Atlantic Monthly*, vol. 274, no. 2, August, pp. 66–70.

Kasperson, Roger E. 1992. "The Social Amplification of Risk: Progress in Developing an Integrative Framework." In *The Social Theories of Risk,* ed. Sheldon Krimsky and Dominic Golding, pp. 153–178. New York: Praeger.

Krier, James E., and Mark Brownstein. 1992. "On Integrated Pollution Control." *Environmental Law,* vol. 22, no. 1, pp. 119–138.

Krier, James E., and Edmund Ursin. 1977. *Pollution and Policy.* Berkeley: University of California Press.

Laden, Francine, and George Gray. 1993. "Toxics Use Reduction: Pros and Cons." In *Risk: Issues in Health and Safety,* vol. 4, pp. 213–234.

Lave, Lester B. 1968. "Safety in Transportation: The Role of Government." *Law and Contemporary Problems,* vol. 33, pp. 512–535.

———— 1981. *The Strategy of Social Regulation.* Washington, D.C.: The Brookings Institution.

Lave, Lester B., and Eric H. Males. 1989. "At Risk: The Framework for Regulating Toxic Substances." *Environmental Science and Technology,* vol. 23, no. 4, pp. 386–391.

Leape, L. L., T. A. Brennan, N. Laird, A. G. Lawthers, A. R. Localio, B. A. Barnes, L. Hebert, J. P. Newhouse, P. C. Weiler, and H. Hiatt. 1991. "The Nature of Adverse Events in Hospitalized Patients: Results of the Harvard Medical Practice II." *New England Journal of Medicine,* vol. 324, no. 6, pp. 377–384.

Litan, Robert, and William Nordhaus. 1983. *Reforming Federal Regulation.* New Haven: Yale University Press.

Loomes, G., and L. McKenzie. 1989. "The Use of QALYs in Health Care Decision Making." *Social Science and Medicine,* vol. 28, pp. 299–308.

Marcus, Alfred A. 1991. "EPA's Organizational Structure." *Law and Contemporary Problems,* vol. 54, no. 4, Autumn, pp. 5–40.

Mastroianni, Anna C., Ruth Faden, and Daniel Federman. 1994. *Women and Health Research: Ethical and Legal Issues of Including Women in Clinical Studies.* Washington, D.C.: National Academy Press.

Melnick, R. Shep. 1983. *Regulation and the Courts: The Case of the Clean Air Act.* Washington, D.C.: The Brookings Institution.

Menell, Peter, and Richard B. Stewart. 1994. *Environmental Law and Policy.* Boston: Little, Brown.

Morgan, M. Granger, and Max Henrion. 1990. *Uncertainty: A Guide to Dealing with Uncertainty in Quantitative Risk and Policy Analysis.* New York: Cambridge University Press.

Motor Vehicle Manufacturers Association v. State Farm Insurance Co., 463 U.S. 29 (1983).

Muir, John. 1988. *My First Summer in the Sierras.* Sierra Club Books, John Muir Library, San Francisco.

Myers, J. P., and T. Colborn. 1991. "Blundering Questions, Weak Answers Lead to Poor Pesticide Policies." *Chemical and Engineering News,* January 7, pp. 40–43.

National Academy of Sciences. 1981. *Risk and Decision Making: Perspectives and Research.* Washington, D.C.

——— 1983. *Risk Assessment in the Federal Government.* Washington, D.C.

Natural Resources Defense Council (NRDC) v. EPA, 824 F.2d 1146 (D.C. Cir. 1987).

Olson, Mancur. 1965. *The Logic of Collective Action.* Cambridge, Mass.: Harvard University Press.

O'Meara, James J., et al. 1994. "A Decision Analysis of Streptokinase plus Heparin as Compared with Heparin Alone for Deep-Vein Thrombosis." *New England Journal of Medicine,* vol. 330, June 30, pp. 1864–1869.

O'Neill, Patrick. 1994. "Surgeon Sees Social Activism as Extension of His Work." *Chapel Hill News,* July 6, p. A1.

Pliskin, Joseph, Donald Shepard, and Milton C. Weinstein. 1980. "Utility Functions for Life Years and Health Status." *Operations Research,* vol. 28, pp. 206–224.

Putnam, Susan, and John D. Graham. 1993. "Chemicals vs. Microbials in Drinking Water: A Decision Sciences Perspective." *Journal of the American Water Works Association,* vol. 85, pp. 57–61.

Rodriguez, Daniel B. 1994. "The Positive Political Dimensions of Regulatory Reform." *Washington University Law Quarterly,* vol. 72, pp. 1–150.

Rosenthal, Alon, George Gray, and John D. Graham. 1992. "Legislating Acceptable Cancer Risk from Toxic Chemicals." *Ecology Law Quarterly,* vol. 19, pp. 269–362.

Rosenthal, Elisabeth. 1993. "Medicine Suffers as Fewer Doctors Join Front Lines." *New York Times,* May 24, p. A1.

Ruckelshaus, William. 1984. *Risk Assessment and Management: Framework for Decision Making.* U.S. Environmental Protection Agency, Washington, D.C.

Safran, D. G., J. D. Graham, and J. S. Osberg. 1994. "Social Supports as a Determinant of Community-Based Care Utilization among Rehabilitatiion Patients." *Health Services Research,* vol. 28, no. 6, pp. 729–750.

Sapolsky, Harvey. 1990. "The Politics of Risk." *Daedalus,* vol. 119, no. 4, Fall, pp. 83–96.

Schneider, Keith. 1993. "Sea-Dumping Ban: Good Politics, But Not Necessarily Good Policy." *New York Times,* March 22, p. A1.

Schroeder, Steven A., and Lewis G. Sandy. 1993. "Specialty Distribution of U.S. Physicians—the Invisible Driver of Health Care Costs." *New England Journal of Medicine,* vol. 328, no. 13, April 1, pp. 961–963.

Shelef, M. 1994. "Unanticipated Benefits of Automotive Emission Control: Reduction in Fatalities by Motor Vehicle Exhaust Gas." *The Science of the Total Environment,* vol. 146/147, pp. 93–101.

Slovic, Paul, Baruch Fischhoff, and Sarah Lichtenstein. 1985. "Regulation of Risk: A Psychological Perspective." In *Regulatory Policy and the Social Sciences,* ed. Roger G. Noll, pp. 241–397. Berkeley: University of California Press.

Stewart, Richard B. 1986. "The Role of the Courts in Risk Management." *Environmental Law Reporter,* vol. 16, August, pp. 10208–10215.

Stewart, Richard B., and Jonathan B. Wiener. 1992. "The Comprehensive Approach to Global Climate Policy: Issues of Design and Practicality." *Arizona Journal of International and Comparative Law,* vol. 9, p. 83.

Sunstein, Cass. 1993. "Valuing Life." *New Republic,* vol. 208, February 15, p. 36.

Suris, Oscar. 1994. "Electric Cars Also Pollute Air, EPA Study Says." *Wall Street Journal,* April 5, p. B1.

Tirpak, Dennis A., and Dilip R. Ahuja. 1990. "Implications of Greenhouse Gas Emissions of Strategies Designed to Ameliorate Other Social and Environmental Problems." EPA Office of Policy Analysis, draft, November 5.

Tversky, A., and D. Kahneman. 1974. "Judgement under Uncertainty: Heuristics and Biases." *Science,* vol. 185, p. 1124.

United Auto Workers (UAW) v. Occupational Safety and Health Administration (OSHA), 938 F.2d 1310 (D.C. Cir. 1991).

United States v. Carroll Towing Co., 159 F.2d 169 (2d Cir. 1947).

United States Environmental Protection Agency (EPA). 1993. "Protection of Stratospheric Ozone." *Federal Register,* vol. 58, May 12, pp. 28094–28192.

Vestigo, James R. 1985. "Acid Rain and Tall Stack Regulation under the Clean Air Act." *Environmental Law,* vol. 15, pp. 711–744.

Viscusi, W. Kip. 1992. *Fatal Tradeoffs: Public and Private Responsibilities for Risk.* New York: Oxford University Press.

Warren, Edward W., and Gary E. Marchant. 1993. "More Good than

Harm: A Hippocratic Oath for Environmental Agencies and Courts." *Ecology Law Quarterly,* vol. 20, pp. 379–440.

Weiner, Jonathan. 1994. "Forecasting the Effects of Health Reform on U.S. Physician Workforce Requirements; Evidence from HMO Staffing Patterns." *Journal of the American Medical Association,* vol. 272, July 20, pp. 222–230.

Weinstein, Milton C., and Harvey Fineberg. 1980. *Clinical Decision Analysis.* Philadelphia: Saunders.

Weyerhauser Co. v. Costle, 590 F.2d 1011 (D.C. Cir. 1978).

Williams, Stephen F. 1993. "Second Best: The Soft Underbelly of Deterrence Theory in Tort." *Harvard Law Review,* vol. 106, pp. 932–944.

Wilson, James Q. 1980. *The Politics of Regulation.* New York: Basic Books.

Wilson, Richard. 1979. "The Environmental and Public Health Consequences of Replacement Electricity." *Energy,* vol. 4, pp. 81–86.

Wolf, Charles. 1988. *Markets or Governments: Choosing Between Imperfect Alternatives.* Cambridge, Mass.: MIT Press.

Contributors

Miriam E. Adams, Sc.D., is Research Associate at the Harvard Center for Risk Analysis.

Paul D. Anderson, Ph.D., is Technical Director, Risk Assessment at Ogden Environmental and Energy Services, Westford, Mass.

Howard Chang, M.D., is Research Fellow in Psychiatry at the Massachusetts Mental Health Center.

Howard Frazier, M.D., is Professor of Health Policy and Management at the Harvard School of Public Health.

John D. Graham, Ph.D., is Professor of Policy and Decision Sciences at the Harvard School of Public Health and Director, Harvard Center for Risk Analysis.

Evridiki Hatziandreau, M.D., Sc.D., is Senior Scientist at Battelle Corporation.

George M. Gray, Ph.D., is Regulatory Toxicologist and Deputy Director, Harvard Center for Risk Analysis.

Susan W. Putnam, Sc.D., is Research Associate at the Harvard Center for Risk Analysis.

Katherine Walker, M.S., is Research Associate at the Harvard Center for Risk Analysis.

Jonathan Baert Wiener, J.D., is Associate Professor of Law and Associate Professor of Environment at Duke University.

Constance Williams, M.D., is Research Fellow at Harvard Medical School.

318

Author Index

Subject Index

Accident risk, 16–17, 32, 33. *See also* Highway safety

Acetaminophen, 3, 39, 40, 265

Acid rain, 8, 212, 240

Administrative Procedures Act (APA), 251, 262, 263, 265

Adverse consequences, 22, 23, 25, 34, 229

Aflatoxins, 14, 25, 186–187

Agranulocytosis, 60, 62–64, 65, 66, 69, 70

AIDS, 125, 134, 143

Air pollution. *See* Pollution: air; emissions

Air traffic, 30, 237

Alcohol, 7, 13, 97, 130, 147

Aldehydes, 130

Aliette (Fosetyl-Al), 181, 185–186, 187–188

Alzheimer's disease, 78

American Association of Motor Vehicle Administrators, 80

American College of Physicians, 46, 48

American Society for International Medicine (ASIM), 244

Americans with Disabilities Act, 84

American Textile Manufacturers Institute, Inc. (ATMI) v. Donovan, 264

American Water Works Association (AWWA), 127, 128, 137, 138, 140, 146

Ames test for mutagenic activity, 182

Ammonia, 40, 138

Amoco-EPA Yorktown Study, 253

Analgesics, 3, 39, 265

Analysis of risk. *See* Risk Tradeoff Analysis (RTA)

Anesthesia, 12–13, 23, 42. *See also* Surgery risk

Anthracnose, 188

Antibiotics, 11, 12, 14

Antidepressants, 14

Antipsychotic drugs, 53, 54, 59, 61, 64, 66, 68, 69

Antiseptics, 12

Anxiety, 44, 46

Aqua Slide 'N Dive Corp. v. Consumer Product Safety Commission, 264

Asbestos, 8, 15, 16, 260–261

Ash, 157, 164, 166

Aspirin, 2, 3, 14, 27, 39, 40, 229, 265

Association of Data Processing Service Organizations v. Camp, 265

Automobiles: safety features, 1, 5, 7, 15, 94, 95, 97, 102, 241; crashworthiness of, 5, 39, 88, 97, 100; downsizing of, 5, 91, 94, 95, 99–

325